Technical Aspects of Focal Therapy in Localized Prostate Cancer

Eric Barret • Matthieu Durand

Editors

Technical Aspects of Focal Therapy in Localized Prostate Cancer

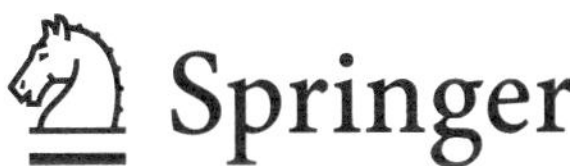 Springer

Editors

Eric Barret
Department of Urology
Institut Montsouris
Paris-Descartes University
Paris
France

Matthieu Durand
Department of Urology
Hôpital Pasteur 2
Centre Hospitalier Universitaire de Nice
University of Nice-Sophia-Antipolis
Nice
France

ISBN 978-2-8178-0556-6   ISBN 978-2-8178-0484-2   (eBook)
DOI 10.1007/978-2-8178-0484-2
Springer Paris Heidelberg New York Dordrecht London

Foreword

Paradigm Shift

A critical change in how localized prostate cancer is managed is likely to take place due to the emerging combination of both new imaging modalities and novel accurate ablative therapies that are aimed at eradicating the controversial index lesion and that radically alter the ways to treat this disease.

Nowadays, prostate cancer may be considered to be a chronic illness that can be treated, focally re-treated, and carefully followed up to control its evolution. With lower focal treatment-related morbidity, in addition to an ambitious dual goal of both organ-sparing and intention-to-treat therapy, the idea of focal treatments sounds appealing to both patients and healthcare providers.

But are we ready for (r)evolution?

Focal therapy has emerged as a new therapy concept in prostate cancer, based on the index lesion concept. Because prostate cancer is multifocal, thinking of eradicating some of the foci is out of the question. Nonetheless, because studies have demonstrated the existence of one most aggressive lesion among the multiple foci that represent a metastatic potential to target and also because salvage focal re-treatment may be considered under certain conditions after primary focal ablation, a new era of localized prostate cancer focal therapy ought to be assessed.

Patient selection remains a critical point to deal with before widely involving patients in a focal therapy protocol. With the extraordinary development of multiparametric MRI and fusion-imaging techniques to improve the targeting of biopsies, standardized selection strategies are needed.

To date, a large therapeutic arsenal has been developed. From among the focal cryotherapy, focal high-intensity focused ultrasound (HIFU), focal brachytherapy, focal photodynamic therapy, focal laser thermal therapy, focal radiotherapy, etc., no one can claim to know what the best ablative energy is, and longer comparative controlled trials are expected.

Regardless of the energy, it is now more crucial than ever to raise the level of knowledge, improving decision-making of suitable focal treatments accordingly. As recommended so far, focal therapy for men with localized prostate cancer must still be considered in the context of controlled clinical trials to compare their use to established intervention and a committed medical community towards the standardization of focal therapies based on scientific evidence-based medicine of efficacy, safety, and reproducibility.

In so doing, this book consists of the experiences of the world's top experts and teams that are involved in focal treatment in localized prostate cancer. All features of patient selection, techniques, and follow-up are addressed to try to meet agreement and commitment to the standardization of the processes.

Congratulations to all these pioneers who work day in and day out for the improved health of their patients, with the search for scientific evidence always in mind.

Paris, France   Guy Vallancien

Contents

Contributors

Y. Ahallal Department of Urology, Institut Montsouris, Paris-Descartes University, Paris, France

Hashim U. Ahmed, PhD, FRCS(Urol), BM, BCh(Oxon) Division of Surgery and Interventional Science, University College London, London, UK

Department of Urology, University College London Hospitals NHS Foundation Trust, London, UK

Maarten Albersen, MD, PhD Department of Urology, University Hospitals Leuven, Leuven, Belgium

Damien Ambrosetti Department of Pathology, Hôpital Pasteur – Centre Hospitalier Universitaire de Nice, University of Nice-Sophia, Antipolis, France

Eric Barret, MD Department of Urology, Institut Montsouris, Paris-Descartes University, Paris, France

Nacim Betrouni Department of Urology, Inserm (French National Institute of Health and Medical Research), U703, Lille, France

Université Lille Nord de France, Lille, France

Franck Bladou, MD H.Black Chair in Surgical Oncology, Chief of Urology Department, Jewish General Hospital, McGill University, Montreal, QC, Canada

Jean-Yves Chapelon Therapeutic Ultrasound Research Laboratory, Inserm U1032, Lyon, France

Department of Urology, Université de Lyon, Lyon, France

Jonathan A. Coleman Urology Service, Department of Surgery, Memorial Sloan-Kettering Cancer Center, New York, NY, USA

Pierre Colin Inserm (French National Institute of Health and Medical Research), U703, Lille, France

Department of Urology, La Louvière Private Hospital, Générale de Santé, Lille, France

Department of Urology, CHU Lille, Univ Lille Nord de France, Lille, France

Jean-Marc Cosset Department of Urology, Institut Mutualiste Montsouris, Paris, France

Department of Oncology/Radiotherapy, Institut Curie, Paris, France

Sebastien Crouzet, MD Department of Urology, Edouard Herriot Hospital, Lyon, France

Therapeutic Ultrasound Research Laboratory, Inserm, U1032, Lyon, France

Université de Lyon, Lyon, France

Urology and Transplantation Department, Edouard Herriot Hospital, Lyon, France

Jean J. M. C. H. de la Rosette Department of Urology, AMC, Amsterdam, The Netherlands

Wahjoe Djatisoesanto, MD, PhD Department of Urology, Airlangga University/ Dr. Soetomo General Hospital, Surabaya, Indonesia

Ian A. Donaldson, MRCS, BMBS Division of Surgery and Interventional Science, University College London, London, UK

Department of Urology, University College London Hospitals NHS Foundation Trust, London, UK

Matthieu Durand, MD Department of Urology, Hôpital Pasteur 2 – Centre Hospitalier Universitaire de Nice, University of Nice-Sophia-Antipolis, Nice, France

Behfar Ehdaie Urology Service, Department of Surgery, Memorial Sloan-Kettering Cancer Center, New York, NY, USA

Health Outcomes Group, Department of Epidemiology and Biostatistics, Memorial Sloan-Kettering Cancer Center, New York, NY, USA

Mark Emberton, FRCS(Urol), MD, MBBS Division of Surgical and Interventional Science, University College London, London, UK

Department of Urology, University College London Hospitals NHS Foundation Trust, London, UK

Alex Freeman, FRCPath, MD, MBBS Department of Histopathology, University College London Hospitals NHS Foundation Trust, London, UK

Albert Gelet Department of Urology, Edouard Herriot Hospital, Lyon, France

Therapeutic Ultrasound Research LaboratoryInserm U1032, Lyon, France

Université de Lyon, Lyon, France

Romain Haider Department of Urology, Hôpital de Pasteur 2 – Centre Hospitalier Universitaire de Nice, University of Nice-Sophia, Antipolis, France

Lukman Hakim, MD Department of Urology, University Hospitals Leuven, Leuven, Belgium

Department of Urology, Airlangga University/Dr. Soetomo General Hospital, Surabaya, Indonesia

Alexandre Ingels Department of Urology, AMC, Amsterdam, The Netherlands

J. Stephen Jones, MD, FACS, MBA Department of Surgery, Glickman Urological and Kidney Institute, Cleveland Clinic, Cleveland, OH, USA

Steven Joniau, MD, PhD Department of Urology, University Hospitals Leuven, Leuven, Belgium

Cyril Lafond Therapeutic Ultrasound Research Laboratory, Inserm U1032, Lyon, France

Université de Lyon, Lyon, France

Petr Macek Department of Urology, General University Hospital and First Faculty of Medicine of Charles University, Prague, Czech Republic

Zeinab Mahate Department of Urology, Hôpital de Pasteur 2 – Centre Hospitalier Universitaire de Nice, University of Nice-Sophia, Antipolis, France

MbChb Medicine with European Studies, University of Manchester, Manchester, UK

John G. Mancini, MD Division of Urologic Surgery, Duke Cancer Institute, Durham, NC, USA

Toru Matsugasumi USC Institute of Urology, University of Southern California, Keck School of Medicine, Los Angeles, CA, USA

Department of Urology, Kyoto Prefectural University of Medicine, Kyoto, Japan

Caroline M. Moore, MD, FRCS (Urol) Division of Surgical and Interventional Science, University College London, London, UK

Department of Urology, University College London Hospitals NHS Foundation Trust, London, UK

Adil Ouzzane Department of Urology, CHU Lille, Univ Lille Nord de France, Lille, France

Inserm (French National Institute of Health and Medical Research), U703, Lille, France

Université Lille Nord de France, Lille, France

Noelle Pierrat Department of Oncology/Radiotherapy, Institut Curie, Paris, France

Thomas J. Polascik, MD Division of Urologic Surgery, Duke Cancer Institute, Durham, NC, USA

Rajan Ramanathan, MD Department of Surgery, Glickman Urological and Kidney Institute, Cleveland Clinic, Cleveland, OH, USA

Raphaële Renard Penna Department of Radiology, Hôpital Pitié Salpétrière, Paris, France

Ashley J. Ridout Division of Surgical and Interventional Science, University College London, London, UK

Department of Urology, University College London Hospitals NHS Foundation Trust, London, UK

Olivier Rouvière Department of Urology, Department of Vascular and Urinary Imaging, Hôpital E. Herriot, Lyon, France
INSERM, Laboratory of Therapeutic Applications of Ultrasound, Lyon, France
Université de Lyon, Université Lyon 1, Lyon, France

Rafael Sanchez-Salas Department of Urology, Institut Montsouris, Paris, France

Thomas Sanzalone Department of Vascular and Urinary Imaging, Hôpital E. Herriot, Lyon, France

Peter T. Scardino Urology Service, Department of Surgery, Memorial Sloan-Kettering Cancer Center, New York, NY, USA
Department of Surgery, Memorial Sloan-Kettering Cancer Center, New York, NY, USA

Arjun Sivaraman Department of Urology, St. John's Medical College, Bangalore, India

Lorenzo Tosco, MD Department of Urology, University Hospitals Leuven, Leuven, Belgium

Osama Ukimura Department of Urology, USC Institute of Urology, University of Southern California, Keck School of Medicine, Los Angeles, CA, USA
Department of Urology, Kyoto Prefectural University of Medicine, Kyoto, Japan

Guy Vallancien Paris Descartes University Consultant at the Institut Montsouris, Paris, France

Willemien Van den Bos, MD Department of Urology, AMC, Amsterdam, The Netherlands

Thomas Van den Broeck, MD Department of Urology, University Hospitals Leuven, Leuven, Belgium

Hein Van Poppel, MD, PhD Department of Urology, University Hospitals Leuven, Leuven, Belgium

Arnaud Villers, MD, PhD Department of Urology, CHU Lille, Univ Lille Nord de France, Lille, France

Inserm (French National Institute of Health and Medical Research), U703, Lille, France

Université Lille Nord de France, Lille, France

Department of Urology, Hôpital Claude Huriez, Lille, France

Victoria Wijeratne Department of Urology, Hôpital de Pasteur 2 – Centre Hospitalier Universitaire de Nice, University of Nice-Sophia, Antipolis, France

MbChb Medicine with European Studies, University of Manchester, Manchester, UK

Rationale for Focal Therapy

Franck Bladou

1.1 Increasing Incidence of Low-Risk Prostate Cancer

Incidence rates for prostate cancer have been increasing for the last three decades, and this is mainly due to earlier diagnoses of asymptomatic diseases by the use of the prostate-specific antigen (PSA) test and PSA screening. In the pre-PSA era, during the decade before 1976, prostate cancer incidence was increasing slowly (2 % per year), when half of all prostate cancers were incidentally detected in transurethral resection chips for benign prostatic hyperplasia treatment or diagnosed by clinical symptoms and digital rectal examination in more advanced diseases [1, 2]. Early detection efforts were associated with a rapid increase in prostate cancer incidence after 1986, from 2 to 12 % per year, with a peak in 1992 (237.2 per 100,000 men in the USA) [3]. In the subsequent 3 years, from 1992 to 1995, a 10 % per year decline occurred. During the following decade (1995–2005), prostate cancer incidence stabilized, but to a higher level (150.5 per 100,000) than those in 1986 (119 per 100,000). USA prostate cancer incidence was estimated at 238,590 in 2013 [4].

In European countries, the incidence of prostate cancer almost doubled from 1995 to 2008, with an age-standardized rate of 47.4–93.4 when PSA testing has been widely used [5]. Meanwhile, the mortality rate decreased in Europe, from an age-standardized rate of 23.5 in 1995 to 20.7 in 2008 [5]. The same trend of mortality rate even before this date occurred in the USA, from 38 per 100,000 in 1995 to 22 per 100,000 in 2006 [6].

Parallel to the increase in prostate cancer incidence, a significant downward risk migration occurred over time, with fewer high-risk diseases (from 40.9 % in 1990 to 14.8 % in 2002) and an increase in low-risk prostate cancers (from 31.2 % in

F. Bladou, MD
H.Black Chair in Surgical Oncology, Chief of Urology Department,
Jewish General Hospital, McGill University,
Pavilion E-941, 3755 Chemin de la Cote Sainte Catherine, Montreal, QC H3T 1E2, Canada
e-mail: fbladou@jgh.mcgill.ca

© Springer-Verlag France 2015
E. Barret, M. Durand (eds.), *Technical Aspects of Focal Therapy in Localized Prostate Cancer*, DOI 10.1007/978-2-8178-0484-2_1

1990 to 47.7 % in 2002) [7]. Early detection of asymptomatic prostate cancer has increased the number of low-risk diseases and, as a consequence, has increased the treatment of such diseases. In prostatectomy series, the proportion of low-risk patients, stratified according to the D'Amico risk group classification for disease progression, in European radical prostatectomy cohorts was up to 66 % in 2004 [8] and up to 75 % in a large series of radical prostatectomies from the USA [9].

1.2   PSA Screening: Facts and Lessons Learned

Overdiagnosis, overtreatment, numbers needed to treat: the price to pay for cost of saving lives.

PSA screening is "Janus-like" (two-faced), where one positive side allows a cancer-specific mortality reduction and the other a negative side, called "overdiagnosis." Overdiagnosis means a diagnosis of prostate cancer with no specific risk for the patient, a cancer that would not progress to symptoms or death. However, due to the lack of pertinent prognostic factors and of precise diagnostic tools, the only certainty that the cancer diagnosed will become a nonthreatening disease is when the patient dies of competitive morbidity while his prostate cancer is not treated or still in place. Most patients and physicians would not take the risk of underdiagnosis and undertreatment with such a lack of crucial information concerning the disease progression risk. The direct drawbacks of overdiagnosis are, therefore, the treatment of all patients, low- and high-risk diseases using the same aggressive treatments, leading to *overtreatment* in a significant proportion of low-risk, nonaggressive prostate cancers (the truly negative side of PSA screening).

The question raised is whether, even when such a dramatic rise in the incidence rate has occurred during the same period of time, the decrease in prostate cancer mortality rates should be attributed to the results of PSA screening. One answer could be the effect of the lead-time in prostate cancer, that is the interval from screen detection to the time of clinical diagnosis, when the tumor would have surfaced without screening. The vast majority of prostate cancers have a low-growth profile, and the lead-time for prostate cancer is estimated to be between 5 and 12 years, depending on the patient's age at screening. For example, in the European Randomized Study of Screening for Prostate Cancer (ERSPC), it has been estimated that for a single screening test, the mean lead-time was 12 years at age 55 and 6 years at age 75 [10].

On the one hand, it has been estimated that more than a million men have been diagnosed and treated for prostate cancer due to the introduction of PSA screening, and therefore the increase in diagnosis has led to an increase in treatment with exposure to known risks of impotence, incontinence, and radiation-induced lesions, particularly in younger males [11]. On the other hand, recent large, randomized clinical trials have shown a significant reduction in metastasis and cancer-specific mortality in the PSA screening group compared to the control group with no screening [12, 13]. It has been estimated, by using projection models, that almost 50 % of the observed decline in prostate cancer mortality in the last decades can be attributed to

PSA screening [14]; it has been also speculated that survival improvement may be due to more effective treatment of early high-risk and advanced prostate cancer patients [15].

Because mortality rates in North America have decreased significantly (by 40 %) since the use of PSA testing in the late 1980s, both in younger populations and in the elderly since 2000, while in other European countries the decrease in the mortality rate was noted only in middle-aged populations, these results suggest that in the USA, PSA screening and aggressive treatments were both offered to the two age groups, whereas in other countries, it was preferred to do PSA testing on men under age 70 and/or the elderly, who were less likely to receive aggressive treatments [16].

Finally, if overdiagnosis is not something negative (knowing that a patient harbors the disease), it bears its own negative consequences, i.e., overtreatment (cancer treated by aggressive management with potential morbidity for a disease that would not otherwise result in symptoms or death, exposing the patient to unneeded side effects): the treatment does more harm for the patient than his disease does, against the background of Hippocrates's "primum non nocere" [first, do no harm] dictum, which is at the root of our daily practice of medicine.

An extensive debate, still ongoing, has led to numerous publications since the initial results of the ERSPC and US Prostate, Lung, Colorectal and Ovarian (PLCO) cancer screening trials were first released in the same issue of the *New England Journal of Medicine* in 2010 [17, 18]. Over 78,000 men in the USA and 240,000 men in Europe have participated in these unique trials, whose initial results after 10–12 years of follow-up are still maturing. However, the published results of these two large studies have motivated the US Preventive Services Task Force (USPSTF) to recommend *against* PSA screening for prostate cancer, creating a storm in the medical community [19, 20]. The results of the two trials are controversial: In the US PLCO trial, there was no significant difference in prostate cancer mortality between the screening and control groups, with a 22 % increase in prostate cancer detection in the screened group. The main drawback of this study was that, in the control group, almost half of the participants had a screening test at some point during the study. In the ERSPC trial, there was a 20 % mortality reduction in the screened group, with a 50–60 % increase in prostate cancer detection in the screened group.

If controversy is still ongoing regarding the pros and cons of PSA screening, data maturation of the two large trials will possibly help to better define the ideal number of patients needed to treat (NTT) and benefit, versus the harm of such screening. If it is clearly demonstrated that PSA screening is efficient enough to detect prostate cancer and even reduce prostate cancer mortality, the actual cost linked to it is the great number of patients needed to treat for each cancer death avoided (48 in the initial ERSPC study results) and its negative consequences –overtreatment [21]. The value of the critical number of NTT has been extensively studied and is still controversial in the literature, with values widely varying – from 48 in the initial ERSPC study to 33 in a second analysis of the same study [12], to 12 in the sub-analysis of the Swedish trial [13], to 5 in the subgroup of men with no life-shortening comorbidities in a post-randomization analysis of the PLCO study [22].

"Number to treat" means the number of patients to expose to the reality of treatment-related morbidity and side effects with potential quality-of-life impairment. The 15-year outcomes of radical prostatectomy and radiation therapy have been recently published from a population-based longitudinal cohort, allowing a close-to-reality picture of patient-reported, disease-specific, health-related, quality-of-life mature outcomes [23]. The prevalence of erectile dysfunction universally affected 90 % of the treated men in this cohort at 15 years, of whom 37–43 % reported being bothered with respect to sexual symptoms. Other publications reported similar results, with 7–14 % of men suffering from urinary incontinence after surgery or radiation therapy [24], 84 % suffering from erectile dysfunction, and 48 % suffering from sexual distress in the prostatectomy group of the Scandinavian Prostate Cancer Group 4 trial at a median follow-up of 12.2 years [25]. It states clearly that men who have undergone prostatectomy or radiotherapy for localized prostate cancer suffer from declines in all functional outcomes throughout early, intermediate, and long-term follow-up.

As always, the controversy is balanced between two extremes – the pros and cons of PSA testing for early detection of prostate cancer. We have the potential to substantially reduce the incidence of prostate cancer and save thousands of lives but at a considerable risk of overtreatment for a large portion of the population. The answer given by the USPSTF against PSA testing has been seen as a negative extreme, as stated in several publications [21, 26, 27], with the feeling that there should not be a black or white answer to this important question. PSA screening, along with information about the risks (overtreatment) and benefits of such a test, should allow to screen and treat only the men at high risk, who are most likely to benefit.

> The field of urology will be judged on how it deals with early detection and treatment of prostate cancer. Let's leave a legacy we can be proud of. [26]

1.3 Active Surveillance: One of the Answers to Overtreatment

Many efforts have been made over the last few decades to decrease the morbidity of whole-gland treatments, in the fields of both urology and radiotherapy. A better selection of ideal candidates for curative treatment is clearly shown in recent series of both surgical and radiation management. Radical prostatectomy procedure has drastically improved in terms of side effects with the introduction of open nerve-sparing procedure, minimally invasive and robot-assisted surgeries. Amongst the main improvements achieved by these procedures are a decreased operative bleeding, a postsurgical recovery improvement, a better urinary continence and erectile function preservation. On the other hand, a more precise delivery of higher doses of radiation to an individual-based target with a better control of organ motion during radiation exposure is one of the improvements made in these fields.

Active surveillance is another important answer to overtreatment, by reducing treatment – and treatment-induced harm – for minimal-risk disease. In the 2000s a few teams in various parts of the world showed that selected patients with initial parameters of low-risk prostate cancer could be followed without any initial treatment and that a treatment could be proposed when there happened to be progression parameters in recurrent prostate biopsy specimens over time. The most mature data on active surveillance comes from Toronto, where a cohort of 453 patients has been followed for more than 10 years with a 10-year actuarial prostate cancer mortality of 3 % [28]. Five patients in this series died of prostate cancer; three of them had initial occult metastasis, one refused treatment, and only one would probably have had a better outcome with initial treatment [21]. The results on conservative management have been supported by those of the Prostate Cancer Intervention versus Observation Trial (PIVOT), which did not show differences in prostate cancer-specific mortality between low-risk patients managed conservatively versus definitively [29].

For these reasons, the National Institutes of Health endorsed active surveillance as an option for all men with low-risk prostate cancer [30] and the NCCN Guidelines favored active surveillance in patients with "very low-risk" prostate cancer (defined as stage T1c, Gleason 6, PSA less than 10 ng/mL with fewer than three positive biopsy cores and less than 50 % of any core involved with cancer, and PSA density of less than 0.15 ng/mL/g) and a life expectancy of less than 20 years, as well as in elderly patients with low-risk disease (stage T1c-2a, Gleason less or equal to 6, PSA less or equal to 10 ng/mL) and less than 10 years' life expectancy.

However, several concerns raised by active surveillance include the initial downgrading of the tumor (almost 30 % of men with initial Gleason scores of $3+3$ harbor higher grade cancer, particularly in the largest glands and among more elderly men) [31]; a lack of definition of optimal criteria for surveillance and treatment decision-making; the risk of disease progression during the surveillance period; the morbidity and cost of recurrent prostate biopsies with an increased risk of severe infection; the quality of life/anxiety of non-treated cancers (knowing that the suicide rate is higher in men diagnosed with prostate cancer [32]); and so forth.

Two large randomized trials are ongoing and will compare active surveillance versus surgical treatment or radiation therapy: in the UK, the ProtecT study (Prostate Testing for Cancer and Treatment trial, ClinicalTrials.gov identifier NCT00632983) and in North America, the START study (Surveillance Therapy Against Radical Treatment trial, ClinicalTrials.gov identifier NCT00499174). Results from these studies will help define the best candidates for active surveillance and analyze the efficacy of such management in this population of men; however, the maturation of these results will take years [33].

1.4 Rationale of Focal Therapy for Localized Prostate Cancer

The increase in prostate cancer incidence, mainly attributed to the use of PSA testing, has resulted in a greater proportion of low-risk cancers occurring in younger men. This population of newly diagnosed prostate cancer men is the one where the risk of complications associated with curative treatments, i.e., incontinence and impotence, has the highest impact. This risk has to be weighted to the small absolute risk reduction of approximately 5 % over 10 years that is associated with surgery, compared to watchful waiting in this population of low-risk disease [34, 35]. Management options for this population therefore lie between the extremes of radical, potentially harmful therapies and active surveillance. On the one hand, there is a maximum chance of cure, together with sexual and/or urinary morbidity, and on the other, a preservation of genitourinary functions with the psychological and health care burdens of absence of treatment and active surveillance.

Focal therapy aims at directing ablative sources of treatment – such as heat, cold, radiation, vascular necrosis – to the only focus of cancer surrounded by the safety margin of a normal gland. Its goals are to control the disease without explicitly eradicating it, to carry out active surveillance of the non-treated gland that could harbor other foci of cancer, and to limit side effects and morbidity of whole-gland treatment while allowing a partial treatment and a decrease of potential anxiety due to the absence of treatment.

This concept follows the one adopted for other malignancies, such as breast, colon, or kidney cancers in selected patients.

Focal therapy, as with every innovation in oncology, raises a lot of questions, hopes, and concerns [36]. In its infancy, this concept's adaptation for prostate cancer has just begun its initial phase study level [37]. Who will be the ideal patients for focal therapy; which source of ablation will emerge from the options available nowadays; what will be the optimal targeting and follow-up (multiparametric prostate MRI being the most advanced tool used to date for this purpose [38]);, what will be the percentage of salvage treatments to perform after focal treatment; what type of salvage options will there be; and how important will the morbidity of such salvage treatments be? These are just a few of the unanswered questions that we will have to address in order to bring focal therapy for prostate cancer to the level of standard treatment options for selected men with localized prostate cancer in the near future – beginning now.

References

1. Meigs JB, Barry MJ, Giovannucci E, et al. High rates of prostate-specific antigen testing in men with evidence of benign prostatic hyperplasia. Am J Med. 1998;104:517–25.
2. Brawley OW. Trends in prostate cancer in the United States. J Natl Cancer Inst Monogr. 2012;45:152–6.
3. Quaglia A, Lillini R, Crocetti E, Buzzoni C, Vercelli M, AIRTUM Working Group. Incidence and mortality trends for four major cancers in the elderly and middle-aged adults: an international comparison. Surg Oncol. 2013;22(2):e31–8.
4. Siegel R, Naishadham D, Jemal A. Cancer statistics, 2013. CA Cancer J Clin. 2013;63(1):11–30.
5. Ferlay J, Parkin DM, Steliarova-Foucher E. Estimates of cancer incidence and mortality in Europe in 2008. Eur J Cancer. 2010;46(4):765–81.
6. Jemal A, Siegal R, Xu J, XU J. CA statistics, 2010. CA Cancer J Clin. 2010;60:277–300.

7. Cooperberg MR, Lubeck DP, Mehta SS, Carroll PR, CaPSURE. Time trends in clinical risk stratification for prostate cancer: implications for outcomes (data from CaPSURE). J Urol. 2003;170(6 Pt 2):S21–5; discussion S26–7. Erratum in: J Urol. 2004 Feb;171(2 Pt 1):811.
8. Budäus L, Spethmann J, Isbarn H, Schmitges J, Beesch L, Haese A, Salomon G, Schlomm T, Fisch M, Heinzer H, Huland H, Graefen M, Steuber T. Inverse stage migration in patients undergoing radical prostatectomy: results of 8916 European patients treated within the last decade. BJU Int. 2011;108(8):1256–61.
9. Gallina A, Chun FKH, Suardi N, Eastham JA, Perrotte P, Graefen M, Hutterer G, Huland H, Klein EA, Reuther A, Montorsi F, Briganti A, Shariat SF, Roehrborn CG, delaTaille A, Salomon L, Karakiewicz PI. Comparison of stage migration patterns between Europe and the USA: an analysis of 11 350 men treated with radical prostatectomy for prostate cancer. BJU Int. 2008;101:1513–8.
10. Draisma G, Boer R, Otto SJ, van der Cruijsen IW, Damhuis RA, Schröder FH, de Koning HJ. Lead times and overdetection due to prostate-specific antigen screening: estimates from the European Randomized Study of Screening for Prostate Cancer. J Natl Cancer Inst. 2003;95(12):868–78.
11. Welch HG, Albertsen PC. Prostate cancer diagnosis and treatment after the introduction of prostate-specific antigen screening: 1986–2005. J Natl Cancer Inst. 2009;101(19):1325–9.
12. Schroder FH, Hugosson J, Roobol MJ, et al. Prostate-cancer mortality at 11 years of follow-up. N Engl J Med. 2012;366:981–90.
13. Hugosson J, Carlsson S, Aus G, et al. Mortality results from the Göteborg randomised population-based prostate-cancer screening trial. Lancet Oncol. 2010;11:725–32.
14. Etzioni R, Tsodikov A, Mariotto A, et al. Quantifying the role of PSA screening in the US prostate cancer mortality decline. Cancer Causes Control. 2008;19:175–81.
15. Kvåle R, Auvinen A, Adami HO, Klint A, Hernes E, Møller B, Pukkala E, Storm HH, Tryggvadottir L, Tretli S, Wahlqvist R, Weiderpass E, Bray F. Interpreting trends in prostate cancer incidence and mortality in the five Nordic countries. J Natl Cancer Inst. 2007;99(24):1881–7.
16. Quaglia A, Parodi S, Grosclaude P, Martinez-Garcia C, Coebergh JW, Vercelli M. Differences in the epidemic rise and decrease of prostate cancer among geographical areas in Southern Europe: an analysis of differential trends in incidence and mortality in France, Italy and Spain. Eur J Cancer. 2003;39:654–65.
17. Schröder FH, Hugosson J, Roobol MJ, Tammela TL, Ciatto S, Nelen V, Kwiatkowski M, Lujan M, Lilja H, Zappa M, Denis LJ, Recker F, Berenguer A, Määttänen L, Bangma CH, Aus G, Villers A, Rebillard X, van der Kwast T, Blijenberg BG, Moss SM, de Koning HJ, Auvinen A, ERSPC Investigators. Screening and prostate-cancer mortality in a randomized European study. N Engl J Med. 2009;360(13):1320–8.
18. Andriole GL, Crawford ED, Grubb 3rd RL, Buys SS, Chia D, Church TR, Fouad MN, Gelmann EP, Kvale PA, Reding DJ, Weissfeld JL, Yokochi LA, O'Brien B, Clapp JD, Rathmell JM, Riley TL, Hayes RB, Kramer BS, Izmirlian G, Miller AB, Pinsky PF, Prorok PC, Gohagan JK, Berg CD, PLCO Project Team. Mortality results from a randomized prostate-cancer screening trial. N Engl J Med. 2009;360(13):1310–9. Erratum in: N Engl J Med. 2009 Apr 23;360(17):1797.
19. Lin K, Lipsitz R, Miller T, Janakiraman S, U.S. Preventive Services Task Force. Benefits and harms of prostate-specific antigen screening for prostate cancer: an evidence update for the U.S. Preventive Services Task Force. Ann Intern Med. 2008;149:192–9.
20. Moyer VA, U.S. Preventive Services Task Force. Screening for prostate cancer: U.S. Preventive Services Task Force recommendation statement. Ann Intern Med. 2012;157(2):120–34.
21. Klotz L. Prostate cancer overdiagnosis and overtreatment. Curr Opin Endocrinol Diabetes Obes. 2013;20(3):204–9.
22. Crawford ED, Grubb 3rd R, Black A, et al. Comorbidity and mortality results from a randomized prostate cancer screening trial. J Clin Oncol. 2011;29:355–61.

23. Resnick MJ, Koyama T, Fan KH, Albertsen PC, Goodman M, Hamilton AS, Hoffman RM, Potosky AL, Stanford JL, Stroup AM, Van Horn RL, Penson DF. Long-term functional outcomes after treatment for localized prostate cancer. N Engl J Med. 2013;368(5):436–45.
24. Sanda MG, Dunn RL, Michalski J, et al. Quality of life and satisfaction with outcome among prostate-cancer survivors. N Engl J Med. 2008;358:1250–61.
25. Johansson E, Steineck G, Holmberg L, et al. Long-term quality-of-life outcomes after radical prostatectomy or watchful waiting: the Scandinavian Prostate Cancer Group-4 randomised trial. Lancet Oncol. 2011;12:891–9.
26. Glass AS, Cooperberg MR, Carroll PR. Early detection of prostate cancer: more information, more clarity. Eur Urol. 2012;62(5):753–5; discussion 755–6.
27. Schröder FH, Hugosson J, Carlsson S, et al. Screening for prostate cancer decreases the risk of developing metastatic disease: findings from the European Randomized Study of Screening for Prostate Cancer (ERSPC). Eur Urol. 2012;62:745–52.
28. Klotz L, Zhang L, Lam A, et al. Clinical results of long-term follow-up of a large, active surveillance cohort with localized prostate cancer. J Clin Oncol. 2010;28:126–31.
29. Wilt TJ, Brawer MK, Jones KM, et al. Radical prostatectomy versus observation for localized prostate cancer. N Engl J Med. 2012;367:203–13.
30. NIH State-of-the-Science Conference. Role of active surveillance in the management of men with localized prostate cancer. 2011. Available at: http://consensus.nih.gov/2011/prostate.htm. Accessed 21 Dec 2011.
31. Lecornet E, Ahmed HU, Hu Y, et al. The accuracy of different biopsy strategies for the detection of clinically important prostate cancer: a computer simulation. J Urol. 2012;188:974–80.
32. Carlsson S, Sandin F, Fall K, Lambe M, Adolfsson J, Stattin P, Bill-Axelson A. Risk of suicide in men with low-risk prostate cancer. Eur J Cancer. 2013;49:1588–99.
33. Fung-Kee-Fung SD, Porten SP, Meng MV, Kuettel M. The role of active surveillance in the management of prostate cancer. J Natl Compr Canc Netw. 2013;11(2):183–7.
34. Bill-Axelsen A, Holmberg L, Mirrja R, et al. Watchful waiting and prostate cancer. NEJM. 2005;352:1977–84.
35. Merrill RM, Stephenson RA. Trends in mortality rates in patients with prostate cancer during the era of prostate specific screening. J Urol. 2000;163:503–10.
36. Eggener SE, Scardino PT, Carroll PR, Zelefsky MJ, Sartor O, Hricak H, Wheeler TM, Fine SW, Trachtenberg J, Rubin MA, Ohori M, Kuroiwa K, Rossignol M, Abenhaim L, International Task Force on Prostate Cancer and the Focal Lesion Paradigm. Focal therapy for localized prostate cancer: a critical appraisal of rationale and modalities. J Urol. 2007;178(6): 2260–7.
37. Ahmed HU, Hindley RG, Dickinson L, Freeman A, Kirkham AP, Sahu M, Scott R, Allen C, Van der Meulen J, Emberton M. Focal therapy for localised unifocal and multifocal prostate cancer: a prospective development study. Lancet Oncol. 2012;13(6):622–32.
38. Dickinson L, Ahmed HU, Allen C, et al. Magnetic resonance imaging for the detection, localisation, and characterisation of prostate cancer: recommendations from a European consensus meeting. Eur Urol. 2011;59:477–94.

Ian A. Donaldson, Mark Emberton,
Alex Freeman, and Hashim U. Ahmed

2.1 Introduction

Prostate cancer is a multifocal disease, but not all of these lesions will cause harm. Recent evidence has been building to suggest that it is the largest and highest-grade cancer which drives the disease to grow, invade, metastasise and lead to premature death (Fig. 2.1). This tumour has been popularly coined the index lesion and, arguably, is central to the entire discipline of focal therapy.

The introduction of PSA has shifted the landscape in which prostate cancer is now detected [1]. Whilst the ability to screen for prostate cancer before it is clinically apparent is of obvious benefit to men who have aggressive disease, there is a real risk of detecting and treating smaller lower-grade cancers that may never cause harm [2]. As such, if not all cancer lesions are clinically significant, one can contemplate changing the management of prostate cancer from treatment directed to the whole gland to treatment directed only to disease that will cause a reduction in either quality or length of life. This represents a radical shift in how we treat the disease, but it certainly is in tune with the paradigm shifts we have witnessed in breast, thyroid, kidney and liver cancers to just name a few. The concept of the index lesion therefore runs to the very core of attempts to reduce the harms of screening

I.A. Donaldson, MRCS, BMBS • M. Emberton, FRCS(Urol), MD, MBBS
H.U. Ahmed, PhD, FRCS(Urol), BM, BCh(Oxon) (✉)
Division of Surgery and Interventional Science,
University College London, London, UK

Department of Urology, University College London Hospitals
NHS Foundation Trust, London, UK
e-mail: hashim.ahmed@ucl.ac.uk

A. Freeman, FRCPath, MD, MBBS
Department of Histopathology, University College London
Hospitals NHS Foundation Trust, London, UK

© Springer-Verlag France 2015
E. Barret, M. Durand (eds.), *Technical Aspects of Focal Therapy
in Localized Prostate Cancer*, DOI 10.1007/978-2-8178-0484-2_2

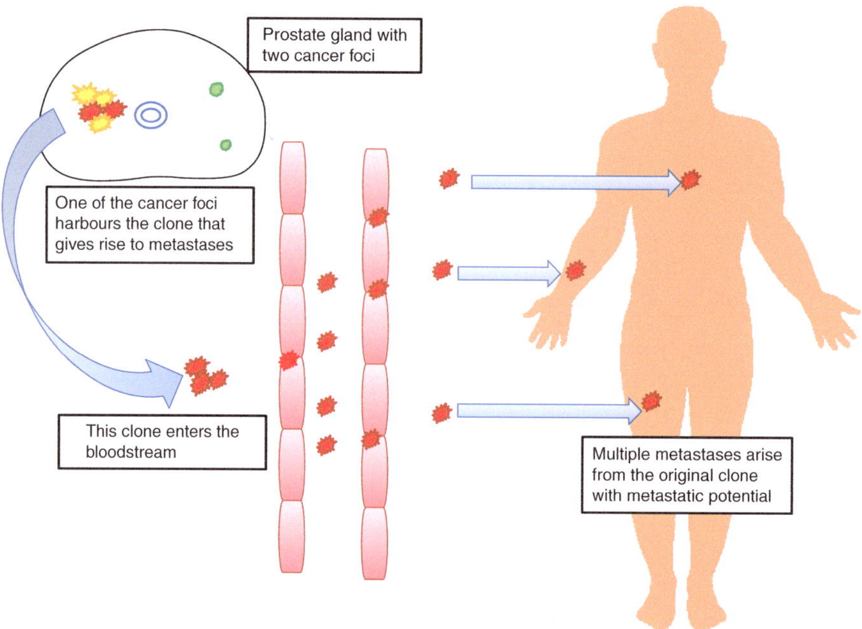

Fig. 2.1 The index lesion hypothesis states that the largest and highest-grade tumour (usually one and the same) is alone capable of metastases

and treatment of prostate cancer, since systematic biopsies which inadvertently detect indolent disease will need to be replaced by targeted precision biopsies directed at a lesion of concern [3].

2.2 Clinically Significant Disease and Tumour Multifocality

Tumour multifocality in solid organs is not a novel phenomenon. It is not only found in prostate cancer (Fig. 2.2), but it is also well recognised at various rates of incidence in the breast, thyroid, lung and even renal cancers. In these cancers physicians have taken an approach to treat only the cancer that will cause harm, leave small indolent tumours (often unknown of) and preserve healthy tissue. In breast cancer, lumpectomy and localised radiotherapy might now be favoured over whole breast adjuvant radiotherapy as recurrences predominantly occur in the area of surgical resection after lumpectomy [4]. The importance of preservation of healthy thyroid tissue is well recognised by colleagues in head and neck oncology leading to renaming the clinically insignificant disease papillary microcarcinoma [5]. The high rates of small lung tumours found at autopsy that would have caused more harm by investigation and treatment are commonly called pseudo-disease in recognition of their non-malignant behaviour. Such a concept is made easier because the diagnostic pathway in those malignancies involves detection of the clinical phenotype, either visually, with palpation or by imaging. In other words, diagnosis and treatment are directed at measurable disease.

In stark contrast to this, prostate cancer is typically detected by a somewhat random deployment of 10–12 transrectal needles, and the disease is confirmed histologically on these microscopic samples. This technique has been deemed adequate as the presence of disease in the prostate was all that was required to inform treatment directed at a whole gland level. By virtue of finding lots of lesions through this

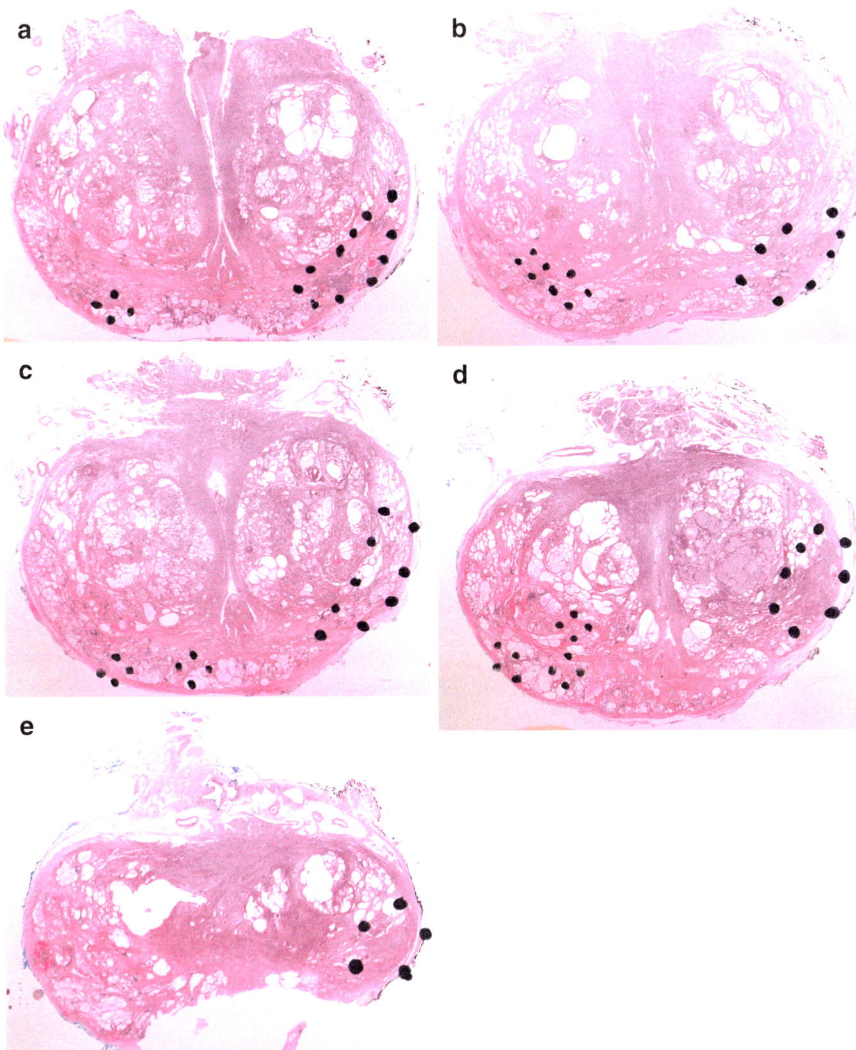

Fig. 2.2 Sections taken from radical prostatectomy specimens (**a–e**) and pathology diagram showing dominant Gleason pattern 4 + 3 lesion with secondary satellite Gleason pattern 3 + 3 prostate cancer (**f**)

Fig. 2.2 (continued)

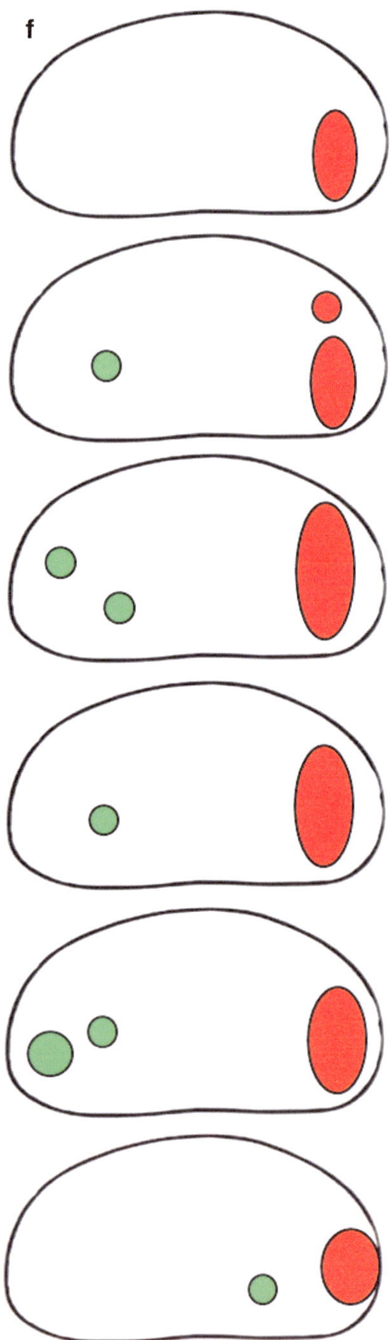

biopsy strategy, the multifocality of the disease has been used as a rationale to treat the entire prostate. However, informed treatment decisions based on biochemical and pathological parameters cannot be made when systematic errors in sampling the prostate can lead to clinically significant disease (disease that will lead to a reduction in quality or quantity of life) being missed or under-sampled or, conversely, clinically insignificant disease (disease that will never cause harm) being oversampled by clustering of the biopsies. Additionally, even when disease in the prostate has been well characterised, it is sometimes difficult to predict the biological behaviour of individual cancers.

Along with multifocality, the idea that within the prostate, separate cancers are behaving differently has long been recognised. In 1963 Halpert et al. surveyed 5,000 autopsies from all causes of death [6]. In their survey they identified the presence of focal and diffuse tumours within the prostate gland. In younger men focal tumours outnumbered diffuse tumours but they were not able to determine whether the focal tumours were precursors of diffuse tumours, or indeed the two types of tumours represented two forms of cancer with different biological behaviour. Thirty years after this publication, Villers et al. from Stanford University published their 3 mm step section analysis of 234 consecutive prostatectomies removed for clinically detected prostate cancer between 1983 and 1989 [7]. In this series a total of 500 adenocarcinomas were identified. A single cancer was found in 117 of the prostates analysed. The remaining 117 specimens contained the clinically detectable lesion plus an additional 266 incidental tumours. Here, despite earlier studies describing diffuse tumours, the authors observed the distribution of normal tissue indicating expansion of the tumour from a single region of the gland.

Examining the Gleason grade of the dominant and secondary lesions in 100 consecutive radical prostatectomies, Karavitakis et al. identified a total of 270 lesions [8]. In the 170 satellite, secondary lesions identified, 87 % were less than 0.5 cc and 99.4 % had a Gleason score of 6 or less. In the 25 specimens where two or more foci of cancer were identified, none contained the higher-grade, more aggressive disease in the secondary lesion.

Considering how size and growth of the index lesion affect outcomes in prostate cancer, Karavitikas et al. examined the extent of positive surgical margins involving the index lesion and secondary lesions [9]. Ninety-five consecutive whole-mount specimens were examined from laparoscopic radical prostatectomy specimens. A total of 269 tumour foci were identified. 2/160 (1.2 %) lesions of volume less than 0.5 cc were involved in the positive surgical margin, whilst 0/132 lesions of volume less than 0.2 cc were involved. In the 19 cases where multifocal cancer displayed a positive surgical margin, the index lesion was the cause in 13 cases and the index lesion plus a satellite lesion in the remaining 6 cases. In the other cases, the satellite lesion had a volume greater than 0.2 cc.

Tumour size was also found to be an important factor in PSA failure in a study by Nelson et al. who analysed 431 consecutive patients undergoing radical prostatectomy for localised prostate cancer [10]. In multivariate analysis tumour volume was found to be an independent predictor of PSA recurrence. The mean tumour volume for PSA recurrence was 6.8 ml.

When Wise et al. compared the impact of small independent cancers and the index lesion on PSA failure in 486 men treated by radical prostatectomy, they found that 83 % of men had multifocal cancer within the prostate [11]. Fifty-eight percent of these smaller secondary cancers were less than 0.5 cc in volume. Factors that independently predicted PSA failure were the presence of any Gleason grade 4 or 5 and the volume of the index lesion. Multiple small cancers appeared to reduce the risk of PSA failure by 14 % for each additional cancer. An explanation for this is that as the index lesion increases in volume, smaller, indolent cancers are assimilated into it. There might also be a paracrine growth inhibition effect between the largest index and smaller secondary lesions, although both of these theories remain to be investigated.

From these studies it starts to become clear that despite being multifocal, individual cancers within the prostate appear to express different behaviour and that perhaps the most aggressive cancer is originating from a single site.

2.3 The Index Lesion

There are two theories that explain multifocality of prostate cancer. One is of monoclonal expansion whereby they arise from the same original cell clone and multifocality is the result of intraprostatic metastasis. The other is of multi-clonal expansion whereby each tumour is a separate independent lesion, genetically distinct, arising in a prostate that is predisposed to cancer through a field effect.

Specifically addressing this question Cheng et al. examined the pattern of allelic loss for a tumour suppressor gene on chromosome 8p and the BRCA1 gene on chromosome 17q in 19 patients with two or more distinct prostate tumours [12]. The pattern of allelic loss was compatible with independent tumour origin in 15 of 18 informative cases. The remaining three were inconclusive and could have been a result of independent origin or monoclonal origin.

This raises the question that if multifocal tumours in the prostate do arise independently, do they exhibit different behaviour and does the index lesion behave in a different manner to the smaller secondary lesions? When one evaluates the evidence with respect to the hallmarks of malignancy, there is striking evidence demonstrating that small low-grade lesions (usually secondary) exhibit few of the traits that would qualify their status as cancer.

Traits that are recognisable in aggressive cancers are an ability to resist cell death, angiogenesis to ensure adequate blood supply and the ability to grow, invade and metastasise. DAD1 is a gene encoding for defender against cell death 1 and displays an antiapoptotic function. True et al. microdissected populations of cells that had Gleason patterns 3, 4 and 5 in 29 specimens [13]. When DAD1 expression was measured, concentrations showed a strong association with Gleason grade, with higher patterns staining more intensely than lower pattern disease.

Prostate cancer cells have an ability to promote new blood vessel formation by production of angiogenic factors such as VEGF, fibroblast growth factor 2 and

COX-2. Raised VEGF and increased microvessel density are related to poor prognosis in prostate cancer, and this association appears more pronounced in high-grade large tumours. Mucci and colleagues established that poorly differentiated tumours showed increased microvessel density [14], and after 20 years of follow-up, men with tumours that had the smallest vessel diameter at inclusion of their study were six times more likely to develop metastatic prostate cancer or die from prostate cancer.

As part of the PELICAN study (Project to Eliminate Lethal Prostate Cancer), Liu et al. analysed 94 separate metastatic deposits from 30 men who died of disseminated prostate cancer [15]. Using copy number analysis and high-resolution genome-wide single nucleotide polymorphism, they were able to show that metastatic prostate cancers have a single clonal origin. Unfortunately they were unable to trace this back to the original prostate lesion for correlation with which lesion caused the metastasis. A new clinical trial – PROGENY – designed to address this has recently opened to prospectively analyse samples taken at the time of prostate biopsy and compare them to any metastatic disease that may develop in the patient's lifetime [16].

However, other studies have provided greater support that low-volume, low-grade lesions do not behave like cancers. Supporting the argument that it is the high-grade lesion that causes lethal prostate cancer is a long-term follow-up study by Eggener and colleagues [17]. At 15 years of follow-up, only 3 out of 9,775 men who had undergone radical prostatectomy for Gleason pattern 3 had died. On review of these three cases, they were all found to have elements of Gleason pattern 4 disease in the whole-mount specimens. Other studies have emerged to demonstrate that low-volume low-grade lesions do not metastasise to lymph nodes [18].

One paper that does counter this argument is from Haffner et al. [19]. In this study they used whole genome sequencing to characterise the lethal cell clone in a single patient who died of metastatic prostate cancer. Interestingly, their analysis revealed that the lethal clone arose from a small, low-grade cancer focus in the primary tumour. However, this study has a number of problems. First, the patient was treated with multiple therapies that might have altered the metastases that eventually were sequenced. Second, the Gleason 6 area supposedly causing metastases was within a larger tumour that covered almost the entire prostate. This Gleason 6 area would in no way be equivalent to a solitary 0.1 cc or 0.2 cc Gleason 6 lesion. Last, even if it is true that this area caused a metastasis, it is likely a rare occurrence as otherwise the one-third of the male population that have small cancer lesions in their prostate would need to undergo radical therapies.

2.4 Clinical Implications

In this chapter we have highlighted the key concepts of the index lesion. In multifocal prostate cancer there is commonly a dominant lesion. This lesion is larger and of higher Gleason grade and appears genetically and histologically distinct. Lower-grade, smaller-volume lesions do not tend to progress, whereas the presence of higher-grade disease and a larger dominant lesion is associated with PSA failure and positive surgical margin and likely to be the source of metastatic disease in the vast majority of cases.

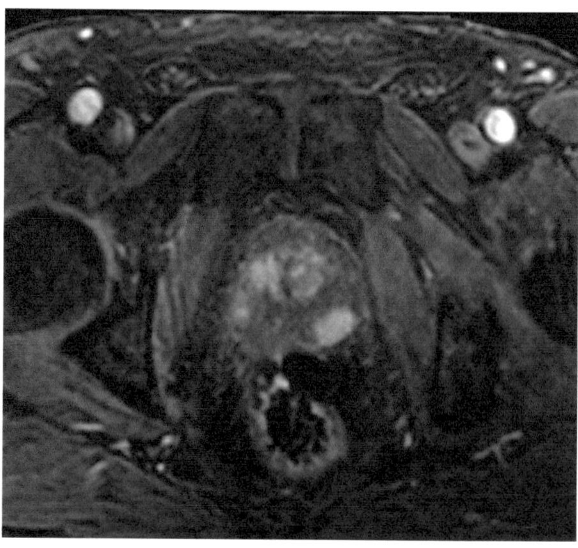

Fig. 2.3 Multiparametric contrast-enhanced MRI demonstrating dominant Gleason 4+3 lesion in the left posterior prostate. Small volume 3+3 detected on right side of the prostate

So what are the clinical implications for this idea? First, random biopsies may no longer be necessary if the index lesion can be identified through imaging (see Fig. 2.3). This may lead to a shift in the way that prostate cancer is diagnosed. There is a growing body of evidence that biopsies directed towards an image-derived target are more efficient and give better representation of the true disease. Second, novel diagnostic tests based on tissue biomarkers or imaging tests should be validated against the presence of clinically significant prostate cancer and not just all cancer. Third, if the index lesion can be detected and characterised with a high degree of accuracy, then therapy directed to just that lesion would not only reduce treatment-related side effects but might prove non-inferior in cancer control to whole gland therapy.

References

1. Cooperberg MR, Moul JW, Carroll PR. The changing face of prostate cancer. J Clin Oncol Off J Am Soc Clin Oncol. 2005;23:8146–51.
2. Wilt TJ, Ahmed HU. Prostate cancer screening and the management of clinically localized disease. BMJ. 2013;325:1–9.
3. Ahmed HU. The index lesion and the origin of prostate cancer. N Engl J Med. 2009;361:1704–6.
4. Vaidya JS, et al. Risk-adapted targeted intraoperative radiotherapy versus whole-breast radiotherapy for breast cancer: 5-year results for local control and overall survival from the TARGIT-A randomised trial. Lancet. 2014;383:603–13.
5. Piersanti M, Ezzat S, Asa S. Controversies in papillary microcarcinoma of the thyroid. Endocr Pathol. 2003;14:183–91.
6. Halpert B, Sheehan EE, Schmalhorst WR, Scott Jr R. Carcinoma of the prostate A survey of 5,000 autopsies. Cancer. 1963;16:737–42.

7. Villers A, McNeal J, Freiha F, Stamey TA. Multiple cancers in the prostate. Morphologic features of clinically recognized versus incidental tumors. Cancer. 1992;70:2313–8.
8. Karavitakis M, et al. Histological characteristics of the index lesion in whole-mount radical prostatectomy specimens: implications for focal therapy. Prostate Cancer Prostatic Dis. 2011;14:46–52.
9. Karavitakis M, Ahmed HU, Abel PD, Hazell S, Winkler MH. Anatomically versus biologically unifocal prostate cancer: a pathological evaluation in the context of focal therapy. Ther Adv Urol. 2012;4:155–60.
10. Nelson BA, et al. Tumour volume is an independent predictor of prostate-specific antigen recurrence in patients undergoing radical prostatectomy for clinically localized prostate cancer. BJU Int. 2006;97:1169–72.
11. Wise AM, Stamey TA, McNeal JE, Clayton JL. Morphologic and clinical significance of multifocal prostate cancers in radical prostatectomy specimens. Urology. 2002;60:264–9.
12. Cheng L, et al. Evidence of independent origin of multiple tumors from patients with prostate cancer. J Natl Cancer Inst. 1998;90(3):233–7.
13. True L, et al. A molecular correlate to the Gleason grading system for prostate adenocarcinoma. Proc Natl Acad Sci. 2006;103(29):10991–6.
14. Mucci LA, et al. Prospective study of prostate tumor angiogenesis and cancer-specific mortality in the health professionals follow-up study. J Clin Oncol. 2009;27:5627–33.
15. Liu W, et al. Copy number analysis indicates monoclonal origin of lethal metastatic prostate cancer. Nat Med. 2009;15:559–65.
16. Prostate Cancer Genomic Heterogeneity (PROGENY). ClinicalTrials.gov NCTT02022371.
17. Eggener SE, et al. Predicting 15-year prostate cancer specific mortality after radical prostatectomy. J Urol. 2011;185:869–75.
18. Ahmed HU, Arya M, Freeman A, Emberton M. Do low-grade and low-volume prostate cancers bear the hallmarks of malignancy? Lancet Oncol. 2012;13:e509–17.
19. Haffner MC, et al. Tracking the clonal origin of lethal prostate cancer. J Clin Invest. 2013;123:2–6.

Definitions and Principles of Focal Therapy

3

John G. Mancini and Thomas J. Polascik

3.1 Introduction: Definition of Focal Therapy

Prostate focal therapy is a term that broadly defines the treatment of prostate cancer by the destruction of a lesion(s) (with cryotherapy, high-intensity focused ultrasound, or any other ablative technique), while sparing a portion of the gland in an effort to minimize morbidity. According to a consensus panel meeting at the Second International Symposium on Focal Therapy and Imaging in Prostate and Kidney Cancer, "Focal therapy is a type of treatment that aims to eradicate known cancer within the prostate and at the same time preserve uninvolved prostatic tissue with the aim of preserving genitourinary function [1]." In essence, the goal is to treat the individual's prostate cancer and avoid as much therapy-related morbidity as possible.

In focal therapy, the surgeon provides a personalized approach to treatment, whereby the lesion of interest is characterized, the extent of disease is determined, and a treatment strategy is individually tailored to the patient. If image-guided therapy strategies are employed to precisely target and destroy the *lesion(s)*, it is conceivable that no two focal therapy treatment strategies will be entirely the same. In concept, if the cancer exists as an isolated *lesion* in the prostate, it can be deliberately treated, leaving the remainder of the prostate intact and unharmed. If a *region* of the prostate (e.g., left side, right side, apex, base, anterior, etc.) is affected, that *region* can be treated, leaving the remainder of the parenchyma untouched.

Disclosure TJP has a consulting agreement with Endo Pharmaceuticals.

J.G. Mancini, MD • T.J. Polascik, MD (✉)
Division of Urologic Surgery,
Duke Cancer Institute, Durham, NC 27710, USA
e-mail: thomas.polascik@duke.edu

© Springer-Verlag France 2015
E. Barret, M. Durand (eds.), *Technical Aspects of Focal Therapy in Localized Prostate Cancer*, DOI 10.1007/978-2-8178-0484-2_3

Focal therapy commences with the identification and characterization of an index lesion, followed by the determination of any additional clinically significant disease, and concludes with the targeting and treatment of that disease while attempting to preserve surrounding normal anatomical structures. Typically, the identification of an index lesion, defined as the tumor responsible for the biologic behavior of the disease, conventionally starts with a 12-core transrectal ultrasound-guided biopsy, with samples obtained from the lateral and medial regions from each side of the apical, mid, and basal thirds of the prostate. The pathological result provides a general idea, albeit not definitive, of those areas of the prostate affected by cancer. In cases where cancer appears to be higher-volume low-risk, intermediate-risk, or low-volume high-risk disease by the D'Amico criteria, focal therapy can be considered [2]. To a lesser degree, the 12-core biopsy may provide some information about those areas that may be unaffected by cancer. For example, if a biopsy core is negative from a particular *region* of the prostate, it does not simply mean that *region* is free of disease.

To determine if additional disease is present after a conventional 12-core TRUS biopsy, multiparametric MRI (mpMRI) is often employed in an attempt to radiographically identify any suspicious areas. If any concerning *lesions* are identified, these can be targeted with an MRI in-bore-guided biopsy or an MRI/TRUS fusion biopsy to confirm the presence of cancer. The contemporary role of mpMRI has been recently reviewed [3]. Alternatively, a repeat TRUS biopsy with either an 18–24-core saturation technique or transperineal 3D mapping biopsy (3DMB) template can be considered. This is important for two reasons – to determine if clinically significant disease exists elsewhere in the prostate and (2) to assess whether an entire region(s) of the prostate appears to be free of disease and therefore can be reasonably spared treatment. There is strong evidence to support additional biopsies, as Mayes et al. have demonstrated that a conventional, office-based biopsy used for the detection of prostate cancer does not predict cancer laterality nor provide the granularity needed to obviate clinically significant disease [4]. Barber et al. evaluated 46 men who underwent radical prostatectomy after only one positive core on sextant or 12-core biopsy and found almost 90 % of those with Gleason 6 or less disease had contralateral disease. The single positive core predicted the laterality of the tumor focus in just 71 % of cases [5]. Therefore, in almost 30 % of cases the index *lesion* is misidentified when relying solely on the 12-core TRUS biopsy and is in actuality on the contralateral side of the prostate. Biopsy approaches where more samples are obtained will increase the number of tissue cores for evaluation, but even with a 3DMB, which can obtain up to 80+ cores, there is no certainty that negative results equal absence of disease in certain areas. However, the aim is to detect clinically significant disease during the evaluation process. There is no consensus on the number of negative cores that would be needed from a specific side or *region* to conclude the patient is free from clinically significant disease.

Once the lesions of interest are pathologically and/or radiologically characterized, they must be targeted and treated in relation to the patient's anatomy, most notably the neurovascular bundles (NVBs). With true image-guided focal therapy, the *lesion* could be pinpointed with definition of its borders and treatment could be precise as to only affect the diseased tissue. The most conservative approach to focal therapy with the current limitations of imaging and treatment remains hemi-ablation whereby the index tumor along with any other secondary lesions within the treated area would be ablated. With hemi-ablation, an entire lobe and its associated NVB are left untreated to preserve patient quality of life, most importantly erectile function and continence. Hemi-ablation has been considered a prototype for focal therapy, placed between active surveillance and radical therapy on the prostate cancer treatment spectrum. It is easily reproducible, as the urethra serves as the natural anatomical structure in the midline, separating the left and right lobes of the prostate, allowing for fashioning of the therapy within one lobe [6]. Hemi-ablation is a technique that can theoretically be reproducible in clinical trials and allow for meaningful comparison between institutions and devices. However, most thought leaders in this field believe we are rapidly moving toward image-guided ablation as the preferred method of delivering focal therapy.

3.2 Principles of Focal Therapy

- *The goals of therapy* are to reduce the risk of prostate cancer mortality, to limit prostate cancer-related morbidity throughout a patient's lifetime, and to preserve quality of life. For example, as the disease progresses and is no longer organ confined, pain from metastasis to the bone or other areas can be lifestyle limiting. By treating the clinically significant disease with focal therapy, prostate cancer-related morbidity can be reduced.
- *Preserving quality of life and functional outcomes* – There is a greater focus on quality of life, as men are living longer and wish to preserve their bodily functions. This becomes especially important for younger men who have an anticipated longer life span. In this respect, focal therapy must improve on quality of life outcomes when compared to whole gland treatment options for clinically significant prostate cancer. There is a very low risk of urinary incontinence as the pad-free continence rate varies between 95 and 100 % as reported in nine studies using validated questionnaires [2]. The continence rate remains very high since the treated prostate remains in situ and the external urinary sphincter is unharmed during therapy. Erectile function can be preserved, especially with nerve-sparing focal therapy approaches. Using validated questionnaires, erectile function sufficient for penetration has been reported in 54–100 % of patients with or without phosphodiesterase-5 inhibitor medication [2]. Additionally, there is little risk of bowel-related morbidity.
- *Avoiding treatment-related morbidity* – Even when compared to nonsurgical treatment options, patients electing to undergo focal therapy can avoid potential quality of life-limiting morbidity. Androgen deprivation therapy or other systemic therapies are used alone or with radiation therapy for treatment. The morbidity of these agents can be avoided with focal therapy that successfully treats the clinically significant cancer. There are no surgical scars, as there would be with an open or robotic prostatectomy. Radiation cystitis and proctitis can be

long-term complications of radiation therapy that are not seen with effective non-radiation focal therapy. Concerns are also voiced about active surveillance potentially missing the window of opportunity for active treatment and cure. When compared to active surveillance, focal therapy provides the patient's freedom from the psychological worry of living with untreated cancer.

- *Combining targeted treatment with active surveillance* – Focal therapy seeks to combine active treatment of the identified clinically significant disease with active surveillance of the remaining unaffected prostate tissue. The goal of focal therapy is to target and destroy clinically significant cancer. This implies that there will be normal prostate tissue as well as the potential for clinically insignificant prostate cancer remaining after treatment. The untreated parenchyma will be placed on active surveillance. There is no consensus on the optimal follow-up regimen after treatment; however, most experts agree that posttreatment surveillance includes a combination of PSA, imaging, and prostate biopsies.
- *Medical management for the untreated domain* – The untreated prostate parenchyma is placed on active surveillance. A chemopreventive strategy, if applicable, can be considered if the side effects of that treatment are minimal.
  - *Tailored treatment* – As stated in this chapter, focal therapy can be tailored to the individual's cancer. The treatment template can be very focused (image-guided index lesion ablation) or very broad (e.g., three-quarter ablation) that can be utilized to eradicate several treatment fields containing several cancer foci.
  - *Avoids overtreatment* – Since focal therapy is applied to the index tumor or perhaps a cancerous region of the prostate, and being that it is not a whole gland therapy, by nature it has the potential to avoid overtreatment.
  - *Patient selection* – The rationale of focal therapy for prostate cancer is to diagnose and treat an organ-confined, clinically significant tumor while sparing the remaining prostate gland that contains either the absence of or biologically insignificant cancer. Generally speaking, various biopsy schemes and imaging techniques are utilized to characterize and define the 3-dimensional location of cancer(s) within the prostate, focusing on detecting the index lesion and other areas of clinically significant disease. It is also necessary to understand and define any zone(s) of the prostate that will not be treated to avoid undertreatment of significant cancer.
  - *Candidacy* – Life expectancy, medical comorbidity, and patient preference are all factors into decision making in prostate cancer management. Age may not be a reliable criterion alone for treatment decisions.
  - *Understanding tumor aggressiveness and metastatic potential* – Prostate cancer specialists need to understand the behavior of each individual prostate cancer focus within the gland. Such an understanding requires a deeper investigation that may include genetic markers of locally aggressive or potentially metastatic prostate cancer. What is the biology and natural history of the individual cancer foci in a cancerous prostate gland? Of patient's multiple tumors, the clinician needs to determine those tumors that require immediate treatment aside from those that are indolent and will not harm the patient during his lifetime.
- *Cancer cure or cancer control?* – The goal of cancer treatment should be to control the disease to such an extent that the (1) disease will not prematurely terminate the

patient's life, (2) the patient will not be noticeably bothered by the signs or symptoms of the disease, and (3) any treatment the patient receives will have a minimal negative effect on their quality of life. Younger healthier men require cure, whereas men with a shorter life expectancy tend to need cancer control.

- *Concept of prostate cancer possibly requiring more than one treatment* – The oncologic goal is to cure or control the cancer, depending on the individual circumstances. Focal therapy combined with active surveillance may convert prostate cancer into a chronic disease that can be intermittently managed with additional treatment should it become necessary.
- *Repeatability* – An advantage of many forms of targeted therapy is that focal ablation can be easily repeated with a low complication rate.
- *"Burn no bridges" concept* – If focal therapy does not provide the anticipated oncologic result, additional treatment may become necessary. As such, focal therapy should not preclude any other treatment options or secondary therapy. To avoid jeopardizing cancer control, it must provide a safety net to rescue those who require more aggressive therapy.
- *Registered to real-time imaging* – Focal therapy requires imaging technology ideally to visualize tumors as well as to monitor the delivery of energy when ablation is performed. The principle is to identify clinically significant tumors with imaging and then focally ablate them along with an adequate surrounding margin of normal tissue.

3.3 Focal Therapy Treatment Strategies

3.3.1 Targeted Focal Ablation

Targeted therapy is indeed true focal therapy, whereby only the lesion(s) identified as malignant is treated and the remainder of the gland is left untreated (Fig. 3.1). In a situation where diagnostic imaging is highly sensitive and specific, and treatment can be performed and outcome monitored in real time with image guidance, targeted therapy would be the ideal treatment. However, at present several limitations exist, mostly related to the challenges of accurately identifying malignancy within the prostate. A transperineal 3DMB can be used to produce a three-dimensional map of the prostate and identify areas that harbor malignancy. This pathological map can then be used to guide focal therapy [7]; however, a fusion of the map with real-time imaging would improve the accuracy of treatment.

MRI has shown promise in identifying malignant lesions within the prostate. Additionally, in-bore MR-guided biopsy and MRI/TRUS fusion biopsies have been performed and yielded satisfactory results [8]. Early studies have demonstrated it is possible that MRI may prove to be a feasible option for targeted image-guided ablative therapy. If the diagnostic accuracy of MRI to detect prostate tumors can be validated in multicenter trials, and possibly serve as a "radiologic signature" of cancer, it may conceivably be possible to evolve to ablative therapy obviating a tissue biopsy. However, at the current time, a histologic biopsy must first be obtained to confirm cancer prior to ablative therapy [9].

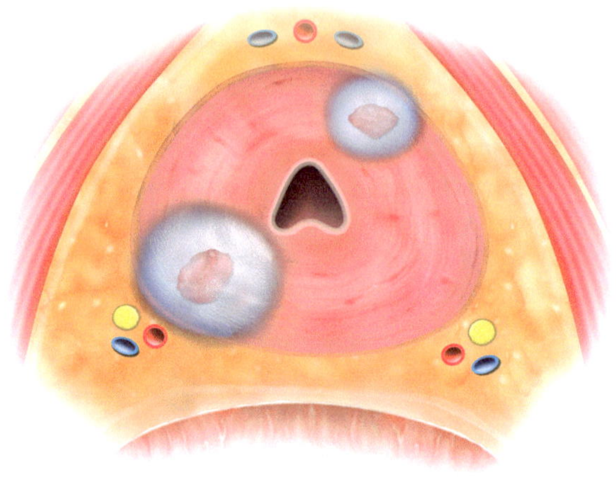

Fig. 3.1 True lesion-targeted focal therapy. The index cancer (*red*) is seen in the right posterior prostate and a nondominant lesion (*red*) is in the left anterior sector of the prostate. Both lesions are completely ablated including a margin of normal, surrounding parenchyma (*blue*). Note sparing of both neurovascular bundles

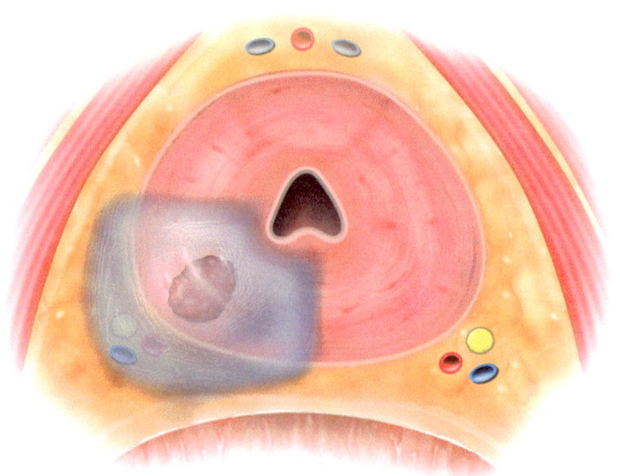

Fig. 3.2 Quadrant ablation. The index cancer (*red*) and other nondominant tumors in the right posterior zone are ablated with intentional extension of the ablation field (*blue*) into the right neurovascular bundle. All other areas of the prostate, including the left neurovascular bundle, are spared

3.3.2 Quadrant Ablation

Quadrant ablation targets and treats a quarter of the prostate that is known to harbor malignancy, leaving the remainder of the prostate untreated (Fig. 3.2). This template is likely the closest to true focal therapy that can be reasonably achieved with many of our current technologies, as it ablates the area of known cancer, as well as broad margin of normal tissue within the zone of treatment. This technique recognizes the inherent inaccuracies of most biopsy strategies and the indistinct boundaries of the tumor. Additionally, by this strategy one or both of the NVBs can be spared depending on the location of the index lesion. Areas of treatment within the category of quadrant ablation can be further refined such that quadrant ablation can represent an area of treatment between image-guided targeted therapy and hemi-ablation.

Fig. 3.3 Hemi-ablation. The index cancer (*red*) is depicted in the right posterior prostate. Illustration shows preservation of a portion of periurethral tissue and intentional extension of ablation field (*blue*) into the right neurovascular bundle. The entire left prostate and neurovascular bundle are spared

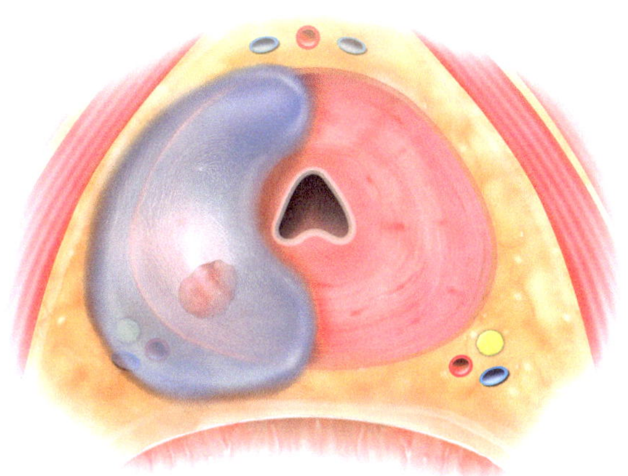

3.3.3 Hemi-ablation

Hemi-ablation, as mentioned previously, was the original prototype for focal therapy and involves destruction of one lobe usually along with the ipsilateral NVB, with preservation of the entire contralateral lobe and NVB, with the urethra serving as the natural boundary for ablation (Fig. 3.3). In this treatment model, all known clinically significant tumor, and normal tissue of either the left or right side of the prostate, is ablated and the contralateral NVB is completely spared. By sparing one NVB, the morbidity of the procedure in terms of erectile dysfunction is markedly reduced.

Nerve-sparing cryotherapy of the prostate for prostate cancer was first described by Onik et al. in 2002, as hemi-ablation of the side of the prostate harbored cancer in a pilot study involving nine men [10]. After 3 years of follow-up, all men had stable PSAs and negative follow-up prostate biopsies. Erectile dysfunction was rare with seven of the nine men (78 %) maintaining potency.

Since that time, several other investigators have reported their results with this approach. Bahn et al. evaluated 73 men at a median follow-up of 3.7 years, who had unilateral, low-intermediate-risk disease confirmed by targeted and systematic biopsy. The authors describe good cancer control and minimal erectile dysfunction after focal therapy. Of the patients, who underwent post-cryotherapy biopsy, 75 % had no evidence of disease. In the 12 cases where post-cryotherapy biopsy was positive, 11 men had cancers identified on the contralateral side and only one was in the treated side. There was no incontinence and 86 % of patients documented erections sufficient for intercourse [11].

3.3.4 Three-Quarter Ablation

Three-quarter ablation is an extension of the hemi-ablation template across the midline only in the anterior region of the contralateral lobe (Fig. 3.4). By this model,

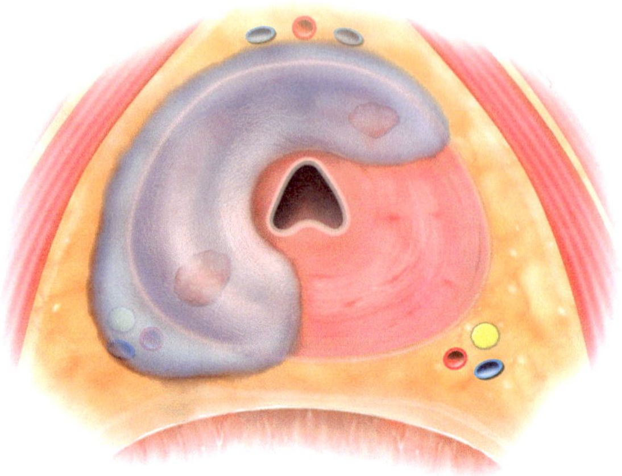

Fig. 3.4 Three-quarter ablation. Illustrated are two cancers (*red*) with the right neurovascular bundle on the side of the index lesion intentionally ablated and the contralateral left side spared. This schema will treat other nondominant tumors residing within the ablation field (*blue*). A rim of periurethral tissue is intentionally protected via a urethral warming device in this example. The treatment on the patient's anterior left side [*right side* of figure] can be extended further posteriorly as needed

three-quarters of the prostate is ablated and one-quarter is spared. This technique provides the benefit of treating unrecognized anterior cancers of the contralateral region. The spared posterolateral region on the side contralateral to the index lesion abuts the NVB, and therefore, erectile function should theoretically be similar as those who were treated with hemi-ablation. An alternative three-quarter ablation model has been described by some authors, whereby the hemi-ablation template is extended across the midline only in the posterior region of the contralateral lobe. Of course, at least one of the NVBs would need to be preserved in the potent man in order to potentially maintain erectile function.

A pathological rationale exists for the three-quarter ablation approach. Of 275 patients with clinically low-moderate-risk features, Polascik et al. found that clinically significant prostate cancer was identified contralateral to a unilaterally positive prostate biopsy (6–16 cores) in radical prostatectomy specimens having such adverse pathological features such as extracapsular extension (ECE) 14.9 %, percent of tumor involvement (PTI) >15 % (8.4 %), Gleason score (GS) >7 (4.7 %), and seminal vesicle involvement (SVI) 2.5 % [12]. Yoon et al. assessed 100 radical prostatectomy specimens with low-risk unilateral disease based on diagnostic biopsy and identified contralateral disease in 65 cases with 13 cases having tumor volumes more than 0.5 ml. The authors found that the more frequent location of inconspicuous lesions on the side contralateral to the positive biopsy was anteriorly in seven cases with six specimens having prostate cancer in the transition zone and one in the

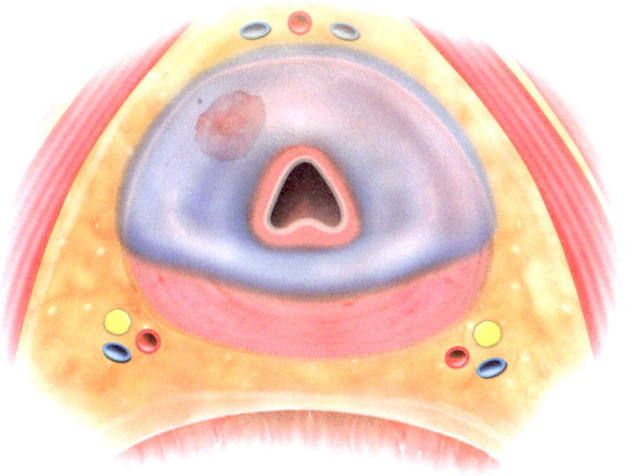

Fig. 3.5 Anterior zone ablation. The index cancer (*red*) is seen in the right anterior zone. Other nondominant lesions [not drawn] identified within the anterior zone will also be treated when in the ablation field (*blue*). Focal therapy is directed toward ablating the entire anterior zone of the prostate. The peripheral zone and both neurovascular bundles are not treated. Note intentional sparing of some periurethral tissue as would occur with cryotherapy as the energy source

anterior horn of the peripheral zone and the transition zone [13]. Finally, Ward et al. evaluated both a hemi-ablation and a three-quarter ablation template on men with biopsy-proven unilateral disease who were treated with radical prostatectomy. If ablative therapy were performed based on the corresponding template, hemi-ablation would have only successfully treated all clinically significant disease in 64 % of patients, whereas three-quarter ablation would have completely treated 81 % of patients [14]. The authors found that if a three-quarter template were applied, it would have encompassed all dominant tumors based on the largest volume cancer.

3.3.5 Anterior Zone Ablation

With the anterior zone template, the bilateral anterior zones are treated and the entire posterior prostate is spared (Fig. 3.5). Both NVBs are spared in this approach as is the prostate abutting the perirectal fat. This would be suitable for unilateral or bilateral anterior tumors. A significant portion of the prostate gland is treated, and therefore, lesions that were not identified on biopsy that fall within the template would be ablated.

Although both NVBs would be spared, however, it remains to be seen whether a bilateral nerve spare would produce less erectile dysfunction than a unilateral nerve-sparing approach.

Conclusion

Focal therapy for prostate cancer holds exciting promise in its ability to effectively treat malignancy, while minimizing the side effects of treatment due to sparing of certain regions of the prostate. The management of prostate cancer may reflect a spectrum, ranging from active surveillance to radical therapy with focal therapy placed squarely in between. From this chapter, it should be understood that focal therapy itself also exists as a spectrum of treatment, from the very precise image-guided targeted therapy to the near whole gland ablation. It is projected that a great deal of research effort will be dedicated to focal therapy in the future in an aim to appropriately select and treat patients, maximizing the curative intent of therapy, while minimizing procedure-related morbidity. As this process continues, it is important to maintain definitions and common terminology, rather than simply labeling everything as "focal therapy," in order to facilitate better communication and collaboration and determine outcomes.

References

1. De la Rossette J, Ahmed H, Barentsz J, et al. Focal therapy in prostate cancer – report from a consensus panel. J Endourol. 2010;24(5):775–80.
2. Valerio M, Ahmed HU, Emberton M, Lawrentschuk N, Lazzeri M, Montironi R, Nguyen PL, Trachtenberg J, Polascik TJ. The role of focal therapy in the management of localized prostate cancer: a systematic review. Kuru t. Journal Urology 2013;190(4):1380–86. doi:10.1016/j.eururo.2013.05.048.
3. Gupta RT, Kauffman CR, Polascik TJ, Taneja SS, Rosenkrantz AB. The state of prostate MRI in 2013. Oncology. 2013;27(4):262–70.
4. Mayes JM, Mouraviev V, Sun L, Tsivian M, Madden JF, Polascik TJ. Can the conventional sextant prostate biopsy accurately predict unilateral prostate cancer in low-risk, localized, prostate cancer? Urol Oncol. 2011;29(2):166–70.
5. Barber T, Pansare V, Nikovaxsky D, et al. Pathologic characteristics of contralateral prostate cancer among patients with a single positive core. J Urol. 2006;175:507.
6. Mouraviev V, Johansen T, Polascik TJ. Contemporary results of focal therapy for prostate cancer using cryoablation. J Endourol. 2010;24(5):827–34.
7. Onik G, Barzell W. Tranperineal 3D mapping biopsy of the prostate: an essential tool in selecting patients for focal prostate cancer therapy. Urol Oncol. 2008;26:506–10.
8. Kuru T, Roethke M, Seidenader J, et al. Critical evaluation of MRI-targeted TRUS-guided transperineal fusion biopsy for detection of prostate cancer. Valerio M: Eur Urol 2014;66(4):732–51. PMID 23608676.
9. Raz O, Haider M, Davidson S, et al. Real-time magnetic resonance imaging-guided focal laser therapy in patients with low-risk prostate cancer. Eur Urol. 2010;58(1):173–7.
10. Onik G, Narayan P, Vaughan D, et al. Focal "nerve-sparing" cryosurgery for treatment of primary prostate cancer: a new approach to preserving potency. Urology. 2002;60(1):109–14.
11. Bahn D, Abreu A, Gill I, et al. Focal cryotherapy for clinically unilateral, low-intermediate risk prostate cancer in 73 men with a median follow-up of 3.7 years. Eur Urol. 2012;62:55–63.
12. Polascik TJ, Mayes JM, Schroeck FR, Sun L, Madden JF, Moul JW, Mouraviev V. Patient selection for hemi-ablative focal therapy of prostate cancer: variables predictive of tumor unilaterality based upon radical prostatectomy. Cancer. 2009;115(10):2104–10.
13. Yoon GS, Wang W, Osunkoya AO, Lane Z, Partin AW, Epstein JI. Residual tumor potentially left behind after local ablation therapy in prostate adenocarcinoma. J Urol. 2008;179:2203–6; discussion 2206.
14. Ward J, Nakanishi H, Pisters L, et al. Cancer ablation with regional templates applied to prostatectomy specimens from men who were eligible for focal therapy. BJU Int. 2009;104(4):490–7.

Patient Selection for Focal Therapy for Prostate Cancer

4

Alexandre Ingels, Willemien Van den Bos,
and Jean J.M.C.H. de la Rosette

4.1 Introduction

The aim of focal therapy is to offer selected patients with prostate cancer (PCa) better control of their disease and lower treatment-related morbidity. Whole-mount prostate treatment is often associated with urinary incontinence (5–20 %), erectile dysfunction (30–70 %), and bowel toxicity (5–10 %) [1, 2]. Treating the correct population by proper patient selection is certainly the cornerstone of this new prostate cancer treatment strategy. Although there are still no high-level evidence studies at the moment, several retrospective or noncontrolled prospective series draw the lines for inclusion and exclusion criteria. The selection has to balance between the risk of overtreatment of nonthreatening disease where active surveillance has proven to be a safe strategy and an inefficient strategy for potentially harmful disease that might require multimodal strategies, including whole-mount prostate treatment (radical prostatectomy or external beam therapy). We base our recommendations on previous and long-running trials and three consensus meetings organized around prostate cancer focal therapy. The main features to focus on are the patient's general health condition, classic prostate cancer criteria for risk stratification, and, more specific to focal therapy, cancer topography into the gland. At the margin of current admitted application of focal therapy but still in the field of patient selection, we mention the role of focal therapy as a salvage treatment after external beam radiation therapy or brachytherapy.

A. Ingels • W. Van den Bos, MD • J.J.M.C.H. de la Rosette (✉)
Department of Urology, AMC, Amsterdam, The Netherlands
e-mail: j.j.delarosette@amc.uva.nl

© Springer-Verlag France 2015
E. Barret, M. Durand (eds.), *Technical Aspects of Focal Therapy
in Localized Prostate Cancer*, DOI 10.1007/978-2-8178-0484-2_4

4.2 Who Is the Best Candidate for Focal Therapy?

Although high-level evidence does not yet determine practice, targeted populations have shifted to a more aggressive disease since the first consensus statement in 2007. At that time, an international task force composed of urologic oncologists, radiotherapists, medical oncologists, epidemiologists, and pathologists, all with a particular interest in prostate cancer, presented expert recommendations for the use of focal therapy. They proposed very selective criteria for treating patients, and focal therapy was just presented as an alternative to active surveillance for low-risk, low-volume PCa [3]. These criteria were a prostate-specific antigen (PSA) concentration <10 ng/mL, no Gleason 4 or 5 pattern on biopsy histology, maximum length of cancer in each core of 7 mm, and less than 33 % of cores positive for cancer (Table 4.1). In fact, even after this consensus statement, many studies have explored the feasibility of focal therapy for more aggressive cancers [7]. Subsequently, other consensuses then agreed to tolerate broader indications including, under certain conditions, intermediate- and high-risk PCa, allowing those technologies to challenge classical radical therapies [4, 8, 9].

Focal therapy can no longer be considered as an alternative to active surveillance for patients reluctant to be part of this strategy. In a recent systemic review, Valerio et al. reported that most studies analyzed had excluded patients with very low-risk disease. Under the scope of 20 studies reporting risk categories, 56 % of men had a low-risk disease ($n=1,109$), 36 % had an intermediate-risk disease ($n=704$), and 8 % had a high-risk disease ($n=164$). Risk categories were not available in 13 other studies. The PSA levels were 3.76–24 ng/mL (overall range, 0.01–82.2 ng/mL), and the median age ranged from 56.5 to 73 (overall range, 47–80) among the studies. Individual Gleason attribution was available in 20 series, with 1,503 men with a Gleason score of ≤6, 521 with a Gleason score of 7, and 82 men with a Gleason score of ≥8. Of the ongoing trials in the primary setting, four are recruiting only men with low-risk disease, seven are recruiting low- through intermediate-risk disease, and one has no risk restriction [7].

Although no randomized controlled trial had confirmed this statement, reports from the literature seem to reveal an empirical orientation of focal therapy toward intermediate-risk patients with at least 10 years' life expectancy. In other words, focal therapy might be a good strategy when the tumor is considered to be clinically significant (Epstein criteria: Gleason >3 + 3, >2 cores positive, >2 mm cancer involvement [10, 11]) so that active surveillance doesn't appear as a safe strategy in terms of oncological outcomes; at this moment, we cannot safely say that it is a safe option for high-risk prostate cancer. Aggressive multimodal treatments, including non-tissue-sparing external beam therapy and radical prostatectomy in association with androgen suppression, are very likely the most relevant options [12, 13] in this situation.

However, patients' general health conditions and classical risk classification criteria (prostate-specific antigen [PSA], Gleason score, clinical stage) are certainly not sufficient to safely indicate focal therapy for prostate cancer. Indeed, the

Table 4.1 Evolution of the concept of focal therapy candidates through consensus panel meetings of 2007 [3], 2010 [4] and 2013 [5]

2007	2010	2013
Clinical		Inclusion criteria
Clinical stage T1 or T2a, PSA <10 ng/mL, PSA density <0.15 ng/mL, PSA velocity <2 ng/mL yearly in the year prior to diagnosis	1 Candidates for focal therapy should ideally undergo transperineal template mapping biopsies, although a state-of-the-art multifunctional MRI with TRUS biopsy at expert centers may be acceptable	Serum PSA: PSA <15 ng/mL, PSA >15 ng/mL should be counseled with caution
Biopsy	2. Candidates for focal therapy should have a life expectancy of 10 or more years	Clinical stage: T1c–T2a
Minimum 12 cores, no Gleason 4 or 5 maximum percentage of cancer in each core (e.g., 20 %), maximum length of cancer in each core (e.g., 7 mm), maximum percentage of total cores with cancer (e.g., 33 %)	3. Patients with previous prostate surgery should be counseled with caution	Pathology: Gleason score 3 + 3, Gleason score 3 + 4
Imaging	4. Patients with previous radiotherapy to the prostate or pelvis should not be treated until more data are available, although the panel accepts that focal salvage therapy may be a possibility in the future	Life expectancy >10 years
Single lesion with a maximum size (e.g., 12 mm), maximum length of capsular contact (e.g., 10 mm)	5. The effects of focal therapy on men with lower urinary tract symptoms are not well known. These men should be counseled with caution	Prostate volume: any. Except in case of HIFU: <40 cc

(continued)

Table 4.1 (continued)

2007	2010	2013
No evidence of extraprostatic extension or seminal vesicle invasion	6. There will be specific attributes that are more related to the energy source than to focal therapy in general. Issues such as prostate size, presence of prostatic calcification, cysts, TUR cavity, access to the rectum, and concurrent inflammation of rectal mucosa may need to be taken into consideration when selecting the optimal therapy	Exclusion criteria
	7. Focal therapy should be limited to patients of low to moderate risk	Previous treatment
	8. Focal therapy should be limited to men with clinical T2a or less N0M0 disease	Previous treatment of the primary cancer within the prostate. Previous hormone treatment for PCa within 6 months before trial. Previous radiation of the pelvis
	9. Focal therapy should be limited to men with radiologic $\leq$ T2b N0M0 disease	Active urinary tract infection
	10. Defining the topography of the cancer is important. Disease that is predominantly apical or anterior in disposition may be technically difficult to manage with existing treatment modalities	Radiologic imaging
	11. The long-term effects of focal therapy on potency/erectile functions are not known. Men should be counseled in this regard before therapy	Prostate imaging reporting and data system score <3; clinically significant cancer is equivocal (Barentsz et al. [6])
		Extracapsular extension or seminal vesicle invasion, lymph node or bone metastasis

specificity of this treatment imposes a thorough analysis of the tumor topography and, in some cases, of the prostate volume (high-intensity focal ultrasound where prostate volume should not exceed 40 mL).

4.3   What Is the Role of a Tumor's Topography in Patient Selection for Focal Therapy?

Spatial location of the tumor within the prostate is certainly of primary importance in selecting a patient for focal therapy. The instinctive idea would be the destruction of any malignant tissue harbored by the gland. This would suggest reserving this strategy for unifocal unilateral tumors. The problem is that multifocality is the common situation in prostate cancer. Meiers et al. reviewed 2,988 patients from 12 contemporary prostatectomy series and found that the incidence of multifocality ranged from 67 to 87 % [14]. Should we exclude this large majority from the focal therapy technology? It has been demonstrated that generally, associated tumors around the main lesion are indolent and will not interfere with disease prognosis. Unlike high-grade, high-volume lesions, small foci harboring Gleason 3 patterns don't meet the criteria of the six hallmarks of cancer as defined by Hanahan and Weinberg [15]. Recently, Ahmed et al. reviewed evidence from the literature emphasizing biomolecular discrepancies between low-volume/low-grade and larger-volume/higher-grade tumors. According to this report, only the larger lesions and those with a Gleason 4 or 5 pattern present the molecular abnormalities to develop self-sufficiency in growth signals, insensitivity to antigrowth signals, resistance to cell death, unlimited replicative potential, sustained angiogenesis and tissue invasion, and metastasis. It calls into question the "cancer status" of these small lesions, and some authors recommend using other designations, such as "indolent lesions of epithelial origin" [16]. This leads to the index lesion concept where prostate cancer is multifocal and composed of a dominant focus (as measured by tumor volume), the so-called "index lesion," responsible of the natural history of the disease and one or more separate, secondary tumor foci of smaller volume [17]. To date, there is no consensus on volume threshold for the significance of an index lesion and total tumor volume.

Among the 25 series reviewed by Valerio et al. [7] using focal therapy in the primary treatment of prostate cancer, 7 included patients with bilateral lesions, 11 were restricted to unilateral lesions, and 7 did not report on this inclusion criterion.

Assessing tumor topography, size, number of foci, and spatial distribution into the prostate is then of primary importance for selecting patients for focal therapy and deciding on the best strategy for tissue preservation: hockey-stick ablation, hemi-ablation, and multifocal or unifocal treatment [7]. The next step is to decide on the best technique to define this tumor topography. Transrectal ultrasound (TRUS)-guided biopsy alone is probably not reliable for deciding on a focal therapy strategy. When compared with a more rigorous sampling method, they often under-grade and understage disease as a result of random and systematic errors in sampling the prostate [18]. TRUS-guided biopsies can miss a clinically significant cancer that would potentially compromise a man's quality or quantity of life. Forty percent of men who test negative on biopsy are estimated to have cancer [19, 20]; one-third of them patients have clinically significant cancer based on lesion volume and presence of high grade [21]. The association of a performant imaging technique, i.e., multiparametric MRI, associated with an intensive sampling strategy such as saturation TRUS-guided biopsies or a transperineal template prostate biopsy (TTPB) is probably the best combination since it allows an accurate estimation of index lesion and total tumor volumes associated with targeted biopsies and an accurate evaluation of the Gleason score. The place of new imaging techniques improving the definition of ultrasound imaging and tumor localization, such as contrast-enhanced ultrasound, elastography, HistoScanning, and MRI/ultrasound fusion imaging, is promising, although high-level evidence is still awaited.

Going back to the literature, most of studies used some form of MRI in combination with biopsy parameters as criteria for selecting patients [7]. In summary, among the 25 studies on focal therapy as a first prostate cancer treatment, two of them used only TRUS-guided biopsies; two used TRUS-guided biopsies and Doppler ultrasound; six used TRUS-guided biopsies combined with MR imaging; and four used TTPB and multiparametric MRI. Preoperative assessment was not reported in 11 studies.

4.4 Focal Therapy as Salvage Treatment?

The place of focal therapy as salvage treatment for cancer recurrence cannot yet be considered a standard option. To the best of our knowledge, only five published series with a total of 115 men treated focused on this strategy [7]. Continence, estimated by a pad-free rate, was achieved in 87.2–100 % of patients. Erectile function was poorly reported, possibly as a result of a poor baseline function. However, in three studies ($n=82$), potency was preserved in 29–40 % of previously potent patients [22–24]. The rate of urethral fistula was significantly higher than in the primary cases. For oncological outcomes, follow-up has a median range of 17–47 months. When considering all patients treated, the positive biopsy rate was 10 %. Only one series reported the presence of residual significant cancer, and it showed a rate of 8 % [24].

Biochemical disease-free rates (bDFS) in the longest series using the Phoenix criteria were 70 and 54 % at 4 and 5 years, respectively [24, 25]. In one series, the bDFS at 2 years was significantly lower at 42 % using the Stuttgart criteria [23]. The second salvage treatment was given to 8–41 % of patients, and metastatic disease was diagnosed in 5–20 %. Overall survival was 100 % in the two series that reported this outcome [24, 26].

According to these controversial outcomes, particularly for the functional aspects and considering the very limited number of patients included in these series, we would not recommend using focal therapy as a routine technique for external beam radiation or brachytherapy failure. This treatment still has to be delivered within the framework of clinical trial evaluations, and patients should be thoroughly counseled when they decide on this option.

4.5   What Should We Learn from the Last Expert Consensus Project?

Although literature on focal therapy as a primary treatment for localized prostate cancer is reaching a level to confirm the feasibility of these techniques, with promising functional and oncological results, all these trials or retrospective studies have different designs with discrepancies in patient selections. This makes it difficult to compare those studies, since the populations under the scope of each particular study differ. Meta-analyses are then irrelevant and it is hard to compare the different techniques of focal therapy. Therefore, an expert panel has been consulted to decide what the uniform, systematic, pre- and posttreatment evaluation with well-defined end points and strict inclusion and exclusion criteria should be. To obtain this consensus on trial design for focal therapy in prostate cancer, a four-staged consensus project based on a modified Delphi process was conducted in which 48 experts in the focal therapy of prostate cancer participated. According to this formal consensus-building method, participants were asked to fill out an iterative sequence of questionnaires to collect data on trial design. Subsequently, a consensus meeting was held on May 28, 2013, in Amsterdam (The Netherlands), at which 13 panelists discussed acquired data, explained the results, and reached their conclusions – which, according to this international multidisciplinary consensus, were that inclusion criteria for candidates in trials should be patients with PSA <15 ng/mL, clinical stages T1c–T2a, Gleason score 3 + 3 or 3 + 4, life expectancy >10 years, and any prostate volume (except HIFU). The optimal biopsy strategy includes TRUS-guided biopsies, to be taken between 6 and 12 months posttreatment. The primary objective should be focal ablation of clinically significant disease with negative biopsies at 12 months posttreatment as the primary end point.

Conclusion

In conclusion, at the moment, no recommendation is based on randomized controlled trials. The data show that focal therapy remains a safe strategy in terms of cancer control at short and middle terms follow-ups and for functional outcomes that are mostly continence and potency. It seems reasonable to offer this option as an alternative to radical treatments, i.e., radical prostatectomy and external beam radiation therapy, to men in good general health (life expectancy >10 years) harboring a prostate cancer with a Gleason grade of 3 + 3 or 3 + 4 on prostate biopsies, a PSA of <15 ng/mL, and possibly an adequate tumor topography on multiparametric MRI evaluation that will allow tissue sparing. Data comparing one technique to another, and determining what technique would be more, relevant for which patient, are still awaited. The new standards recommended by the last consensus meeting should allow more reproducible trials in the future and make it easier to compare studies and develop statistically powerful meta-analyses.

Take-Home Message   Focal therapy for prostate cancer cannot be addressed only to active surveillance candidates any more. Patients with intermediate-risk localized PCa with a Gleason 3 + 4 and/or PSA between 10 and 15 ng/mL are also very likely to benefit from this strategy when tumor topography allows it.

References

 1. Sanda MG, Dunn RL, Michalski J, Sandler HM, Northouse L, Hembroff L, et al. Quality of life and satisfaction with outcome among prostate-cancer survivors. N Engl J Med. 2008;358(12):1250–61.
 2. Wilt TJ, MacDonald R, Rutks I, Shamliyan TA, Taylor BC, Kane RL. Systematic review: comparative effectiveness and harms of treatments for clinically localized prostate cancer. Ann Intern Med. 2008;148(6):435–48.
 3. Eggener SE, Scardino PT, Carroll PR, Zelefsky MJ, Sartor O, Hricak H, et al. Focal therapy for localized prostate cancer: a critical appraisal of rationale and modalities. J Urol. 2007;178(6):2260–7.
 4. De la Rosette J, Ahmed H, Barentsz J, Johansen TB, Brausi M, Emberton M, et al. Focal therapy in prostate cancer-report from a consensus panel. J Endourol. 2010;24(5):775–80.
 5. Van den Bos W, Muller BG, Ahmed H, Bangma CH, Barret E, Crouzet S, et al. Focal therapy in prostate cancer: international multidisciplinary consensus on trial design. Eur Urol. 2014;65(6):1078–83.
 6. Barentsz JO, Richenberg J, Clements R, Choyke P, Verma S, Villeirs G, et al. ESUR prostate MR guidelines 2012. Eur Radiol. 2012;22(4):746–57.
 7. Valerio M, Ahmed HU, Emberton M, Lawrentschuk N, Lazzeri M, Montironi R, et al. The role of focal therapy in the management of localised prostate cancer: a systematic review. Eur Urol. 2014;66(4):732–51.
 8. Langley S, Ahmed HU, Al-Qaisieh B, Bostwick D, Dickinson L, Veiga FG, et al. Report of a consensus meeting on focal low dose rate brachytherapy for prostate cancer. BJU Int. 2012;109 Suppl 1:7–16.
 9. Ahmed HU, Akin O, Coleman JA, Crane S, Emberton M, Goldenberg L, et al. Transatlantic consensus group on active surveillance and focal therapy for prostate cancer. BJU Int. 2012;109(11):1636–47.
10. Epstein JI, Walsh PC, Carmichael M, Brendler CB. Pathologic and clinical findings to predict tumor extent of nonpalpable (stage T1c) prostate cancer. JAMA. 1994;271(5):368–74.
11. Epstein JI. Prognostic significance of tumor volume in radical prostatectomy and needle biopsy specimens. J Urol. 2011;186(3):790–7.
12. Bolla M, Van Tienhoven G, Warde P, Dubois JB, Mirimanoff R-O, Storme G, et al. External irradiation with or without long-term androgen suppression for prostate cancer with high metastatic risk: 10-year results of an EORTC randomised study. Lancet Oncol. 2010;11(11):1066–73.
13. Boorjian SA, Karnes RJ, Viterbo R, Rangel LJ, Bergstralh EJ, Horwitz EM, et al. Long-term survival after radical prostatectomy versus external-beam radiotherapy for patients with high-risk prostate cancer. Cancer. 2011;117(13):2883–91.
14. Meiers I, Waters DJ, Bostwick DG. Preoperative prediction of multifocal prostate cancer and application of focal therapy: review 2007. Urology. 2007;70(6 Suppl):3–8.
15. Hanahan D, Weinberg RA. The hallmarks of cancer. Cell. 2000;100(1):57–70.
16. Esserman L, Shieh Y, Thompson I. Rethinking screening for breast cancer and prostate cancer. JAMA. 2009;302(15):1685–92.
17. Wise AM, Stamey TA, McNeal JE, Clayton JL. Morphologic and clinical significance of multifocal prostate cancers in radical prostatectomy specimens. Urology. 2002;60(2):264–9.
18. Barzell WE, Melamed MR, Cathcart P, Moore CM, Ahmed HU, Emberton M. Identifying candidates for active surveillance: an evaluation of the repeat biopsy strategy for men with favorable risk prostate cancer. J Urol. 2012;188(3):762–7.
19. Taira AV, Merrick GS, Bennett A, Andreini H, Taubenslag W, Galbreath RW, et al. Transperineal template-guided mapping biopsy as a staging procedure to select patients best suited for active surveillance. Am J Clin Oncol. 2013;36(2):116–20.
20. Djavan B, Ravery V, Zlotta A, Dobronski P, Dobrovits M, Fakhari M, et al. Prospective evaluation of prostate cancer detected on biopsies 1, 2, 3 and 4: when should we stop? J Urol. 2001;166(5):1679–83.

21. Lecornet E, Ahmed HU, Hu Y, Moore CM, Nevoux P, Barratt D, et al. The accuracy of different biopsy strategies for the detection of clinically important prostate cancer: a computer simulation. J Urol. 2012;188(3):974–80.
22. Eisenberg ML, Shinohara K. Partial salvage cryoablation of the prostate for recurrent prostate cancer after radiotherapy failure. Urology. 2008;72(6):1315–8.
23. Ahmed HU, Cathcart P, McCartan N, Kirkham A, Allen C, Freeman A, et al. Focal salvage therapy for localized prostate cancer recurrence after external beam radiotherapy: a pilot study. Cancer. 2012;118(17):4148–55.
24. De Castro Abreu AL, Bahn D, Leslie S, Shoji S, Silverman P, Desai MM, et al. Salvage focal and salvage total cryoablation for locally recurrent prostate cancer after primary radiation therapy. BJU Int. 2013;112(3):298–307.
25. Nguyen PL, Chen M-H, D'Amico AV, Tempany CM, Steele GS, Albert M, et al. Magnetic resonance image-guided salvage brachytherapy after radiation in select men who initially presented with favorable-risk prostate cancer: a prospective phase 2 study. Cancer. 2007;110(7):1485–92.
26. Shariat SF, Raptidis G, Masatoschi M, Bergamaschi F, Slawin KM. Pilot study of radiofrequency interstitial tumor ablation (RITA) for the treatment of radio-recurrent prostate cancer. Prostate. 2005;65(3):260–7.

Role and Technique of Transrectal Ultrasound for Focal Therapy

5

Osamu Ukimura and Toru Matsugasumi

5.1 Introduction

Prostate cancer death rates in the United States declined in the early 1990s [1]. Many physicians have pointed out that the introduction of prostate-specific antigen (PSA)-based prostate cancer screening was followed by subsequent dramatic reductions in prostate cancer mortality. Although few have mentioned the role of transrectal ultrasound (TRUS) in contributing to this phenomenon, it is noteworthy that systematic prostate biopsy guided by TRUS, reported by Hodge in 1989 [2], spreads simultaneously with the widespread use of PSA. Unfortunately, however, current routine practitioners (mainly urologists) may not use TRUS as an important tool for image-targeted biopsy and intervention but only for simple delivery of the prostate biopsy needle toward the sextant portion of the prostate, even though TRUS-guided targeted biopsy from TRUS suspicious lesions is highly recommended in the guidelines of multiple organizations worldwide [3]. Modern TRUS technology has significantly evolved and is absolutely not at the same level as it was a decade ago. Nowadays, since prostate biopsy continues to rely on real-time TRUS image guidance and TRUS is the most effective imaging modality in the outpatient clinic in the urological field, we must rethink the contemporary role and techniques of TRUS to improve the management of prostate cancer. Especially, new technology related with modern TRUS, such as the multiparametric functions of TRUS, real-time three-dimensional imagery, simultaneous biplane TRUS, US contrast enhancer,

O. Ukimura (⊠) • T. Matsugasumi
Department of Urology, USC Institute of Urology, Keck School of Medicine,
University of Southern California, Los Angeles, CA, USA

Department of Urology, Kyoto Prefectural University of Medicine, Kyoto, Japan
e-mail: ukimura@med.usc.edu

© Springer-Verlag France 2015
E. Barret, M. Durand (eds.), *Technical Aspects of Focal Therapy
in Localized Prostate Cancer*, DOI 10.1007/978-2-8178-0484-2_5

image fusion technology, various ablative energy techniques available using TRUS guidance, multi-planar display, and device tracking systems, would support the several specific aims of focal therapy for prostate cancer.

The diagnostic and staging process of prostate cancer has multiple steps. In addition to both digital rectal examination (DRE) and PSA, improved quality of imaging to visualize suspicious lesions is vital to enhance detection as well as to better characterize the cancer. Evolving functions of TRUS have significantly contributed to this. Modern imaging can improve the process of prostate cancer diagnosis and staging, through the ability to localize and characterize lesions and to guide precise targeting [4]. Every effort to decrease sampling error has been critical for the precise characterization of prostate cancer, as routine prostate biopsy in current practice may be called "image-blinded" prostate biopsy [3]. Also, importantly, although some criticize that imaging is operator dependent, it has to be said that any interventional procedure or surgery is operator dependent. Especially, in image-guided surgery such as the focal therapy of prostate cancer, imaging technique is in fact an essential part of the surgical technique. Preoperative accurate localization of the cancer and intraoperative precise targeting of it are vital for establishing an effective focal therapy of the prostate cancer [5, 6]. Intraoperative TRUS guidance remains the most effective imaging modality to guide intraprostatic targeting and has been most familiar in urological outpatient practice as well as in the urological operation room.

This chapter focuses on the contemporary role of TRUS for the effective management of prostate cancer with focal therapy.

5.2 Technical Aspects of TRUS

5.2.1 Cancer Diagnosis, Characterization, and Staging

TRUS has improved knowledge of prostate zonal anatomy and internal prostate architecture. The technique is operator dependent, as the quality of this modality is related to the operator's knowledge and experience. The majority of prostate cancers originate from the peripheral zone [7], in which typical clinically significant nodules can be characterized as a hypoechoic appearance in comparison to the homogeneous echotexture of normal glandular tissue in the peripheral zone. Ultrasonographers define brighter ultrasound images from a stronger ultrasound reflector (due to its heterogeneous structure) as *hyperechoic*, while darker ultrasound images from a weaker ultrasound reflector (due to its homogeneous structure) are known as *hypoechoic*; and lesions with an ultrasound appearance similar to the adjacent tissue are referred to as *isoechoic*. As a higher Gleason score cancer has less normal glandular structure, the ultrasound image of the lesion is likely to be more hypoechoic from benign glands, although the issue is that the prostate has several benign structures with a hypoechoic appearance which mimic hypoechoic cancer.

Biopsies taken from TRUS suspicious lesions are almost twice as likely to show cancer as when no lesion is visible [8]. These cancers in targeted biopsy from TRUS-visible lesions have a significantly higher grade (Gleason score 7 or greater) when compared to those from TRUS-invisible lesions (69 % vs. 28 %, $p<0.001$). Similarly, biopsies from TRUS-visible lesions had a greater median percent of the core involved with the cancer in comparison to TRUS-invisible lesions (50 % vs. 10 %, $p<0.001$). Therefore, the cancers in targeted biopsy from TRUS-visible lesions are more clinically significant. In a Canadian clinical setting study ($n=982$), logistic regression analysis revealed that a TRUS-visible lesion is the most important independent predictor of prostate cancer detection (odds ratio [OR], 2.47; 95 % confidence interval [CI], 1.91–3.2), followed by DRE (OR, 2.29; 95 % CI, 1.72–3.06; $p<0.01$), as well as of high-grade cancer detection [9].

On the other hand, diffuse tumors and clinically insignificant small tumors may obscure the normal glandular tissue or appear isoechoic because of the lack of contrast with adjacent normal glandular tissue. The difference of the echotexture of a lesion in ultrasound is dependent on how much different the anatomical structure of the lesion is from that of the adjacent tissue. The transition zone of the prostate is the origin of benign prostatic hyperplasia (BPH) and approximately 15–20 % of prostate cancers [10]. Fibromuscular tissue in the anterior fibromuscular stroma and BPH nodules in the transition zone are also likely to be characterized as hypoechoic. Therefore, the challenge is to diagnose the transition zone cancer with a single use of conventional grayscale TRUS. When there is ultrasound interference such as prostatic calculi or calcified corpora amylacea, the anterior part of the interface has poor image resolution due to the acoustic shadow from the interface.

The hypoechoic appearance of an area is often multiple in a prostate and is not a specific sign of cancer. Various benign prostate tissues of age-related physiological changes and zone-dependent biological differences mimic the cancerous hypoechoic lesion. These include BPH nodules, prostatic inflammation, glandular ectasia, cystic lesions, and so on. Importantly, the operator must be careful about the anisotropic effect (mimicking hypoechoic, but being an artifact), which is often seen in the posterior-lateral edge of the prostate. When an ultrasound beam hits the prostate lateral border in a tangential direction near the neurovascular bundle, a significant part of the ultrasound beam may be reflected in other directions, resulting in the attenuation of the ultrasound beam reflected back to the probe; this causes the posterior-lateral edge of the prostate to mimic the hypoechoic area as an artifact.

Taken together, the obvious limitation of conventional grayscale TRUS in identifying the hypoechoic lesion is that it is highly dependent on operator experience and ultrasound technology. However, in the hands of an expert in TRUS, the higher-grade and larger cancer can be more often visualized by grayscale TRUS, to better characterize clinically significant cancer [4, 5, 11]. As such, cooperation with the uroradiologist or expert ultrasonographer in TRUS imaging would be essential for establishing a meaningful clinical team for a focal therapy program [12].

The higher the frequency of the ultrasound beam, the higher the resolution is in the image but with less penetration in ultrasound wave delivery. For prostate imaging, an ultrasound frequency of 8–12 MHz is typically used for TRUS in consideration of the balance between ultrasound penetration depth (to allow visualization of the entire prostate) and to achieve a reasonable resolution of the image. In order to improve the image resolution with an additional signal, the introduction of a novel US technique using the nonlinear acoustic effects of US interaction either within the prostate or with the use of microbubble contrast agents has opened new prospects for grayscale US in native tissue and also for contrast imaging [13]. In physics, the ultrasound wave becomes distorted through the tissue, and additional frequencies that did not exist in the original wave form are generated. The multiples of the fundamental frequency are called harmonics, and the second harmonic frequency is used for construction of harmonic imaging. Tissue harmonic imaging uses higher frequencies generated on propagation of the US beam through the prostate to improve image visibility of the hypoechoic structure. Nowadays, the use of harmonic grayscale imagery has become routine practice during grayscale TRUS for the experienced ultrasonographer. On the other hand, using contrast harmonic imaging in addition to grayscale harmonic US, Halpern et al. reported that contrast-enhanced TRUS with intermittent harmonic imaging provides a statistically significant improvement in discrimination between benign and malignant biopsy sites ($p<0.05$) [14].

Integration of the different functions of imaging potentially enhances diagnostic accuracy. Based on the concept that cancerous tissue has more neovascular supply to feed the cancer cells than normal tissue, the use of color or power Doppler TRUS has become a routine TRUS procedure to enhance the diagnostic accuracy of TRUS with the visualization of increased blood flow in the suspicious lesion [4, 15]. Sauvain et al. reported that targeted biopsy from increased blood flow in any part of the prostate was useful to detect isoechoic areas or lesions in patients with first negative biopsy results, as 57 % (41/72) of patients who had first negative biopsies and power Doppler TRUS-guided targeted biopsy were revealed as having a cancer by targeted biopsy [15]. Nelson et al. [16] also reported that a linear trend of increasing Gleason score was demonstrated with abnormal lesions on grayscale ($P<0.001$) and Doppler ($P<0.005$) images, where flow signs were strongly associated with Gleason 8–10 lesions. Furthermore, use of contrast agents enhances the Doppler function to identify a suspicious lesion, due to the increased ultrasound reflectors in the vasculature in the lesion. Mitterberger reported in 690 men who underwent contrast-enhanced color Doppler targeted biopsy that contrast-enhanced color Doppler targeted biopsy detected cancers with higher Gleason scores (6.8 vs. 5.4, $P<0.003$) and had a better cancer detection rate (11 %, 379/3,417 vs. 5.7 %, 400/6,900, $p<0.001$) than systematic biopsy [17]. Interestingly, Morelli et al. reported that vardenafil-enhanced power Doppler ultrasound enables excellent visualization of the microvasculature associated with cancer and can improve the detection rate compared to contrast-enhanced power Doppler ultrasound and the random systematic technique [18]. Analysis of the three methods including (a) vardenafil-enhanced power Doppler ultrasound-guided biopsy, (b) contrast-enhanced power Doppler ultrasound-guided biopsy, and (c) conventional random systematic biopsy showed significantly higher detection in the use of vardenafil (41.2 % vs. 22.7 % and 8.1 %, $p<0.005$ and <0.001, respectively). These new techniques suggest that the expanded vasculature or increased ultrasound reflector in the lesion can enhance the diagnostic accuracy of Doppler TRUS. When comparing the Doppler study before and after targeted focal therapy, Ukimura et al. reported that the preoperatively documented signs of increased blood flow in the biopsy-proven cancer decreased or disappeared (and were likely accompanied with shrinking or the disappearance of hypoechoic appearance) suggesting the technical success of targeted focal therapy [4]. When the recent emerging TRUS technologies including Doppler, contrast, harmonic, elastography, computer analysis (such as HistoScanning), or image fusion with other imaging modalities could be integrated in a platform, the so-called multiparametric TRUS would have a key role for prostate imaging to facilitate the focal therapy of prostate cancer [5].

TRUS is also able to visualize the nodule with macroscopic signs of clinical T3 disease, which are associated with the ultrasound signs of bulging mass, discontinuity of capsular echo, disappearance of fat layer in the Denonvilliers space, and involvement of adjacent neurovascular bundles or seminal vesicles by the hypoechoic nodule [19]. Quantitative measurement of the TRUS-measured contact length of the biopsy-proven cancer has the ability to predict microscopic extraprostatic disease [20, 21]. Ukimura et al. reported that in 189 prostatectomy specimens, the contact length, maximum length (mm.) of the portion of the peripheral zone cancer that was in contact with the fibromuscular rim (prostate capsule), was more significantly related to extraprostatic extension than tumor volume, PSA level, and tumor grade. For men who are clinically candidates for radical prostatectomy and have peripheral zone hypoechoic cancers, the combination of ultrasound contact length and PSA value is the best predictor of microscopic extraprostatic extension [20].

TRUS can be used to direct the biopsy sampling from the suspicious area of the extraprostatic disease. Lee et al. reported that among 100 men with systematic biopsy-proven clinically T1–T2 prostate cancer who presented for an opinion for prognosis and treatment options, 27 % were upstaged to pathological T3–T4 disease by TRUS-directed staging biopsy [22]. Okihara et al. reported that among 244 possible candidates of prostatectomy who had a diagnostic biopsy Gleason score of 8 or higher and/or indications of extraprostatic extension (including the seminal vesicles and neurovascular bundles) by DRE or TRUS and underwent staging biopsies using an 18-gauge needle, 31 % (75/244) had positive staging biopsies to provide histological confirmation of locally advanced disease [23].

TRUS-directed staging biopsy has the ability to diagnose histological extracapsular extension and objectifies prognosis and choice of treatment [4, 22, 23].

5.2.2 Novel Techniques of TRUS for Cancer Mapping and Image Fusion

The major challenge for both active surveillance and focal therapy is precise mapping of baseline cancer location and extent. A significant debate continues over the optimal screening biopsy template as well as staging biopsy strategy prior to focal therapy. It is our belief that the key to refining optimal biopsy protocols is not to simply increase the number of cores taken, but rather to improve the quality of each biopsy by real-time image-guided targeting and to document each individual biopsy location to revisit the exact location of the known cancer during possible future interventions [24].

Conventional systematic random biopsies of the prostate are delivered randomly with estimation toward the prostatic sextant template. Current practice with conventional systematic random biopsy, even when extended, does not confidently map out all existing cancers [25, 26].

As the landmark report by Stamey et al. suggested, it is generally accepted that tumors less than 0.5 ml do not contain high-grade cancer and thus could be deemed as clinically insignificant [27]. In order to achieve potential diagnosis of all clinically significant cancer, several groups have proposed transperineal template 5-mm grid-based three-dimensional (3D) mapping ("saturation" biopsy) and introduced this strategy to avoid missing any clinically significant cancer in the prostate prior to focal therapy [28–30]. However, concerns have been raised with this grid-based saturation biopsy method, including the cost, potential biopsy-related complications, and further overdiagnosis of indolent cancer. Furthermore, since a grid-based delivery technique simply relies on the mathematical documentation of points on a grid outside the prostate, there are potential errors between the extraprostatic grid-based documentation and intraprostatic reality of the sampled 3D volume, due to prostatic swelling, needle bending, and/or deformation and shift of the prostate during multiple insertions of the needle. As such, a comprehensive but maximally invasive saturation biopsy method may yield maximum cancer detection but illustrates the limitations of grid-based mathematical 3D mapping biopsy when one simply increases the numbers of biopsies to increase detection [27].

Importantly, more sophisticated 3D cancer mapping strategies require computer-assisted technology including the image capture of real-time TRUS for the 3D volume of the prostate and its reconstruction into a 3D computer model, which can be supported by using either the tracking technology of a 2D TRUS probe or 3D TRUS image-based tracking of the prostate [24]. These emerging technologies also allow the novel and promising opportunity for image fusion-guided prostate biopsy between real-time TRUS and any other imaging modality such as multiparametric MRI that is acquired prior to the time of biopsy.

There are several technologies for tracking the TRUS probe in order to reconstruct a 3D computer model of the prostate, including the use of a magnetic tracker, an optical tracker, or robotic mechanical tracking. Generally, these intend to track the location of a 2D end-fire TRUS probe to image and then to reconstruct 3D prostate volume data, in order to register the 3D volume data of a preoperatively acquired prostate (such as by MRI) onto the real location of the prostate at the time of biopsy. This is because the image fusion of the preoperatively acquired MRI data with TRUS requires reliable registration between preoperative and intraoperative conditions. However, there are various challenges to achieve precise registration between the preoperative and the intraoperative reality of the prostate. The intraoperative reality of the prostate may change once the patient moves or when the prostate is deformed or shifted on needle insertion. Real-time monitoring and adjustment of such intraoperative change in location or shape of the prostate with the preoperative condition are essential to achieve reliable image fusion. For this, the most reliable approach is to track the prostate using real-time 3D TRUS and, second, using simultaneous biplane TRUS, since these new TRUS technologies can determine a specific point with coordinates of (x1, y1, z1) in the space of the prostate by documentation of either real-time 3D volume data or cross-sectional two plane (axial and sagittal) data, respectively. In order to achieve precise image fusion, the capability of determining the spatial location of intraprostatic specific points with coordinates of (x, y, z) between preoperative data and intraoperative data is necessary. In contrast, the use of a single end-fire TRUS probe cannot determine an intraprostatic specific point with coordinates of (x, y, z) [31–33]. As long as it uses the tracking system of a single plane TRUS probe, it may have significant error in image fusion once the patient moves or the prostate deforms or shifts at the time of biopsy, since such a tracking system can *track the TRUS probe itself but is unlikely to track the prostate*. Using a real-time 3D TRUS probe or a simultaneous biplane TRUS probe can *track the prostate itself*; therefore, these likely achieve a more precise image fusion. Taken together, the use of an image-based tracking system with a 3D TRUS probe or a simultaneous biplane TRUS probe is likely to achieve more precise monitoring and registration of reality of the prostate than the use of a single end-fire TRUS probe with any tracking system. Furthermore, since the prostate is a mobile organ and prostate shape is deformable between preoperative and intraoperative conditions, the use of image fusion with a nonrigid, i.e., elastic, image fusion technique is vital to achieve precise image fusion between them. An image-based tracking system using real-time 3D TRUS with elastic image fusion seems the most reliable registration and localizing system to document biopsy trajectory overlaid onto the image suspicious lesion [31–33].

On the other hand, in order to achieve precise real-time targeting into the suspected lesion, real-time simultaneous parallel display of the real-time TRUS and virtual MRI target is attractive [34, 35]. Since at the time of needle insertion through the prostate it is deformable, real-time 2D TRUS monitoring of such deformation is vital. In the display with both real-time TRUS and virtual fused MRI image, the operator must rely on the real-time TRUS image, but must not look at the virtual, i.e., image-fused image of the MRI, which is not real. The real-time TRUS is more important, since the TRUS image is real and the fused MRI target is virtual. In the authors' experience, an MRI highly suspicious lesion (categorized as "Score 5" = clinically significant disease) is highly likely to be present and, in the scoring systems of MRI [36], is almost always visible in routine grayscale TRUS. However, when the MR suspected lesion is completely invisible (isoechoic) on TRUS or when a concerted effort has not been made to interpret the real-time US image, biopsy accuracy becomes challenging because real-time guidance then relies exclusively on a virtual image [37, 38]. The operator of MR/US fusion should make every effort to minimize the potential error at each step of the process.

5.2.3 Intraoperative and Postoperative TRUS Monitoring for Focal Therapy When the Cancer Is Visible or Even When It Is Invisible

Contemporary multiparametric TRUS with high-frequency, grayscale, harmonic, Doppler, contrast-enhanced, elastography, and/or computer-assisted analysis ultrasound can display a substantial percentage of biopsy-proven cancers due to a change in the intensity of the returning echoes. Furthermore, in addition to the use of a single 2D image, the use of simultaneous biplane TRUS or 3D TRUS with multiplanar functions improves the acquisition of the 3D volume data of the prostate to retrospectively review any angled tomography and also enables quantitative measurement of the anatomical details in the 3D view to improve reproducibility in measurement and 3D localization of the target without confusion based on possible differences between preoperative and intraoperative conditions.

Image visibility enhanced the precision of targeting and accurate spatial mapping of cancer to help identify more appropriate candidates for focal therapy [4]. When comparing TRUS-visible and TRUS-invisible index lesions using grayscale plus power Doppler study, the cancer-involved core length was 6.1 vs. 1.5 mm ($P<0.001$), respectively; furthermore, the percent of core with involved cancer was 48 vs. 16 % ($P<0.001$), and the mean Gleason score was 7.0 vs. 6.2 ($P<0.001$).

Image visibility of a cancer lesion opens up exciting possibilities including (1) precise biopsy with recorded trajectory, (2) precise therapeutic targeting of the lesion plus margin, and (3) "per-lesion" follow-up after focal therapy [37]. For focal therapy to be successful, we must know where the cancer is. Even if a random biopsy-diagnosed cancer is invisible on imaging (using multiparametric TRUS or even using multiparametric MRI), if that biopsy trajectory is digitally recorded in computerized data, we can now compute the 3D intraprostatic location of the cancer lesion. However, if biopsy trajectories were not recorded, accurately "revisiting" a biopsy-proven cancer lesion would not be feasible. As such, for tissue-preserving targeted focal therapy, sophisticated imaging and/or precise geographically recorded biopsies are necessary, if we want to treat both visible and invisible lesions. When the biopsy-proven cancer lesion was visible with imaging, retargeting of the lesion could be achieved with image guidance. The real challenge is retargeting the cancer-proven lesion that is not identifiable by available imaging. In this situation, we must rely on the (x, y, z) coordinates recorded from the previous biopsy session by computerized techniques to guide the delivery of the retargeting biopsy or ablative probe toward the intended target plus a potential safety margin around the target.

Use of multiparametric TRUS as well as multiparametric MRI data with the aid of MRI/ultrasonography fusion would probably contribute to more sophisticated diagnosis and appropriate treatment of prostate cancer [31–35]; however, given that an imaged lesion is likely to be underestimated or overestimated compared with the true lesion [20, 39, 40], lesion-targeted therapy (instead of hemi-ablative therapy) needs to account for an additional safety margin by calculating the prediction error in imaging studies to ensure that the focal therapeutic zones cover the entire cancer lesion.

To preserve the accuracy of a planned intervention, any image-guided intervention system would require the capture of real-time imaging to constantly update the 3D planning model. The critical importance of real-time TRUS monitoring and corresponding real-time 3D planning model is supported by the successful practices in some of the most investigated real-time TRUS-guided therapeutic modalities, including TRUS-guided cryosurgery, brachytherapy, HIFU (high-intensity focused ultrasound), and photodynamic therapy.

The initial 3D planning models for these technologies have been developed to be adjustable during any time of the intervention, based on the comparison of initially referenced reconstructed 3D images and real-time TRUS imaging. This capability is considered a key feature in achieving the precision and efficacy necessary for focal therapy. In fact, the prostate is a mobile deformable organ and can be swollen or shift from within during the intervention. During therapy guided by real-time TRUS, the real-time image becomes the actual eyes through which the surgeon looks at the surgical field within the prostate. Due to needle insertion or energy delivery into the prostate, the prostate potentially swells and shifts [41]. If at least multiple treatment secession is necessary, without real-time modification of the 3D targeting plan according to the intraoperative swelling and shift during treatment, targeted focal therapy may potentially leave untreated gaps between two adjacent treatment zones. Based on the real-time TRUS monitoring of possible changes in 3D shape of the prostate, intraoperative adjustment of the treatment plan has an impact on achieving precise therapeutic targeting.

Techniques of postoperative follow-up are still evolving in focal therapy. TRUS can document the shrink of the prostate in size in the treated area as well as the disappearance of the biopsy-proven lesion after focal therapy [4]. Documentation of the evidence of the decreased blood flow or change from enhanced to unenhanced signatures between pre- and post-focal therapy could be important evidence for suggesting technical success or possible cancer cell death. Since TRUS is the main imaging technique to visualize and monitor the postoperative change in the urological outpatient clinic allowing surveillance of prostate biopsy to target the preoperatively confirmed cancer lesion as well as the possible multifocal unknown disease in the untreated area, TRUS continues to be of significant importance in the follow-up.

Conclusion

In conclusion, real-time TRUS remains an essential technology to support the diagnosis and characterization of cancer, intraoperative targeting and monitoring, and follow-up surveillance after focal therapy. For developing protocol for meaningful focal therapy of prostate cancer in urological field, the era of TRUS renaissance may come (Figs. 5.1, 5.2, 5.3, and 5.4).

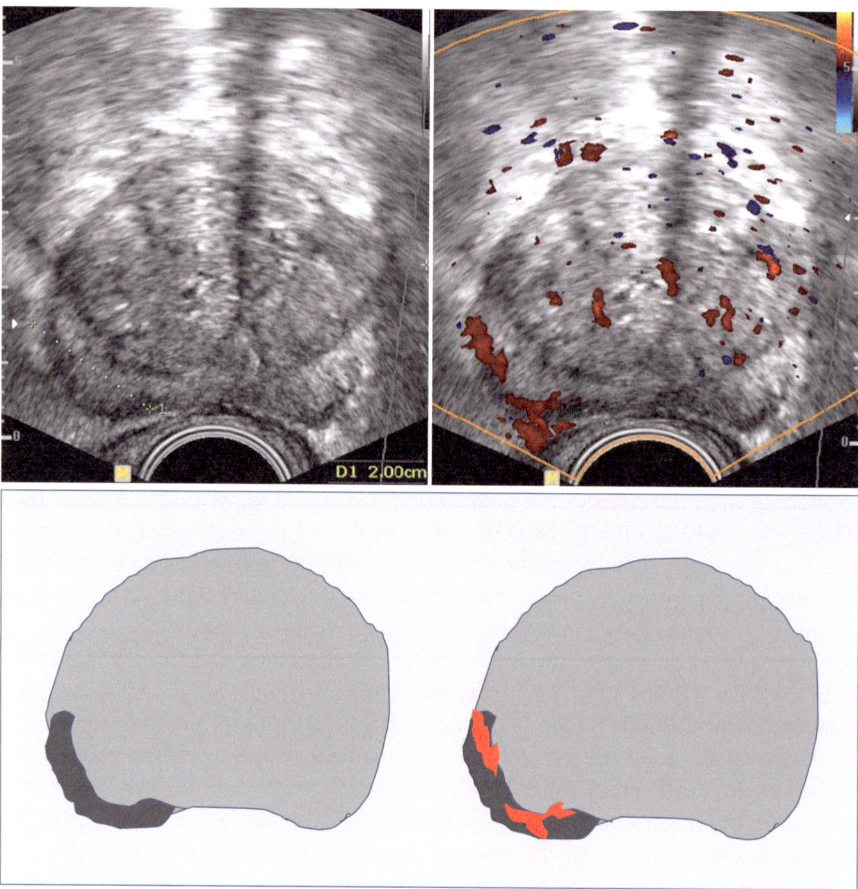

Fig. 5.1 Case 1: A 66-year-old man having PSA value of 7.47 ng/ml and TRUS-measured prostate volume of 51 g. TRUS with Doppler study identified hypoechoic suspicious lesion in right posterior-lateral aspects with suspicious focal increased blood flow. TRUS-guided targeted biopsy revealed Gleason 3+4=7 cancer in the TRUS-visible lesion with 9 mm cancer core length

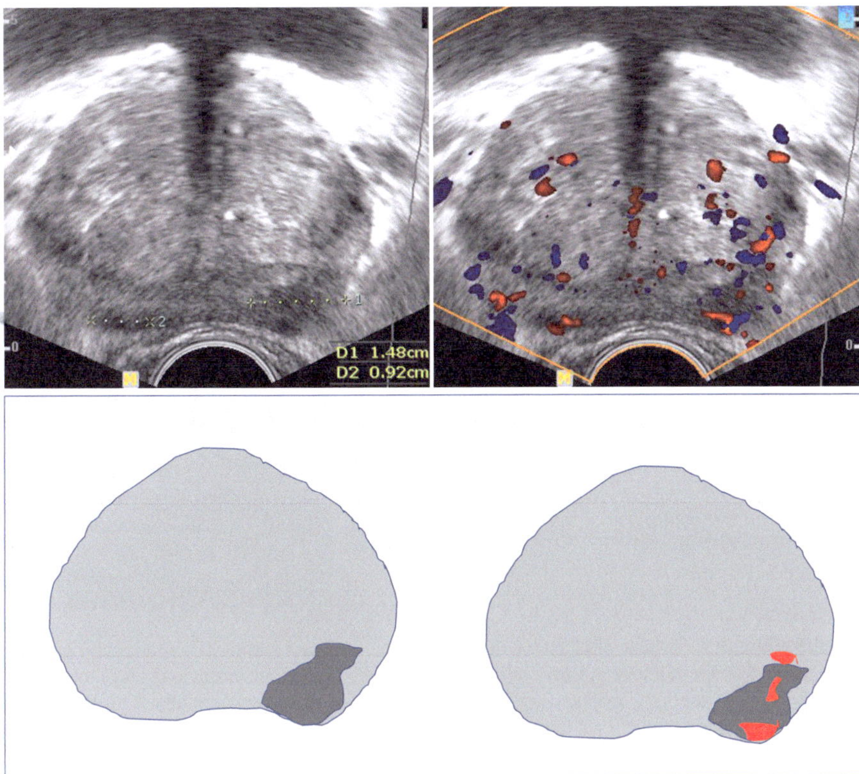

Fig. 5.2 Case 2: A 68-year-old man having PSA value of 3.5 ng/ml and TRUS-measured prostate volume of 53 g. TRUS with Doppler study identified hypoechoic suspicious lesion in left posterior-lateral aspects with suspicious focal increased blood flow. TRUS-guided targeted biopsy revealed Gleason 3 + 3 = 6 cancer in the TRUS-visible lesion with 4 mm cancer core length

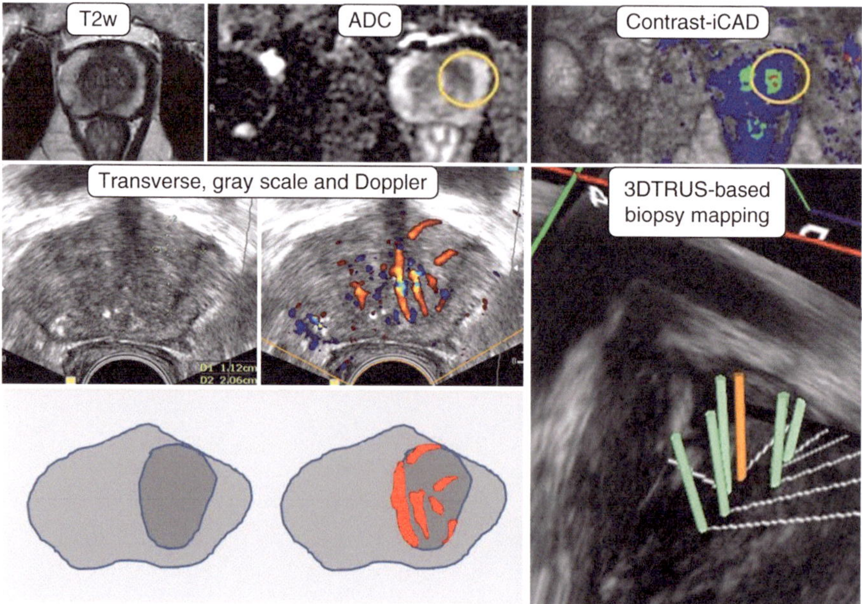

Fig. 5.3 Case 3: A 58-year-old man having PSA value of 4.2 ng/ml and TRUS-measured prostate volume of 38 g. Pre-biopsy multiparametric MRI suggested moderate suspicious lesion in the left transition zone in the ADC map and contrast-enhanced i-CAD color-coded image. This lesion corresponded with remarkable focal increased flow in TRUS Doppler study. Targeted biopsy from the TRUS Doppler-visible and ADC/contrast MR-visible lesion revealed Gleason 3 + 3 = 6 cancer with 12 mm cancer core length. Digitally documented 3D TRUS-based mapping biopsy could indicate the precise location of biopsy-proven cancer in the 3D space of the prostate

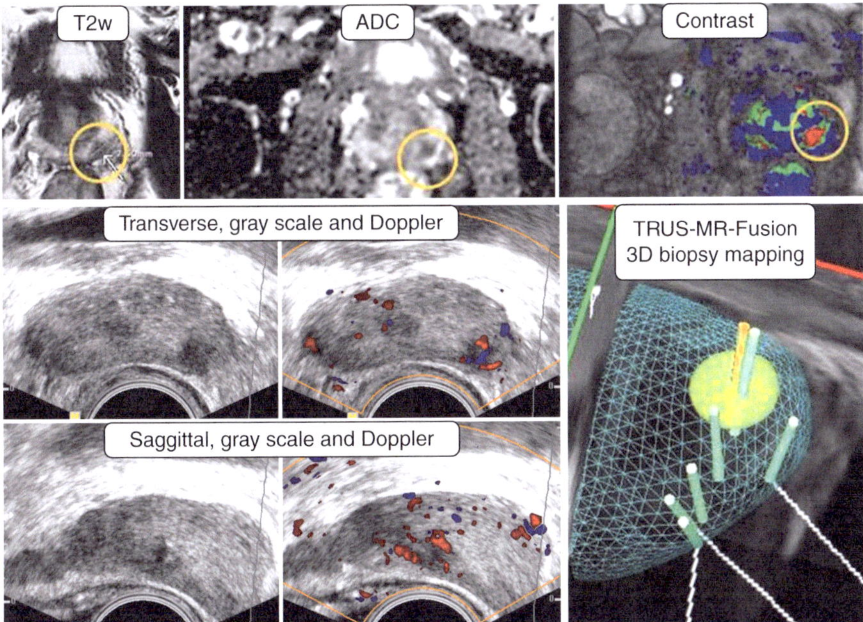

Fig. 5.4 Case 4: A 59-year-old man having PSA value of 4.1 ng/ml and TRUS-measured prostate volume of 28 g. Pre-biopsy multiparametric MRI suggested highly suspicious lesion in the left peripheral zone in all three functions of MRI including T2-weighted, ADC map, and contrast-enhanced i-CAD color-coded image. This lesion corresponded with remarkable hypoechoic lesion with highly suspicious focal increased flow in TRUS Doppler study. MR/US fusion targeted biopsy from the TRUS-visible and MR-visible lesion revealed Gleason 4 + 3 = 7 cancer with 11 mm cancer length

References

1. Howlader N, Noone AM, Krapcho M, et al. SEER cancer statistics review, 1975–2009 (Vintage 2009 populations). http://seer.cancer.gov/csr/1975_2009_pops09/. Accessed 20 Aug 2012.
2. Hodge KK, McNeal JE, Terris MK, Stamey TA. Random systematic versus directed ultrasound guided transrectal core biopsies of the prostate. J Urol. 1989;142(1):71–4.
3. Ukimura O, Coleman J, de la Taille A, Emberton M, Epstein J, Freedland S, Giannarini G, Kibel A, Montironi R, Ploussard G, Roobol M, Scattoni V, Jones S. Contemporary role of systematic prostate biopsies: indications, technique, implications on patient care. Eur Urol. 2013;63(2):214–30.
4. Ukimura O, Abreu AL, Gill IS, Shoji S, Hung AJ, Bahn D. Image-visibility of cancer to enhance targeting precision and spatial mapping biopsy for focal therapy of prostate cancer. BJU Int. 2013;111(8):E354–64.
5. Bahn D, de Castro Abreu AL, Gill IS, Hung AJ, Silverman P, Gross ME, Lieskovsky G, Ukimura O. Focal cryotherapy for clinically unilateral, low-intermediate risk prostate cancer in 73 men with a median follow-up of 3.7 years. Eur Urol. 2012;62(1):55–63.

6. Ahmed HU, Hindley RG, Dickinson L, Freeman A, Kirkham AP, Sahu M, Scott R, Allen C, Van der Meulen J, Emberton M. Focal therapy for localised unifocal and multifocal prostate cancer: a prospective development study. Lancet Oncol. 2012;13(6):622–32.

7. McNeal JE. The zonal anatomy of the prostate. Prostate. 1981;2(1):35–49.

8. Toi A, Neill MG, Lockwood GA, Sweet JM, Tammsalu LA, Fleshner NE. The continuing importance of transrectal ultrasound identification of prostatic lesions. J Urol. 2007;177:516–20.

9. Trottier G, Roobol MJ, Lawrentschuk N, et al. Comparison of risk calculators from the prostate cancer prevention trial and the European randomized study of screening for prostate cancer in a contemporary Canadian cohort. BJU Int. 2011;108:E237–44.

10. McNeal JE, Redwine EA, Freiha FS, Stamey TA. Zonal distribution of prostatic adenocarcinoma. Correlation with histologic pattern and direction of spread. Am J Surg Pathol. 1988;12(12):897–906.

11. Shinohara K, Scardino CSS, Wheeler TM. Pathologic basis of the sonographic appearance of the normal and malignant prostate. Urol Clin North Am. 1989;16(4):675–91.

12. Ukimura O, Gill IS, Reply from Authors re: Mark Emberton. Tissue preservation may offer a harm-reduction strategy for men with early prostate cancer. Eur Urol. 2012;62:64–6. Eur Urol. 62:66–7.

13. Lencioni R, Cioni D, Bartolozzi C. Tissue harmonic and contrast-specific imaging: back to gray scale in ultrasound. Eur Radiol. 2002;12(1):151–65.

14. Halpern EJ, Ramey JR, Strup SE, Frauscher F, McCue P, Gomella LG. Detection of prostate carcinoma with contrast-enhanced sonography using intermittent harmonic imaging. Cancer. 2005;104(11):2373–83.

15. Sauvain JL, Palascak P, Bourscheid D, Chabi C, Atassi A, Bremon JM, Palascak R. Value of power doppler and 3D vascular sonography as a method for diagnosis and staging of prostate cancer. Eur Urol. 2003;44(1):21–30.

16. Nelson ED, Slotoroff CB, Gomella LG, Halpern EJ. Targeted biopsy of the prostate: the impact of color Doppler imaging and elastography on prostate cancer detection and Gleason score. Urology. 2007;70:1136–40.

17. Mitterberger M, Pinggera GM, Horninger W, Bartsch G, Strasser H, Schäfer G, Brunner A, Halpern EJ, Gradl J, Pallwein L, Frauscher F. Comparison of contrast enhanced color Doppler targeted biopsy to conventional systematic biopsy: impact on Gleason score. J Urol. 2007; 178(2):464–8.

18. Morelli G, Pagni R, Mariani C, Minervini R, Morelli A, Gori F, Ferdeghini EM, Paterni M, Mauro E, Guidi E, Armillotta N, Canale D, Vitti P, Caramella D, Minervini A. Results of vardenafil mediated power Doppler ultrasound, contrast enhanced ultrasound and systematic random biopsies to detect prostate cancer. J Urol. 2011;185(6):2126–31.

19. Lee F, Torp-Pedersen ST, Siders DB, Littrup PJ, McLeary RD. Transrectal ultrasound in the diagnosis and staging of prostatic carcinoma. Radiology. 1989;170:609–15.

20. Ukimura O, Troncoso P, Ramirez EI, Babaian RJ. Prostate cancer staging: correlation between ultrasound determined tumor contact length and pathologically confirmed extraprostatic extension. J Urol. 1998;159(4):1251–9.

21. Ukimura O, Magi-Galluzzi C, Gill IS. Real-time transrectal ultrasound guidance during laparoscopic radical prostatectomy: impact on surgical margins. J Urol. 2006;175(4):1304–10.

22. Lee F, Bahn DK, Siders DB, Greene C. The role of TRUS-guided biopsies for determination of internal and external spread of prostate cancer. Semin Urol Oncol. 1998;16(3):129–36.

23. Okihara K, Kamoi K, Lane RB, Evans RB, Troncoso P, Babaian RJ. Role of systematic ultrasound-guided staging biopsies in predicting extraprostatic extension and seminal vesicle invasion in men with prostate cancer. J Clin Ultrasound. 2002;30:123–31.

24. Ukimura O, Hung A, Gill IS. Innovations in prostate biopsy strategies for active surveillance and focal therapy. Curr Opin Urol. 2011;21(2):115–20.

25. Tareen B, Godoy G, Sankin A, et al. Can contemporary transrectal prostate biopsy accurately select candidates for hemi-ablative focal therapy of prostate cancer? BJU Int. 2009;104:195–9.
26. Falzarano SM, Zhou M, Hernandez AV, et al. Can saturation biopsy predict prostate cancer localization in radical prostatectomy specimens: a correlative study and implications for focal therapy. Urology. 2010;76:682–7.
27. Stamey TA, Freiha FS, McNeal JE, et al. Localized prostate cancer. Relationship of tumor volume to clinical significance for treatment of prostate cancer. Cancer. 1993;71(3 Suppl):933–8.
28. Crawford ED, Wilson SS, Torkko KC, et al. Clinical staging of prostate cancer: a computer-simulated study of transperineal prostate biopsy. BJU Int. 2005;96:999–1004.
29. Barzell WE, Melamed MR. Appropriate patient selection in the focal treatment of prostate cancer: the role of transperineal 3-dimensional pathologic mapping of the prostate: a 4-year experience. Urology. 2007;70(6 Suppl):27–35.
30. Onik G, Miessau M, Bostwick DG. Three-dimensional prostate mapping biopsy has a potentially significant impact on prostate cancer management. J Clin Oncol. 2009;27:4321–6.
31. Ukimura O, Desai M, Palmer S, Valencerina S, Gross M, Abreu A, Aron M, Gill IS. Three-dimensional elastic registration system of prostate biopsy location by real-time 3-dimensional transrectal ultrasound guidance with magnetic resonance/transrectal ultrasound image fusion. J Urol. 2012;187:1080–6.
32. Delongchamps NB, Peyromaure M, Schull A, Beuvon F, Bouazza N, Flam T, Zerbib M, Muradyan N, Legman P, Cornud F. Prebiopsy magnetic resonance imaging and prostate cancer detection: comparison of random and targeted biopsies. J Urol. 2013;189(2):493–9.
33. Cornud F, Brolis L, Delongchamps NB, Portalez D, Malavaud B, Renard-Penna R, Mozer P. TRUS-MRI image registration: a paradigm shift in the diagnosis of significant prostate cancer. Abdom Imaging. 2013;38:1447–63.
34. Ukimura O, Hirahara N, Fujihara A, Yamada T, Iwata T, Kamoi K, Okihara K, Ito H, Nishimura T, Miki T. Technique for a hybrid system of real-time transrectal ultrasound with preoperative magnetic resonance imaging in the guidance of targeted prostate biopsy. Int J Urol. 2010;17(10):890–3.
35. Pinto PA, Chung PH, Ratinehad AR, et al. Magnetic resonance imaging/ultrasound fusion guided prostate biopsy improves cancer detection following transrectal ultrasound biopsy and correlates with multiparametric magnetic resonance imaging. J Urol. 2011;186:1281–5.
36. Dickinson L, Ahmed HU, Allen C, Barentsz JO, Carey B, Futterer JJ, Heijmink SW, Hoskin P, Kirkham AP, Padhani AR, Persad R, Puech P, Punwani S, Sohaib A, Tombal B, Villers A, Emberton M. Scoring systems used for the interpretation and reporting of multiparametric MRI for prostate cancer detection, localization, and characterization: could standardization lead to improved utilization of imaging within the diagnostic pathway? J Magn Reson Imaging. 2013;37(1):48–58.
37. Ukimura O, Gill IS. Reply from authors re: Mark Emberton. Tissue preservation may offer a harm-reduction strategy for men with early prostate cancer. Eur Urol. 2012;62:64–6. Eur Urol. 62:66–7.
38. Ukimura O. Editorial comment. J Urol. 2013;189(1):91–2.
39. Mazaheri Y, Hricak H, Fine SW, et al. Prostate tumor volume measurement with combined T2-weighted imaging and diffusion-weighted MR: correlation with pathologic tumor volume. Radiology. 2009;252:449–57.
40. Dudea SM, Giurgiu CR, Dumitriu D, et al. Value of ultrasound elastography in the diagnosis and management of prostate carcinoma. Med Ultrason. 2011;13:45–53.
41. Shoji S, Uchida T, Nakamoto M, Kim H, de Castro Abreu AL, Leslie S, Sato Y, Gill IS, Ukimura O. Prostate swelling and shift during high intensity focused ultrasound: implication for targeted focal therapy. J Urol. 2013;190(4):1224–32.

Magnetic Resonance Imaging for Patient Selection for Focal Therapy

Raphaële Renard Penna

6.1 Introduction

Over the past decade, magnetic resonance (MR) imaging (MRI) has become more useful for the workup and follow-up of prostate cancer, with the addition of new techniques (diffusion-weighted MR imaging, dynamic contrast-enhanced MRI, and MR spectroscopy) and technological advances (improvement in coil design and 3-T imaging systems). MRI has the potential to provide information about tumor volume, location, and local extension.

The role of imaging before treatment is to characterize cancer already diagnosed by biopsy, determine the tumor location if it is visible, and guide biopsy protocol if necessary. MRI has to assess the prostate volume and exclude patients with intermediate- or high-risk cancer that would be inappropriate for focal therapy. MRI can help to identify patients suitable for focal therapy, to plan and implement focal treatment, and to monitor for cancer recurrence and progression.

6.2 MR Imaging Techniques

Both 1.5- and 3-T scanners are currently used for prostate cancer diagnosis, with the latter becoming increasingly available and generally preferred because of a higher signal-to-noise ratio and better structural and functional detail. Coil technology includes a pelvic phased-array coil with or without an endorectal coil. The debate over whether there is a need for an endorectal coil is still ongoing, but for detection and localization indications, the use of a phased-array coil is sufficient.

R. Renard Penna
Department of Radiology, Hôpital Pitié Salpétrière, Paris, France
e-mail: raphaele.renardpenna@gmail.com

© Springer-Verlag France 2015
E. Barret, M. Durand (eds.), *Technical Aspects of Focal Therapy in Localized Prostate Cancer*, DOI 10.1007/978-2-8178-0484-2_6

6.3   Anatomic T2-Weighted Imaging

High spatial resolution T2-weighted imaging is acquired in the axial, coronal, and sagittal planes. T2-weighted MRI is generally used to depict prostate anatomy. The normal peripheral zone has high T2 signal intensity similar to or greater than the signal of adjacent periprostatic fat. On T2-weighted images, prostate cancer can appear as an area of low signal intensity within the high signal intensity of a normal peripheral zone (Fig. 6.1a). A limitation of T2-weighted imaging is that focal areas of low signal intensity in the peripheral zone do not always represent cancer. Benign abnormalities such as chronic prostatitis atrophy, scars post-irradiation or hormonal treatment effects, and post-biopsy hemorrhage, may mimic tumor tissue. Cancer in the transition zones is more difficult to discern because of the presence of BPH. However, helpful signs for detection of malignancy in this zone have been reported to be homogeneously low signal intensity, ill-defined irregular edges, and lenticular shape.

6.4   Dynamic Contrast-Enhanced Imaging (DCE Imaging)

Dynamic contrast-enhanced MR imaging consists of a series of fast T1-weighted sequences covering the entire prostate before and after the rapid injection of a bolus of a low-molecular-weighted gadolinium chelate. Assessment of signal intensity changes can be performed qualitatively, semiquantitatively, and quantitatively. Numerous qualitative and quantitative methods to summarize the large amounts of DCE MRI data have been suggested. Qualitatively, the characteristics of the dynamic uptake and washout curves can be used to generate images that can be overlaid over the corresponding high spatial resolution anatomic images; quantitatively, the MR data are fit to mathematical models of the tissue behavior. Cancers often demonstrate early nodular enhancement before the rest of the parenchyma and early washout of signal intensity. This pattern is highly predictive of prostate cancer but is not pathognomonic (Fig. 6.1b, b'). Some prostate cancers are mildly or moderately hypervascular and thus are not detectable with this method. It was found that dynamic contrast-enhanced MR imaging at 3 T had comparable sensitivity (73 %) and specificity (77 %) in prostate cancer localization. When dynamic contrast-enhanced pelvic phased-array MR imaging was used in combination with T2-weighted imaging, a negative predictive value of 0.85 for 0.2 cm^3 lesions and 0.95 for 0.5 cm^3 lesions was found [1].

This characteristic makes dynamic contrast-enhanced MR imaging a sensitive technique for prostate cancer localization [2].

One of the limitations of dynamic contrast-enhanced MR imaging is related to discrimination of cancer from prostatitis in the peripheral zone and BPH nodules in the transition zone.

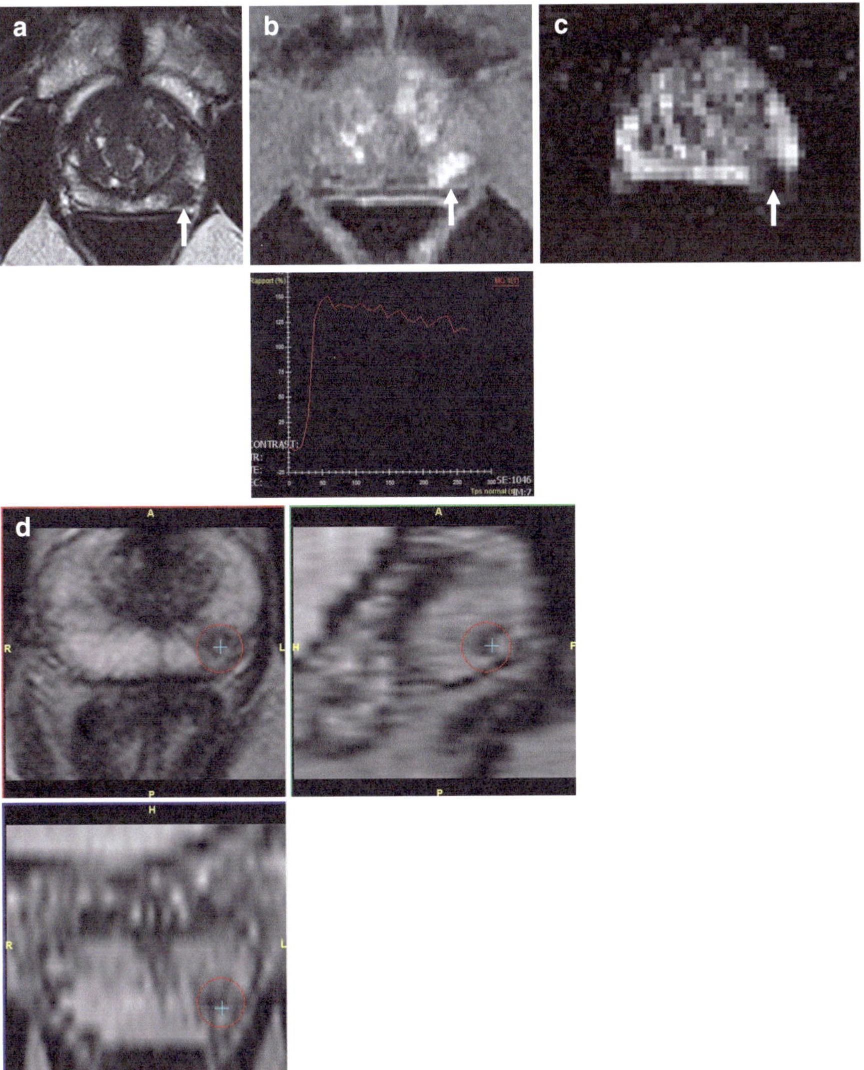

Fig. 6.1 (**a–c**) Axial pre-biopsy multiparametric MR images of prostate show an 8-mm lesion (score 5 of 5) (*arrow*). (**d**) Tagging (*red circle*) of a suspicious focus in left peripheral zone. (**e**) Transfer into the three-dimensional transrectal ultrasonography (3D TRUS) by organ-based registration (Koelis, La Tronche, France). This is an elastic registration that allows to take into account prostate movement and prostate deformation of the patient. After registration, MRI-suspicious areas are highlighted by colored tags (*Green*, negative cores; *Orange*, high-grade PIN, *Red*, cancer). In this example, only targeted cores are cancerous. (**f**) MRI for assessment of treatment effects after ablative therapy. The image from dynamic contrast-enhanced acquisition at day 10 after focal HIFU shows focal zone of nonenhancement within left prostate (*solid arrow*) consistent with treatment-related necrosis. (**g**) 6 months MRI after focal HIFU. Markedly decreased size of left prostate lobe and loss of zonal differentiation. Dynamic contrast-enhanced acquisition shows no enhancement (*arrow*). Biopsies were negative

Fig. 6.1 (continued)

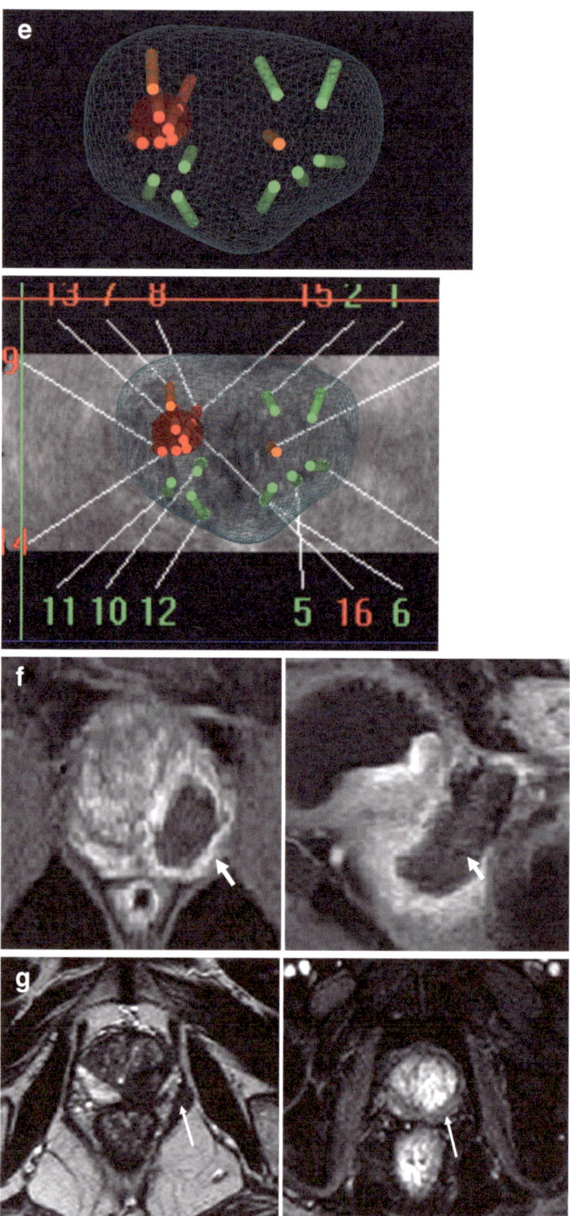

6.5 Diffusion Imaging (DW Imaging)

Of all functional imaging, DW imaging is the most practical, fast, and simple in use. Diffusion-weighted MRI (DWI) is a noninvasive technique with which variations in the Brownian movement of water molecules are depicted and quantified with an apparent diffusion coefficient (ADC). Water diffusion in biological tissues correlates inversely with tissue cellularity and the integrity of cell membranes.

For prostate cancer, b values between 500 and 2,000 s/mm² are typically used. Healthy prostate tissue in the peripheral zone allows extensive diffusion of water molecules within the gland tubules and thus has a high ADC. Prostate cancer tissue destroys the normal glandular structure of the prostate and replaces ducts with a higher cellular density. Cancerous lesions will generally have restricted diffusion with lower ADCs than surrounding healthy prostate tissue and so will appear hypointense on ADC maps, but hyperintense on the diffusion-weighted, high b-value image. On ADC maps, therefore, prostate cancer often shows lower ADC in comparison to surrounding healthy peripheral zone (Fig. 6.1c). DW imaging does reflect cellular density, which makes the technique potentially suitable for prostate cancer aggressiveness.

6.6 Mutiparametric Imaging

A multiparametric MR imaging consists of T1- and T2-weighted imaging combined with one or more functional MR imaging techniques. Minimal requirements for a multiparametric MR imaging protocol include a combination of T1- and T2-weighted MR imaging with DW and dynamic contrast-enhanced MR imaging.

6.7 Role of MRI in Focal Therapy

6.7.1 Detection

Recently, sensitivities and specificities of 70–90 % and 61–89 %, respectively, have been reported with negative predictive values of between 85 and 95 % for clinically significant cancer [3].

It was shown that the use of T2-weighted imaging combined with diffusion-weighted imaging improved sensitivity in the detection of significant prostate cancer (0.81 vs 0.54) and negative predictive value (0.88 vs 0.77) compared with T2-weighted imaging alone [4].

In a recent evaluation of multiparametric MR imaging at 3 T (76), Delongchamps et al. [5] found sensitivity of 80 % and specificity 97 % in the peripheral zone and sensitivity of 53 % and specificity of 83 % in the transition zone. They concluded that adding diffusion-weighted imaging and dynamic contrast-enhanced imaging to T2-weighted imaging increased MR performance for cancer detection but failed to improve performance in the transition zone.

6.7.2 Tumor Volume

Accurate noninvasive measurement of prostate cancer tumor volume could substantially improve the determination of tumor prognosis and assist in the selection of appropriate treatment.

Studies [6, 7] have shown that pathologic tumor volume correlates with pathologic stage, pathologic Gleason grade, margin status, and disease progression after radical prostatectomy. Tumors smaller than about 0.5 cm^3 and with no Gleason pattern 4 or 5 cancer are considered to be clinically insignificant and potentially appropriate for deferred therapy.

The volume of high-grade adenocarcinoma appears to be an important prognostic factor; as tumor volume increases, the frequency and volume of high-grade tumor increase.

There is poor correlation between tumor volumes measured at T2-weighted imaging alone, with an overestimation most of the time.

Mazaheri et al. have shown that prostate tumor volume measurements with T2 and DW1 are accurate and well correlated with pathologic tumor volume and Gleason grade [8]. Prostate cancer tumor volume measurements obtained with combined T2-weighted and DW MR imaging may help determine tumor prognosis and assist in the selection of appropriate treatment.

6.7.3 Tumor Location

The ability to accurately localize tumors within the prostate becomes of particular importance for the selection of patients who are appropriate candidates for focal ablation.

Accurate definition of prostate cancer location helps improve cancer detection in targeting prostate biopsies with MR imaging guidance and improves guidance of minimally invasive focal therapies.

Sensitivity and especially specificity of T2-weighted MR imaging prostate cancer localization vary, ranging from 54 to 91 % and 27 to 91 %, respectively [4, 9].

Localization accuracy with dynamic contrast-enhanced MR imaging increased to 72–91 %, as compared with 69–72 % for anatomic T2-weighted MR imaging only [2, 10]. The addition of DW imaging to T2-weighted MR imaging significantly improved sensitivity to 81 % (sensitivity for T2- weighted MR imaging alone, 54 %), whereas specificity was slightly lower for T2-weighted MR imaging combined with DWI (84 %) than for T2-weighted MR imaging alone (91 %) in this prospective prostatectomy-referenced study [4].

6.7.4 Tumor Grade

Accurate determination of patient prognosis is important when one is treating patients with unifocal prostate cancer. The Gleason score has been shown to be an important prognostic factor for predicting biochemical failure (PSA progression), systemic recurrence, and overall patient survival.

Patients with well-differentiated tumors (Gleason score 2–6) generally have a favorable prognosis, while those with high-grade tumors (Gleason score 7–10) have higher rates of progression [11].

Results for ADC as a possible marker of cancer aggressiveness are very promising: In a retrospective study of 3-T DW imaging ($b = 0$, 50, 500, and 800 s/mm^2) by

Hambrock et al. [12], cancers with a Gleason score of 2–3 components were discerned from cancers with Gleason score of 4–5 components, with an Az of 0.90. Furthermore, in a study of 1.5-T DW imaging ($b = 0$ and 600 s/mm^2) in 110 patients with 197 tumors, ADC values are negatively correlated with Gleason grades in peripheral zone prostate cancers of patients who underwent radical prostatectomy.

6.8   MRI-Guided Biopsy Protocol

The best predictor of tumor aggressiveness in prostate cancer is the Gleason score, which can be obtained only with histopathologic analysis of biopsy samples. Prostate biopsy, usually performed with a core needle inserted transrectally with real-time US guidance, remains an essential component of the diagnostic workup. But biopsy alone has been found insufficient for more than one-third of cases. Studies have consistently shown that at biopsy, tumor burden is undersampled, numerous tumor foci are missed, and the volume, grade, and stage of disease are underrepresented [13].

MRI-guided prostate biopsy can potentially improve prostate cancer detection, because multiparametric MR imaging-guided biopsy can be targeted toward previously determined regions that are suspicious for cancer (Fig. 6.1a–e).

Fused MR imaging- and transrectal US-guided prostate biopsy combine the advantages of each procedure in a single technique and offer a promising alternative to targeted prostate biopsies by directing the biopsy needle toward the regions with an abnormal MR imaging appearance. In a recent series of 583 patients, Rais-Bahrami et al., using MRI-guided software-based MR/ultrasound fusion, targeted biopsies of MRI lesions in addition to systematic 12-core biopsies, demonstrated strong associations with cancer detection in patients with Gleason 7 or greater (OR 3.3, $p < 0.001$) and Gleason 8 or greater (OR 4.2, $p < 0.0001$) cancers [14].

Numerous studies have shown the role of performing prostate MRI to improve tumor visualization that allows targeted imaging-guided biopsies [15–17]. This not only would avoid biopsy-related artifact but also has the potential for improving the yield of subsequent biopsy sessions by allowing targeting of suspicious regions on MR images. In this way, the combination of MRI and biopsy can more accurately select low-risk patients for focal therapy, thereby avoiding undertreatment of high-risk prostate cancer and controlling the cancer with a minimal impact on the patients' quality of life [15, 18].

6.9   MRI for Guidance of Targeted Minimally Invasive Ablative Therapy

Currently, ablative therapy procedures for prostate cancer, including cryoablation, HIFU, and vascular-targeted photodynamic therapy, are principally performed within a traditional operating room. MRI-guided therapy has precisely localized some tumor foci and can be used to guide the placement of the laser fiber to the tumor focus via a transperineal or transrectal approach (Fig. 6.2a).

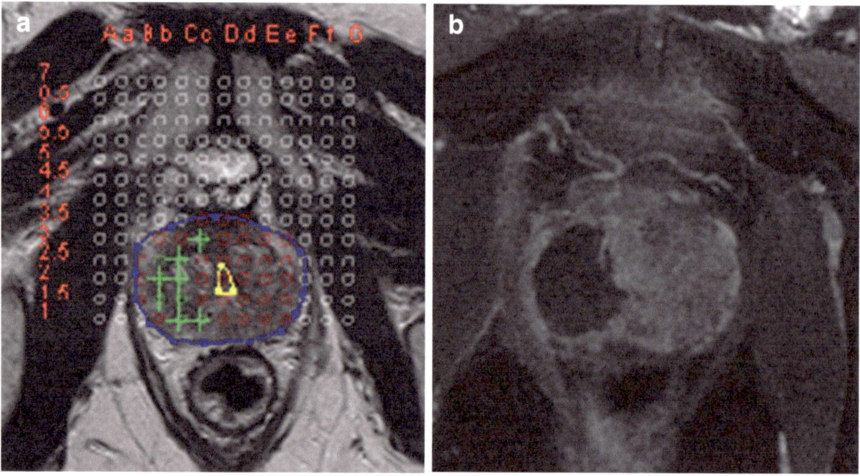

Fig. 6.2 (**a**) MRI guides the placement of the laser fiber on the right side of the prostate before photodynamic therapy. (**b**) 10 days MRI shows focal zone of nonenhancement within right lobe of the prostate, and no complication

MRI can be used to decide what kind of treatment – focal, hemiablation, or subtotal – should be used:

Focal treatment: when extended biopsy indicates the presence of a unifocal tumor and MRI is able to localize the tumor (Fig. 6.1a–g)

Hemiablation: when biopsy identifies a multifocal tumor that is confined to one lobe of the prostate, suggesting unilateral disease, MRI is useful for evaluating the contralateral lobe for evidence of a tumor that may have gone undetected on biopsy, rather than for direct visualization of the tumor itself.

6.10 MRI for the Assessment of Treatment Effects After Ablative Therapy

MRI contrast-enhanced imaging is performed immediately after therapy to confirm successful tissue necrosis (day 10). Findings from the initial posttreatment MRI are useful for assessing the efficacy of the ablative therapy in causing tissue destruction. Thus, MRI shortly after ablation provides feedback regarding the completeness of treatment (Figs. 6.1f and 6.2b).

6.11 MRI for the Assessment for Residual or Recurrent Tumor After Ablative Therapy

By 6 months after ablative therapy, a characteristic appearance of the prostate on MRI has been described [19]. The area of necrosis observed on the immediate posttreatment scan will usually have regressed and disappeared, becoming replaced

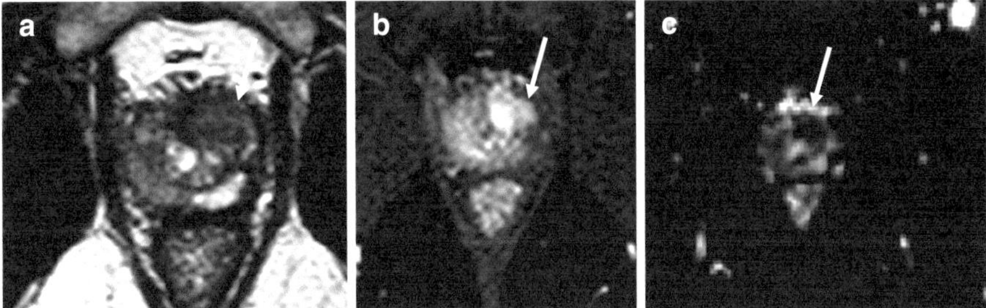

Fig. 6.3 A 59-year-old man with prostate cancer. The patient had undergone total gland ablation with cryotherapy more than 6 months before MRI. (**a**) Axial T2-weighted image shows expected changes of ablation procedure, including markedly decreased size of prostate and loss of zonal differentiation. There is a well-circumscribed area of decreased T2 signal intensity within the left anterior prostate (*arrow*). (**b**) The image from dynamic contrast-enhanced acquisition shows corresponding avid enhancement in left anterior prostate (*arrow*). (**c**) Axial apparent diffusion coefficient (ADC) map shows corresponding decreased ADC value in this region (*arrow*). Subsequent biopsy from the left revealed Gleason 3 + 4 tumor; all biopsy cores from the right were negative

by fibrosis (Fig. 6.1g). By this time, the volume of the prostate will have decreased significantly compared with the prostatic volume before treatment (Fig. 6.1a, g). The remaining prostatic parenchyma typically shows decreased T2 signal intensity, with loss of differentiation of the boundary between the peripheral zone and central gland as well as poor visualization of the prostatic capsule.

MRI may be used to detect areas suspicious for residual or recurrent tumor that may then undergo targeted biopsy. The literature to date most strongly supports dynamic contrast-enhanced imaging as having the highest sensitivity for the detection of tumors in this setting (Figs. 6.1g and 6.3a–c) [19, 20].

Conclusion

A vital key to the success of selective focal ablation of the prostate is proper patient selection. The latter is dependent on a staging procedure that can exclude patients whose cancer is outside the area destined to be treated, while precisely locating the targeted area to be selectively ablated. Prostate MRI is a reliable imaging modality essential to properly identify candidates for focal therapy, confidently target lesions, evaluate results, and monitor for treatment failure.

References

1. Villers A, Puech P, Mouton D, Leroy X, Ballereau C, Lemaitre L. Dynamic contrast enhanced, pelvic phased array magnetic resonance imaging of localized prostate cancer for predicting tumor volume: correlation with radical prostatectomy findings. J Urol. 2006;176:2432–7.
2. Kim CK, Park BK, Kim B. Localization of prostate cancer using 3T MRI: comparison of T2-weighted and dynamic contrast-enhanced imaging. J Comput Assist Tomogr. 2006;30:7–11.
3. Arumainayagam N, Ahmed HU, Moore CM, et al. Multiparametric MR imaging for detection of clinically significant prostate cancer: a validation cohort study with transperincal template prostate mapping as the reference standard. Radiology. 2013;268:761–9.

4. Haider MA, van der Kwast TH, Tanguay J, et al. Combined T2-weighted and diffusion-weighted MRI for localization of prostate cancer. AJR Am J Roentgenol. 2007;189:323–8.

5. Delongchamps NB, Rouanne M, Flam T, et al. Multiparametric magnetic resonance imaging for the detection and localization of prostate cancer: combination of T2-weighted, dynamic contrast-enhanced and diffusion-weighted imaging. BJU Int. 2011;107:1411–8.

6. McNeal JE. Cancer volume and site of origin of adenocarcinoma in the prostate: relationship to local and distant spread. Hum Pathol. 1992;23:258–66.

7. McNeal JE, Villers AA, Redwine EA, Freiha FS, Stamey TA. Capsular penetration in prostate cancer. Significance for natural history and treatment. Am J Surg Pathol. 1990;14:240–7.

8. Mazaheri Y, Hricak H, Fine SW, et al. Prostate tumor volume measurement with combined T2-weighted imaging and diffusion-weighted MR: correlation with pathologic tumor volume. Radiology. 2009;252:449–57.

9. Turkbey B, Pinto PA, Mani H, et al. Prostate cancer: value of multiparametric MR imaging at 3 T for detection – histopathologic correlation. Radiology. 2010;255:89–99.

10. Futterer JJ, Heijmink SW, Scheenen TW, et al. Prostate cancer localization with dynamic contrast-enhanced MR imaging and proton MR spectroscopic imaging. Radiology. 2006;241:449–58.

11. Meiers I, Waters DJ, Bostwick DG. Preoperative prediction of multifocal prostate cancer and application of focal therapy: review 2007. Urology. 2007;70:3–8.

12. Hambrock T, Somford DM, Huisman HJ, et al. Relationship between apparent diffusion coefficients at 3.0-T MR imaging and Gleason grade in peripheral zone prostate cancer. Radiology. 2011;259:453–61.

13. Scattoni V, Zlotta A, Montironi R, Schulman C, Rigatti P, Montorsi F. Extended and saturation prostatic biopsy in the diagnosis and characterisation of prostate cancer: a critical analysis of the literature. Eur Urol. 2007;52:1309–22.

14. Rais-Bahrami S, Siddiqui MM, Turkbey B, et al. Utility of multiparametric magnetic resonance imaging suspicion levels for detecting prostate cancer. J Urol. 2013;190(5):1721–7.

15. Moore CM, Robertson NL, Arsanious N, et al. Image-guided prostate biopsy using magnetic resonance imaging-derived targets: a systematic review. Eur Urol. 2013;63:125–40.

16. Portalez D, Mozer P, Cornud F, et al. Validation of the European Society of urogenital radiology scoring system for prostate cancer diagnosis on multiparametric magnetic resonance imaging in a cohort of repeat biopsy patients. Eur Urol. 2012;62:986–96.

17. Puech P, Rouviere O, Renard-Penna R, et al. Prostate cancer diagnosis: multiparametric MR-targeted biopsy with cognitive and transrectal US-MR fusion guidance versus systematic biopsy – prospective multicenter study. Radiology. 2013;268(2):461–9.

18. Ridout AJ, Kasivisvanathan V, Emberton M, Moore CM. Role of magnetic resonance imaging in defining a biopsy strategy for detection of prostate cancer. Int J Urol. 2014;21(1):5–11.

19. Rouviere O, Girouin N, Glas L, et al. Prostate cancer transrectal HIFU ablation: detection of local recurrences using T2-weighted and dynamic contrast-enhanced MRI. Eur Radiol. 2010;20:48–55.

20. Kim CK, Park BK, Lee HM, Kim SS, Kim E. MRI techniques for prediction of local tumor progression after high-intensity focused ultrasonic ablation of prostate cancer. AJR Am J Roentgenol. 2008;190:1180–6.

Prostate Histoscanning

7

Petr Macek

Histoscanning (HistoScanning™) is an ultrasound-based computer-assisted technology for tissue differentiation. The technology was developed by Advanced Medical Diagnostics in Belgium. The first information on histoscanning use comes from a report on the characterization of ovarian masses [3], but the use of histoscanning for prostate cancer diagnosis was initially published in 2008 [1]. Prostate histoscanning (PHS) is designed to distinguish between benign and malignant tissue in solid organs; it uses one compound of ultrasound (US) energy, the backscattered waves (the so-called native radiofrequency data), which is processed using three tissue characterization algorithms [5].

Data are acquired by transrectal ultrasonography with a transducer magnetically attached to a rotation holder (Fig. 7.1). The ultrasound scanner is connected to a dedicated computer system with special software – the workstation (Fig. 7.2). The histoscanning workstation is currently approved for use only with BK Medical ultrasound scanners. Data acquisition is first carried out by holding the probe holder in a steady position, with the patient on his side or in the lithotomy position. During acquisition, the holder rotates so that the attached probe scans the prostate with a sagittal view from right to left by 179°, scanning 1 frame per 0.2°. All of the frames are joined together to create a three-dimensional (3-D) image of the prostate and its vicinity, both in the ultrasound scanner and in the workstation. The data is processed by the workstation computer in several steps with the interaction of an operator, who marks the borders of the prostate in the three planes, and the machine creates a volume of interest, which is basically an outline of the prostate's borders. This can then be fine-tuned by the operator, and in the next step, the computer will perform the tissue characterization processing. This results in a 3-D model of the prostate,

P. Macek
Department of Urology, General University Hospital and First Faculty
of Medicine of Charles University, Prague, Czech Republic
e-mail: macekp@gentlemail.com

© Springer-Verlag France 2015
E. Barret, M. Durand (eds.), *Technical Aspects of Focal Therapy
in Localized Prostate Cancer*, DOI 10.1007/978-2-8178-0484-2_7

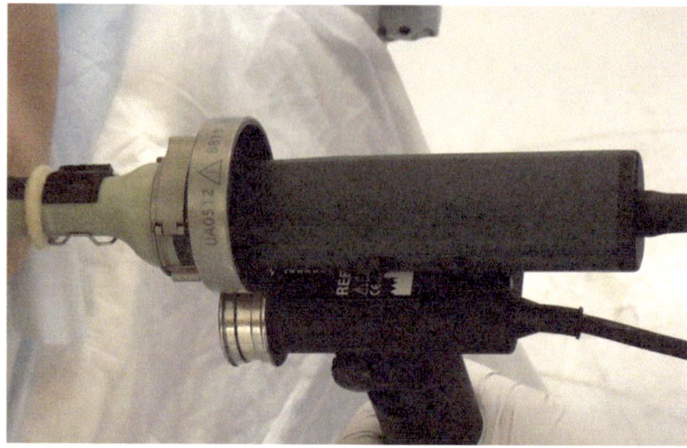

Fig. 7.1 Transrectal probe attached to a magnetic rotation holder during data acquisition (Source: author)

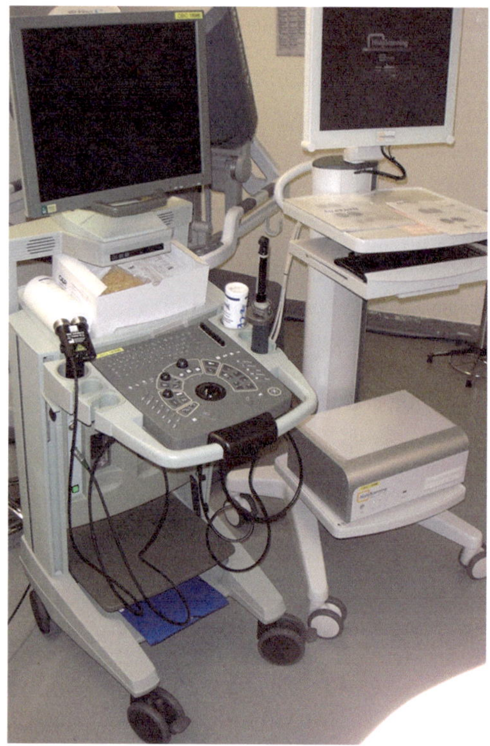

Fig. 7.2 Demonstration of histoscanning equipment – an ultrasound scanner BK Pro Focus UltraView, with transrectal probe and magnetic rotation holder, connected to a HistoScanning™ workstation (Source: author)

with color-highlighted suspicious areas (Fig. 7.3). The minimum volume of tissue that is individually characterized is 0.04 ml [6]. Lesions of interest are marked by the software. Usually, lesions equal to or greater than 0.1 ml are marked. Manual fine adjustment of the lesions, by adding or removing certain areas according to the operator's judgment, can be done as well. Therefore, unlike elastography, histoscanning is not now a real-time imaging because the data acquisition and processing usually take a few minutes, and the results are viewed on the screen afterward. Data

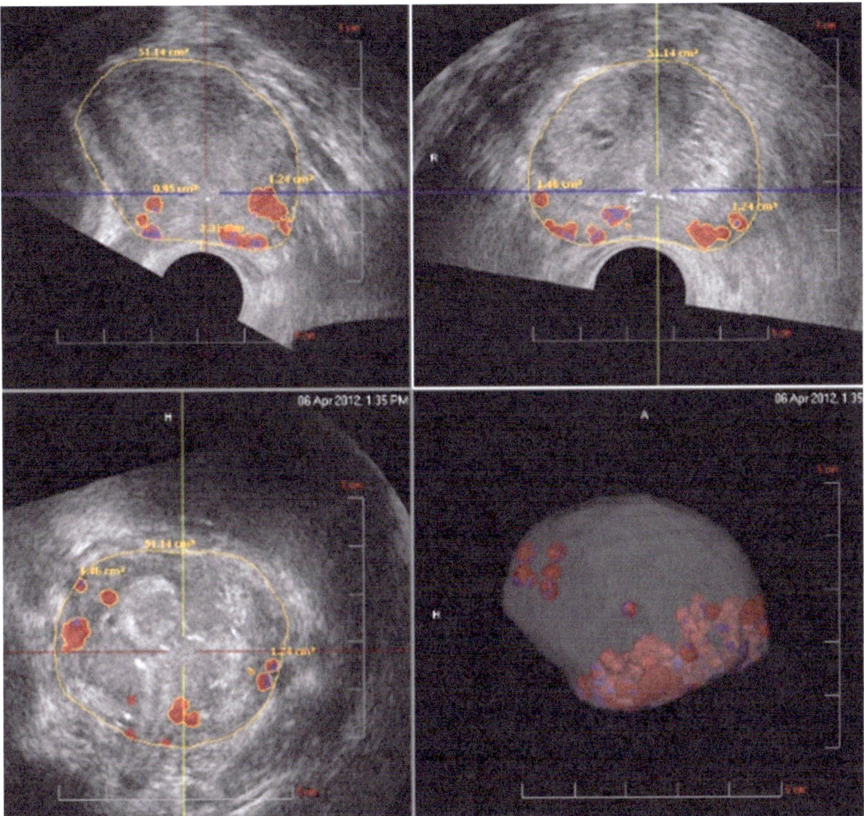

Fig. 7.3 An example of histoscanning analysis with a 3D prostate model, together with color-highlighted suspicious areas, and the corresponding three plane views which can be used for scrolling through the prostate, in order to achieve an appropriate spatial distribution of lesions (Source: author)

processing usually takes more time with large prostates. If a biopsy is planned, cognitive (= visual) lesion guidance is necessary. The newly introduced biopsy software module ("HistoScanning™ True Targeting") can help with transrectal biopsy navigation (Fig. 7.4).

Initial studies on PHS yielded very promising results of prostate cancer detection, with PHS-navigated prostate biopsies, with a radical prostatectomy specimen used as a reference standard [1, 2, 9]. Reports by Braeckman et al found a 100 % concordance with prostate cancer multifocality and laterality [1], and later 100 % sensitivity and 82 % specificity, for the diagnosis of prostate cancer lesions of 0.5 ml and higher within the prostate [2]. Sensitivity and specificity of 92 and 72 %, respectively, for lesions of 0.2 ml within six regions (= sextants) of the prostate, were reported later [9]. The latter results are encouraging, because if we virtually divide the prostate into six regions and look at them as potential target areas for focal

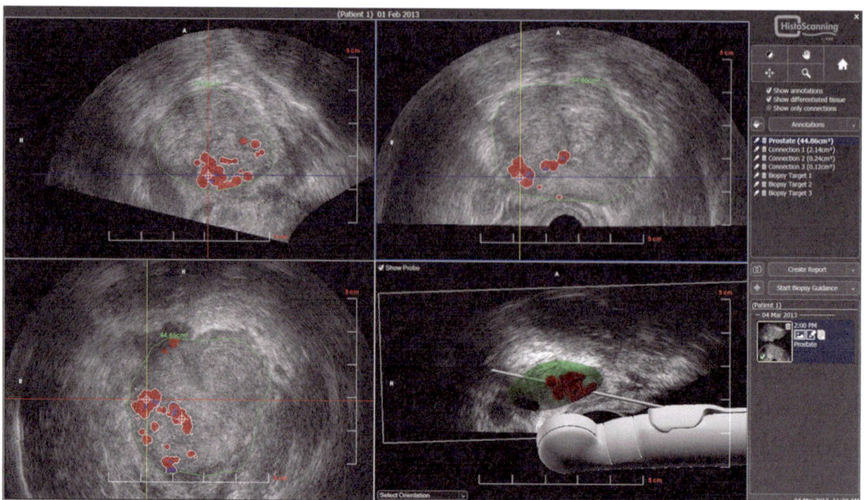

Fig. 7.4 A screenshot of HistoScanning™ True Targeting software for image-guided prostate biopsies. The volume of interest (the prostate outline) is marked *green*, and the biopsy target is one of the *red* marked lesions with a cross. Once the biopsy needle is inserted, the software will automatically detect and save it, along with the needle trajectory of the tissue sampling (Images courtesy (CLI-103) of Dr. Johan G. Braeckman, Universitair Ziekenhuis Brussel (UZB), Belgium)

treatment, it becomes an interesting concept. Very similar results for prostate cancer detection within the six regions with a 94 % sensitivity and an 80 % specificity were also reached by other groups [7]. But it is necessary to point out that various types of transrectal probes were used in the different studies. Therefore, it might be difficult to reach a unifying conclusion on which would be the best one for such situations, since so far there is no direct probe comparison [10].

The concept of focal therapy is linked to the minimization of side effects and, among other concerns, an impact on erectile function. A study by Salomon et al found that PHS may be helpful in the estimation of the probability of positive surgical margins, reporting that the presence of a 0.2 ml lesion in the lateroposterior part of the prostate resulted in a 3.7 times greater probability of the positive surgical margins [8]. This finding, together with the previously reported correct lateralization of prostate cancer, can be potentially usable for focal treatment planning with regards to the laterality of treatment and the neurovascular bundle-sparing treatment.

Biopsy or treatment planning can be done well ahead of the planned intervention, or just before it, because complete data acquisition and processing usually takes 5–10 min for an experienced operator. This, however, also emphasizes the fact that PHS is an operator-dependent ultrasound-based technology. Therefore, the examiner needs to be familiar with transrectal ultrasonography and the appropriate anatomy. It is estimated that approximately 80 cases of PHS need to be worked on in order to overcome the learning curve and improve results [6]. For optimal results, data acquisition is the key point of histoscanning analysis. One of the maneuvers that can affect the results is the distance between the ultrasound probe and the posterior border of the prostate, where 3–4 mm seems optimal (according to my personal experience). In large prostates, two overlapping scans can be done in order to get the best picture of each part of the prostate [8]. Although there are already ideas of the potential use of PHS as a screening tool [4], we should remain realistic for now and first solve the issue of PSA screening.

Besides an already well-documented use of PHS with a transrectal biopsy, a transperineal biopsy with histoscanning guidance was also reported, with an increased detection rate for transperineal- vs. transrectal- guided biopsies (82 % vs. 54 %) with the same number of cores [6]. This experience with the combination of PHS and transperineal approaches is especially valuable, because it is typically used in focal therapy.

Prostate histoscanning is a very promising technology for the future, with a potential for targeted prostate biopsies as well as for focal therapy. But certainly more information is needed, because at present most papers exclude patients with a major calcification (>5 mm) – which are not uncommon. Additionally, we do not have any reliable data on the results of patients with chronic prostatitis or following transurethral prostate interventions (i.e., TURP or laser treatment).

There are currently two benefits of PHS for focal therapy: It is possible to provide a very accurate description of a spatial distribution of lesions in the prostate, even by topography. Histoscanning, which seems to be fairly accurate, is also able to provide information about the size of the lesion. The concordance between the total cancer volume measured by histoscanning and on the whole-mount section specimen was within $r=0.97$ for lesions above 0.1 ml [2]. This is especially helpful in the treatment planning, because the treatment plan can be prepared before the intervention, together with an estimate of the number of needles necessary and the depth of insertion, for cryoablation, or focal high-intensity focused ultrasound planning, with possible better nerve sparing.

Additionally, for the suitably trained urologist, all steps of the treatment may remain in his/her hands and take less time, for example, when compared to the use of MRI targeting, which is quite time-consuming. We should also not forget the initial costs of the ultrasound/histoscanning system, when compared to the very expensive MRI-safe equipment necessary for MR targeting. Another future application of PHS lies in the monitoring of the lesion size, or its characteristics, following treatment. Although there are currently no papers reporting the use of PHS following focal therapy, this is an especially attractive option, because at least some patients could potentially be spared from follow-up biopsies.

References

1. Braeckman J, Autier P, Garbar C, Marichal MP, Soviany C, Nir R, Nir D, Michielsen D, Bleiberg H, Egevad L, Emberton M. Computer-aided ultrasonography (HistoScanning): a novel technology for locating and characterizing prostate cancer. BJU Int. 2008;101(3):293–8.
2. Braeckman J, Autier P, Soviany C, Nir R, Nir D, Michielsen D, Treurnicht K, Jarmulowicz M, Bleiberg H, Govindaraju S, Emberton M. The accuracy of transrectal ultrasonography supple-

mented with computer-aided ultrasonography for detecting small prostate cancers. BJU Int. 2008;102(11):1560–5.

3. Cachin F, Geissler B, Ronayette H, Autier P, Maublant J. Les avancées de l'imagerie? TEP-Scan, Echo-doppler, Histo-scanner. Oncologie. 2005;7(7):537–44.

4. De Coninck V, Braeckman J, Michielsen D. Prostate HistoScanning: a screening tool for prostate cancer? Int J Urol. 2013. doi:10.1111/iju.12148.

5. Govindaraju SK, Ahmed HU, Sahu M, Emberton M. Tissue characterisation in prostate cancer using a novel ultrasound approach. Br J Medi Surg Urol. 2008;1(3):98–106.

6. Hamann MF, Hamann C, Schenk E, Al-Najar A, Naumann CM, Jünemann K-P. Computer-aided (HistoScanning) biopsies versus conventional transrectal ultrasound-guided prostate biopsies: do targeted biopsy schemes improve the cancer detection rate? Urology. 2013;81(2):370–5.

7. Nunez-Mora C, Garcia-Mediero JM, Patino P, Orellana C, Garrido A, Rojo A, Rendon D. Utility of Histoscanning prior to prostate biopsy for the diagnosis of prostate adenocarcinoma. Actas Urol Esp. 2013. doi:10.1016/j.acuro.2013.01.003.

8. Salomon G, Spethmann J, Beckmann A, Autier P, Moore C, Durner L, Sandmann M, Haese A, Schlomm T, Michl U, Heinzer H, Graefen M, Steuber T. Accuracy of HistoScanning for the prediction of a negative surgical margin in patients undergoing radical prostatectomy. BJU Int. 2013;111(1):60–6.

9. Simmons LA, Autier P, Zat'ura F, Braeckman J, Peltier A, Romic I, Stenzl A, Treurnicht K, Walker T, Nir D, Moore CM, Emberton M. Detection, localisation and characterisation of prostate cancer by Prostate HistoScanningTM. BJU Int. 2012;110(1):28–35.

10. Macek P, Barret E, Sanchez-Salas R, Galiano M, Rozet F, Ahallal Y, Gaya JM, Durant M, Mascle L, Giedelman C, Lunelli L, Validire P, Nesvadba M, Cathelineau X. Prostate histoscanning in clinically localized biopsy proven prostate cancer: an accuracy study. J Endourol. 2014;28(3):371–6. doi:10.1089/end.2013.0419.

Elastography for Prostate Cancer

8

Petr Macek

Elastography (EG) is a method of evaluating tissues on the basis of stiffness (in other words: elasticity). EG does not assess the anatomy, rather the quality of a tissue, because it is presumed that the quality of a malignant tissue differs from that of a benign one – the malignant tissue is stiffer [18]. The principles of EG were first described in 1987 [15], and its application in imaging and in its detection of prostate cancer were first reported in 2002 [10]. Although it has existed for several years, its use has recently become more frequent. There are several ways for tissue excitation to create strain (compression, energy pulses, or vibrations), and various types of imaging, such as ultrasound or magnetic resonance, can be used to detect the tissue strain. Ultrasound is the most common medical imaging used in this application, and tissue stiffness is visualized through an elastogram.

The understanding of tissue properties and their distribution within the prostate improves the detection of prostate cancer lesions and enables more accurate targeting for tissue acquisition (targeted prostate biopsy) and/or potentially a more accurate navigation for targeted therapy, a very promising option.

To obtain an elastogram, the tissue quality is assessed by measuring (or observing) tissue stiffness as a function of strain and by following an application of force to the tissue [4]. In general, there are two types of possible force that can be used to generate strain in the tissue: quasi-static and dynamic. There are several characteristics that all EG techniques have in common, besides the characterization of tissue stiffness. Image processing is based on a measurement of time-dependent tissue displacement, and ultrasound is used to "observe" the tissue deformation. The acquired information is then converted into an elastogram, where different colors are assigned to the various degrees of tissue stiffness [4] that is characterized by a

P. Macek
Department of Urology, General University Hospital and First Faculty
of Medicine of Charles University, Prague, Czech Republic
e-mail: macekp@gentlemail.com

© Springer-Verlag France 2015
E. Barret, M. Durand (eds.), *Technical Aspects of Focal Therapy
in Localized Prostate Cancer*, DOI 10.1007/978-2-8178-0484-2_8

parameter called Young's modulus (E), which is directly related to tissue quality [13]. An elastogram is usually viewed simultaneously with a B-mode image in the form of an overlay.

For the imaging of prostate cancer, two main elastography techniques are used: strain EG (SE) and shear-wave EG (SWE) [11]. SE, also called real-time EG (RTE), is quasi-static in nature. The force used to generate tissue strain is an active external compression of tissue surface (reference), which is basically a pressure "palpation" on the prostate surface [12]. The second technique is SWE, which is dynamic in nature. The force used to generate tissue strain is represented by low-frequency ultrasound waves (10–2,000 Hz) that generate low-speed (1–50 m/s) transverse propagation waves called shear waves; hence, any external force on the tissue is unnecessary [11, 12].

It is up to the potential user to decide which technology is preferable. Both, however, allow color characterization of the tissue quality and a measurement of the strain, with some quantification. Benign tissue typically has a low stiffness signal (Fig. 8.1) [5]. In benign prostatic hyperplasia, the peripheral zone should remain basically the same, but an enlarged transitional zone may seem to become stiffer; moreover, calcifications that are frequently encountered in benign prostatic hyperplasia increase tissue stiffness. The suspicion of a malignant lesion would typically be hypoechoic and stiff (Fig. 8.2) [11].

The general advantages of elastography imaging include the procurement of mainly additional information on the tissue characteristics for decision-making and related lesion targeting (i.e., biopsy or therapy), which can be adjusted accordingly. Potentially, focal therapy guidance may be possible. The great benefit when compared to magnetic resonance is that elastography is always real time, with absolute operator control. There are, of course, drawbacks; the main one still lies in the person as an operator, as do most ultrasound methods [1], and it has been reported that users with more than 500 elastographic liver studies have had better results [9]. For

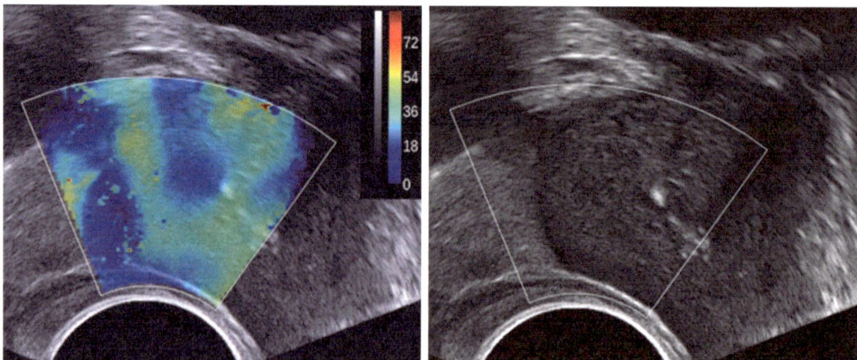

Fig. 8.1 Elastogram (*left*) of the prostate, with the corresponding gray-scale image (*right*), demonstrating benign characteristics of the tissue. The tissue is homogeneous isoechoic with a blue color, indicating a low stiffness (= high elasticity) as can be seen on the attached scale (Source: author)

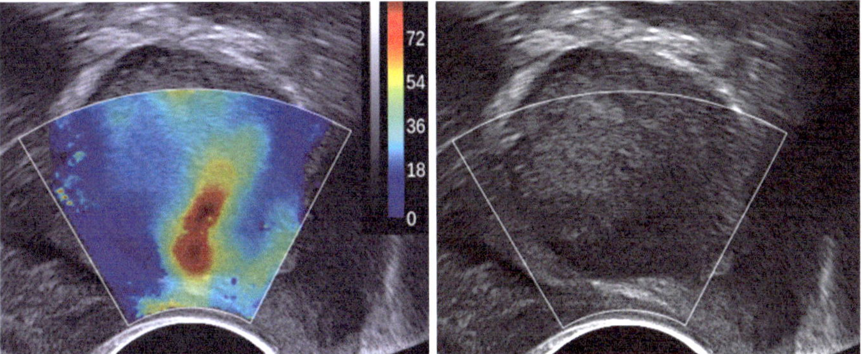

Fig. 8.2 Elastogram (*left*) of the prostate, with the corresponding gray-scale image (*right*), demonstrating a red lesion within the peripheral zone of the prostate, which is hypoechoic and with a high stiffness (= low elasticity), indicating the high likelihood of a cancer presence. The patient's PSA was 7.48 and biopsies from this area revealed an adenocarcinoma Gleason score of 3 + 3 (Source: author)

prostate elastography, 3–6 months seem to be necessary to achieve consistent results [16]. In strain elastography, the force control (i.e., the degree of probe pressure on the tissue) directly affects the final result. On the contrary, due to a different principle of force generation in shear-wave elastography, the maximum probe stability seems to be important, and it is necessary to stabilize the probe for approximately 2–4 s to get a good image [11]. From a technical point of view, color coding and setting are not standardized among the various manufacturers, although limits may usually be customized for individual studies.

8.1   Quasi-Static (= Strain) Elastography

Strain elastography (real-time elastography) was the first of the two elastography methods that are currently available for prostate imaging, as seen in Fig. 8.3. There are several manufacturers with systems based on this technology (alphabetically): BK Medical, Echosens, Esaote, GE Healthcare, Hitachi Aloka, Phillips, Siemens, and Toshiba. But only some have probes for transrectal imaging. Active, gentle compressions of the prostate surface by transducer are typically used. To achieve the best results, some manufacturers provide an on-screen visual control of applied force for correction (Fig. 8.4).

Salomon et al. reported results of RTE with a positive predictive value, a negative predictive value, and an accuracy of 87.8, 59, and 76 %, respectively [18]. Results presented by Brock et al. showed sensitivity and specificity of 60.8 and 68.4 %, respectively, with RTE detecting prostate cancer in 51.1 % of the patients sampled with RTE, compared with 39.4 % of comparable patients utilizing a gray-scale ultrasound guidance only [8]. But Taverna et al. found RTE's sensitivity, specificity, positive and negative predictive values of 24.4, 65.7, 21.9 and 68.6 %, respectively [21].

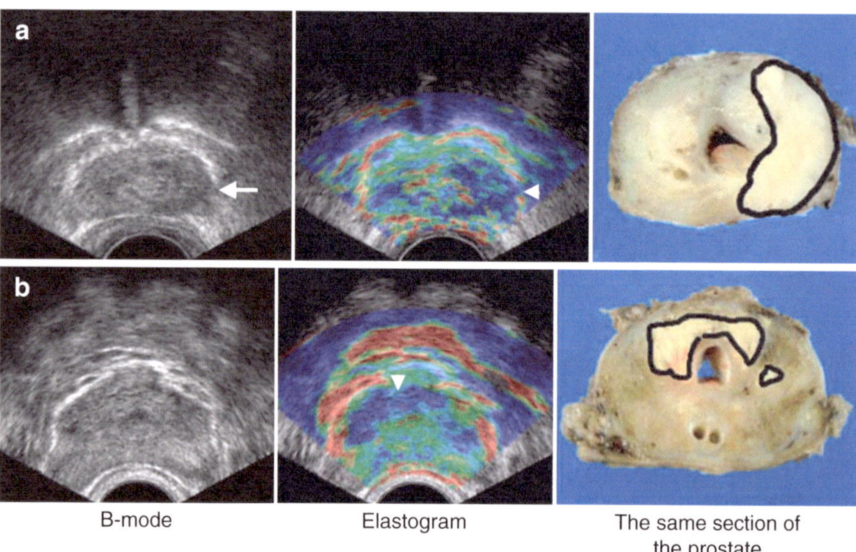

Fig. 8.3 Example of images obtained by real-time elastography (ultrasound scanner EUB-6500; Hitachi Medical, Tokyo, Japan, with 7.5 MHz transrectal probe) with corresponding B-mode images and pathology sections (**a**-case 1, **b**-case 2). For both cases, the areas with the blue-colored signal within the prostate are suspicious of the presence of cancer, with corresponding pathology sections where the cancer areas are marked (Reproduced from Tsustumi et al. [23], with permission of the publisher)

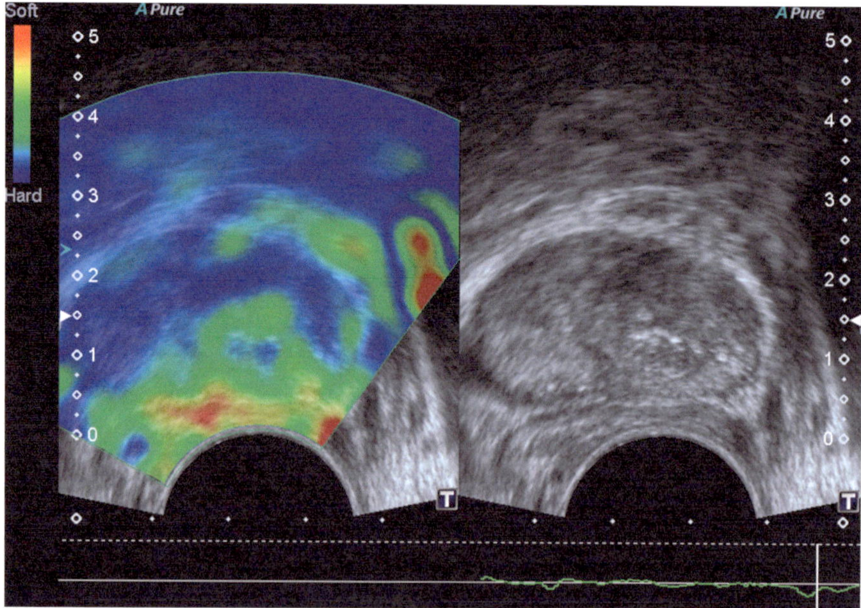

Fig. 8.4 Example of images obtained by real-time elastography (ultrasound scanner Toshiba Aplio 500 with 3–11 MHz transrectal probe). Please note tissue stiffness range of the left side indication that harder tissue is blue with corresponding gray-scale image. The pressure graph can be seen on the *bottom*, providing an indicator of correct pressure on the tissue (Image courtesy of Audioscan Ltd., an exclusive representative of Toshiba Medical Systems for Czech Republic)

The latter study also reported an overall accuracy of 53.9 %, with a twofold increase in prostate cancer detection per number of cores in RTE-targeted versus systematic biopsies (positive 15 % targeted vs. 7.8 % systematic cores), but only seven of 102 patients were true-positive RTE. Therefore, they concluded that systematic biopsies should not be omitted at this point in time if there is a clinical suspicion of prostate cancer [21]. On the other hand, Aigner et al. found that the cancer detection rate per core was 4.7 times greater for RTE-targeted biopsy compared to a systematic one, and they believe that RTE may be helpful in decreasing the total number of biopsy cores [3].

Meta-analysis by Teng et al. looked at the real-time elastography techniques, and for patients with a suspicion of prostate cancer, the pooled sensitivity was 62 % (95 % CI 55–68 %) and the pooled specificity was 79 % (74–84 %); however, the threshold of positivity was defined by color only, with no specified pressure limit [22]. Another meta-analysis performed by Aboumarzouk et al. found that for patients with a radical prostatectomy specimen histopathology report used as a reference standard, the sensitivity of RTE ranged from 71 to 82 % and specificity ranged from 60 to 95 %, with an area under curve (AUC) of 0.865. They also found that the patients with a positive RTE imaging have a 20 times higher chance of having prostate cancer [1]. The same meta-analysis looked at the spatial distribution of areas where RTE had the best performance, because it is a crucial piece of information if focal therapy is to be considered. There was, unfortunately, a significant inconsistence, because some of the studies found the best detection rates in the basal regions, others in the mid-gland, and some anteriorly.

One of the key points of an ideal prostate cancer diagnostic method is the detection of a significant prostate cancer. However, at this moment there is mixed information about RTE's ability to distinguish between high-grade and low-grade prostate cancer. Some say it is not currently possible [21], whereas others have shown that the sensitivity of RTE is increasing with greater Gleason scores that show 42.6, 65.4, and 80.4 % for scores less than 7, equal to 7, and greater than 7, respectively [25]. It also seems that the lesion size is important, and Zhu et al. also reported that the sensitivity of RTE for lesions of less than and over 5 mm was 22.6 and 77.8 %, respectively [25]. On the other hand, an inverse correlation of RTE sensitivity and Gleason scoring has been shown as well [23].

At this moment, we should only consider RTE as the source of an additional piece of information to the gray scale of ultrasound in the detection of prostate cancer. Also, the current statement by the Consensus Panel on the role of transrectal ultrasound in focal therapy is that no current ultrasound technique can alone, and accurately, visualize prostate cancer suitable for focal therapy and that multi-core prostate biopsies are still necessary [19]. This is supported by Walz et al. who reported that a combination of RTE and a 12-core biopsy led to the correct identification of 85 % of index prostate cancer lesions that could be treated [24].

Issues that have not been solved satisfactorily include the performance of RTE in patients with chronic prostatitis, or following previous treatment, either with radiotherapy, or any form of previous local and/or focal approach, such as the high-intensity focus of ultrasound or cryotherapy. Similar to multiparametric magnetic resonance, the idea of a multi-parametric ultrasound was introduced, combining elastography and a contrast-enhanced ultrasound. Such an approach decreased the false-positive rate from 34.9 to 10.3 %, together with an increased positive predictive value of 65.1–89.7 % [7]. This clearly looks promising, but it is too early to see if it will become a viable option.

So far, there are no reports on a combination of transrectal elastography imaging combined with a transperineal prostate biopsy, or, as mentioned previously, with focal therapy. And although B-mode ultrasound imaging is used for the real-time monitoring of focal treatment, such as a high-intensity focused ultrasound, cryotherapy, a vascular targeted therapy, and, potentially, also for electroporation [6], we do not have any data on the real-time monitoring of focal treatment by elastography. Preliminary information on the use of elastography for real-time treatment application monitoring has so far come from the experience with liver elastography [17].

8.2   Shear-Wave Elastography

Shear-wave elastography (SWE) was introduced in 2002 and its use for prostatic tissue characterization was presented in 2007 [14]. Although there is more than one manufacturer with shear-wave technology implemented into its ultrasound machines, there is currently only one (Supersonic Imagine) offering an application for prostate cancer diagnosis.

The information on SWE comes mostly from reports about liver and breast imaging, with so far not many reports about prostate imaging [2, 5]. However, its ease of use makes it a very promising technology and the results are very hopeful. Similar to RTE, the results of shear-wave imaging are expressed by colors, but unlike RTE, values of Young's modulus in kilopascals (kPa) are readily available (Fig. 8.5). Identical to RTE, it is also possible to simultaneously visualize gray-scale images with a parallel elastogram. Initial reports presented sensitivity, specificity, and positive and negative predictive values of 96.2, 96.2, 69.4, and 99.6 %, respectively, if 37 kPa was used as a cutoff point between benign and malignant tissue. The mean of Young's modulus of malignant tissues was 58 kPa (range 30–110 kPa) [5]. Even higher values were reported by Ahmad et al. with a mean of 134 kPa (range 43–216 kPa), which was approximately twice the values of benign tissue with a mean of 75 kPa. The latter paper reported 90 % sensitivity, 88 % specificity, and positive and negative predictive values of 93 and 83 % [2]. Besides an assessment of tissue quality by Young's modulus, it is also possible to compare the regions of interest in the prostate, because it takes into account an individual's prostate properties and differences between the peripheral zone and other parts of the prostate. The ratio for benign parts is 1.5 ± 0.9 and 4.0 ± 1.9 for malignant ones [11].

It seems that SWE might be slightly easier to perform because there is no need to create a specific pressure on the prostate [20]. Nevertheless, good knowledge of prostate ultrasound and biopsies remains essential [11, 5]. The limitations of SWE include a smaller size of the region of interest, which means that very large prostates require a stepwise approach, and anterior areas of such a prostate are not well covered [11].

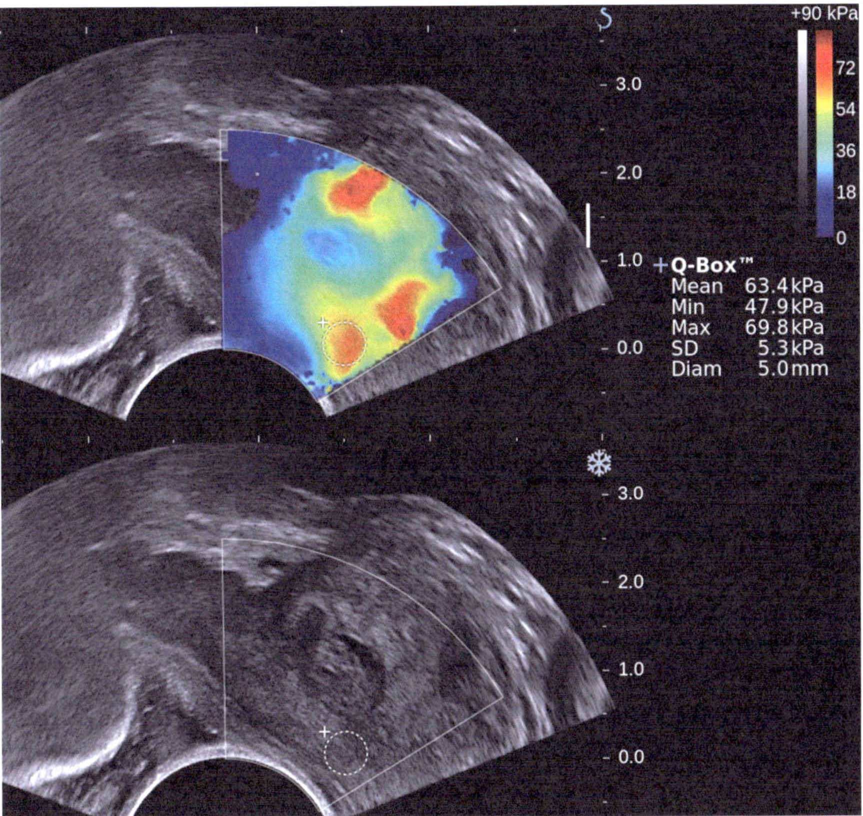

Fig. 8.5 Example of images obtained by shear-wave elastography (SWE), with corresponding gray-scale images, demonstrating a lesion within the peripheral zone of the prostate, spreading anteriorly, with a homogeneous isoechoic signal (ultrasound scanner Aixplorer; Supersonic Imagine, Aix-en-Provence, France, with 3–12 MHz probe, scanned at 11 MHz). The lesion had a red to yellow color with a mean value of Young's modulus (Q-box values on the right with a corresponding scale) of 63 kPa. Even higher values were in the *red area* above (not shown). Please also note a centrally located nodule of the tissue on the gray-scale image, which could be suspicious too. The *blue color*, however, corresponds to a very low stiffness and it is an example of a benign signal. The patient's PSA was 15.94, and all biopsies from this side of the prostate were positive for an adenocarcinoma Gleason score of 3+4 (Source: author)

Although one report found differences among Young's moduli of various Gleason scores for prostate cancer, this relationship between tissue stiffness and greater Gleason scores was not linear [2]. Therefore, as with RTE, there is not sufficient information on whether or not SWE is able to identify significant cancers.

At present, there are no papers reporting the results of SWE-guided prostate biopsies, or focal therapy with SWE guidance. My personal unpublished experience with SWE-guided biopsies shows interesting results, but no conclusions can be made so far. It seems that not needing specific pressure on the prostate makes lesion targeting easier, and this may be applicable in the future with the joint use of very stable transrectal imaging by SWE and transperineal needle guidance.

References

1. Aboumarzouk OM, Ogston S, Huang Z, Evans A, Melzer A, Stolzenberg JU, Nabi G. Diagnostic accuracy of transrectal elastosonography (TRES) imaging for the diagnosis of prostate cancer: a systematic review and meta-analysis. BJU Int. 2012;110(10):1414–23.
2. Ahmad S, Cao R, Varghese T, Bidaut L, Nabi G. Transrectal quantitative shear wave elastography in the detection and characterisation of prostate cancer. Surg Endosc. 2013. doi:10.1007/s00464-013-2906-7.
3. Aigner F, Pallwein L, Junker D, Schafer G, Mikuz G, Pedross F, Mitterberger MJ, Jaschke W, Halpern EJ, Frauscher F. Value of real-time elastography targeted biopsy for prostate cancer detection in men with prostate specific antigen 1.25 ng/ml or greater and 4.00 ng/ml or less. J Urol. 2010;184(3):913–7.
4. Bamber J, Cosgrove D, Dietrich CF, Fromageau J, Bojunga J, Calliada F, Cantisani V, Correas JM, D'Onofrio M, Drakonaki EE, Fink M, Friedrich-Rust M, Gilja OH, Havre RF, Jenssen C, Klauser AS, Ohlinger R, Saftoiu A, Schaefer F, Sporea I, Piscaglia F. EFSUMB guidelines and recommendations on the clinical use of ultrasound elastography. Part 1: basic principles and technology. Ultraschall in der Medizin (Stuttgart, Germany: 1980). 2013;34(2):169–84.
5. Barr RG, Memo R, Schaub CR. Shear wave ultrasound elastography of the prostate: initial results. Ultrasound Q. 2012;28(1):13–20.
6. Bozzini G, Colin P, Nevoux P, Villers A, Mordon S, Betrouni N. Focal therapy of prostate cancer: energies and procedures. Urol Oncol. 2013;31(2):155–67.
7. Brock M, Eggert T, Palisaar RJ, Roghmann F, Braun K, Loppenberg B, Sommerer F, Noldus J, von Bodman C. Multiparametric ultrasound of the prostate: adding contrast enhanced ultrasound to real-time elastography to detect histopathologically confirmed cancer. J Urol. 2013;189(1):93–8.
8. Brock M, von Bodman C, Palisaar RJ, Loppenberg B, Sommerer F, Deix T, Noldus J, Eggert T. The impact of real-time elastography guiding a systematic prostate biopsy to improve cancer detection rate: a prospective study of 353 patients. J Urol. 2012;187(6):2039–43.
9. Castera L, Foucher J, Bernard PH, Carvalho F, Allaix D, Merrouche W, Couzigou P, de Ledinghen V. Pitfalls of liver stiffness measurement: a 5-year prospective study of 13,369 examinations. Hepatology (Baltimore, MD). 2010;51(3):828–35.
10. Cochlin DL, Ganatra RH, Griffiths DF. Elastography in the detection of prostatic cancer. Clin Radiol. 2002;57(11):1014–20.
11. Correas JM, Tissier AM, Khairoune A, Khoury G, Eiss D, Helenon O. Ultrasound elastography of the prostate: state of the art. Diagn Interv Imaging. 2013;94(5):551–60.
12. Cosgrove D, Piscaglia F, Bamber J, Bojunga J, Correas JM, Gilja OH, Klauser AS, Sporea I, Calliada F, Cantisani V, D'Onofrio M, Drakonaki EE, Fink M, Friedrich-Rust M, Fromageau J, Havre RF, Jenssen C, Ohlinger R, Saftoiu A, Schaefer F, Dietrich CF. EFSUMB guidelines and recommendations on the clinical use of ultrasound elastography. Part 2: clinical applications. Ultraschall in der Medizin (Stuttgart, Germany: 1980). 2013;34(3):238–53.
13. Gennisson JL, Deffieux T, Fink M, Tanter M. Ultrasound elastography: principles and techniques. Diagn Interv Imaging. 2013;94(5):487–95.
14. Hoyt K, Parker KJ, Rubens DJ. Real-time shear velocity imaging using sonoelastographic techniques. Ultrasound Med Biol. 2007;33(7):1086–97.
15. Krouskop TA, Dougherty DR, Vinson FS. A pulsed Doppler ultrasonic system for making noninvasive measurements of the mechanical properties of soft tissue. J Rehabil Res Dev. 1987;24(2):1–8.
16. Pallwein L, Mitterberger M, Gradl J, Aigner F, Horninger W, Strasser H, Bartsch G, zur Nedden D, Frauscher F. Value of contrast-enhanced ultrasound and elastography in imaging of prostate cancer. Curr Opin Urol. 2007;17(1):39–47.
17. Rivaz H, Fleming I, Assumpcao L, Fichtinger G, Hamper U, Choti M, Hager G, Boctor E. Ablation monitoring with elastography: 2D in-vivo and 3D ex-vivo studies. Med Image Comput Comput-Assist Interv. 2008;11(Pt 2):458–66.

18. Salomon G, Kollerman J, Thederan I, Chun FK, Budaus L, Schlomm T, Isbarn H, Heinzer H, Huland H, Graefen M. Evaluation of prostate cancer detection with ultrasound real-time elastography: a comparison with step section pathological analysis after radical prostatectomy. Eur Urol. 2008;54(6):1354–62.
19. Smeenge M, Barentsz J, Cosgrove D, de la Rosette J, de Reijke T, Eggener S, Frauscher F, Kovacs G, Matin SF, Mischi M, Pinto P, Rastinehad A, Rouviere O, Salomon G, Polascik T, Walz J, Wijkstra H, Marberger M. Role of transrectal ultrasonography (TRUS) in focal therapy of prostate cancer: report from a consensus panel. BJU Int. 2012;110(7):942–8.
20. Smeenge M, de la Rosette JJ, Wijkstra H. Current status of transrectal ultrasound techniques in prostate cancer. Curr Opin Urol. 2012;22(4):297–302.
21. Taverna G, Magnoni P, Giusti G, Seveso M, Benetti A, Hurle R, Colombo P, Minuti F, Grizzi F, Graziotti P. Impact of real-time elastography versus systematic prostate biopsy method on cancer detection rate in men with a serum prostate-specific antigen between 2.5 and 10 ng/mL. ISRN Oncology. 2013. doi:10.1155/2013/584672.
22. Teng J, Chen M, Gao Y, Yao Y, Chen L, Xu D. Transrectal sonoelastography in the detection of prostate cancers: a meta-analysis. BJU Int. 2012;110(11 Pt B):E614–20.
23. Tsutsumi M, Miyagawa T, Matsumura T, Kawazoe N, Ishikawa S, Shimokama T, Shiina T, Miyanaga N, Akaza H. The impact of real-time tissue elasticity imaging (elastography) on the detection of prostate cancer: clinicopathological analysis. Int J Clin Oncol. 2007;12(4):250–5.
24. Walz J, Marcy M, Pianna JT, Brunelle S, Gravis G, Salem N, Bladou F. Identification of the prostate cancer index lesion by real-time elastography: considerations for focal therapy of prostate cancer. World J Urol. 2011;29(5):589–94.
25. Zhu Y, Chen Y, Qi T, Jiang J, Qi J, Yu Y, Yao X, Guan W. Prostate cancer detection with real-time elastography using a bi-plane transducer: comparison with step section radical prostatectomy pathology. World J Urol. 2012. doi:10.1007/s00345-012-0922-1.

Assessment of Tissue Destruction After Focal Therapy

9

Olivier Rouvière and Thomas Sanzalone

9.1 Introduction

Thermoablation techniques (using either high-intensity focused ultrasound (HIFU) or interstitial laser), vascular-targeted photodynamic therapy (VTP), or cryotherapy have in common the induction of necrosis of a given target area within the prostate with a good spatial accuracy. Thus, they seem ideal tools for the focal treatment of prostate cancer.

Treatment planning is of course a crucial phase of all these ablative techniques. It needs to take into consideration the location and size of the target tumor(s), the size of the safety margin to be applied (based on known imprecision of tumor volume estimation and on the spatial accuracy of the treatment targeting), and the position of structures to be preserved (e.g., neurovascular bundles, external sphincter, rectal wall). Imaging is likely to play a major role in this planning, given the good results recently obtained in detecting and localizing prostate cancer foci, especially with multiparametric magnetic resonance imaging (MRI).

Once the position and volume of the area to be destroyed have been defined, the next step is to make sure that it is correctly targeted during treatment. This can be done visually or may need an image fusion if the target volume has been defined on MRI and the treatment is performed under ultrasound (US) guidance. But this is not enough. Ideally, one must also monitor the energy deposition within the target

O. Rouvière (✉)
Department of Vascular and Urinary Imaging, Hôpital E. Herriot, Lyon, France

INSERM, Lab TAU, Laboratory of Therapeutic Applications of Ultrasound, U1032, Lyon F-69003, France

Department of Urology, Université de Lyon, Université Lyon 1, Lyon F-69003, France
e-mail: olivier.rouviere@chu-lyon.fr

T. Sanzalone
Department of Vascular and Urinary Imaging, Hôpital E. Herriot, Lyon, France

© Springer-Verlag France 2015
E. Barret, M. Durand (eds.), *Technical Aspects of Focal Therapy in Localized Prostate Cancer*, DOI 10.1007/978-2-8178-0484-2_9

volume. This step depends on the ablative technique and the image guidance used. During cryotherapy, the size and position of the ice ball can be monitored in real time using ultrasound (US) or magnetic resonance (MR) guidance. Heat deposition during thermoablation can be monitored in real time using MR thermometry. However, when thermoablation procedures are performed under US guidance, they usually rely on mathematical or theoretical modeling rather than true monitoring. VTP procedures also rely on theoretical modeling.

The last step is to assess, at the end of the treatment, whether the target volume has been destroyed as planned. This step has often been neglected in the past, at least for whole-gland treatments. Indeed, until recently there was no accurate US-based method that could show, in the operating room, the volume of tissue destruction after US-guided thermoablation or VTP. As for cryotherapy, the extent of the ice ball is usually considered a surrogate of the ablated volume, even if it indicates the volume of tissue submitted to freezing (below 0 °C) and not the volume of tissue submitted to lethal temperatures (below −20 °C).

The advent of focal treatment questions this attitude. Does it really make sense to submit the patient to high-technology imaging and therapeutic procedures and not to perform quality control at the end of the treatment? Would not an accurate assessment of tissue destruction – with the possibility of immediate re-treatment in case of unsatisfactory results – be a crucial key for the final success of focal therapies? Should we – and can we – do better? In this chapter, we review the recent advances in the assessment of tissue destruction after thermal ablation, VTP, and cryotherapy, and examine whether this is feasible in the operating room on a routine basis.

9.2 High-Intensity Focused Ultrasound and Laser Treatments

9.2.1 Should We Assess Tissue Destruction Immediately After Treatment?

The histological lesion induced by High-Intensity Focused Ultrasound (HIFU) or interstitial laser treatments is the same. In both cases there is a sharp delineation between treated and untreated areas. Treated areas show a central core of coagulation necrosis surrounded by a peripheral rim of hemorrhage, edema, and partial necrosis [1–8]. Experimental data obtained in canine and human prostates with HIFU showed that the central core of coagulation was homogeneous and that the peripheral zone of edema and incomplete necrosis surrounding this coagulation core was thin (less than 3 mm), emphasizing the spatial accuracy of these therapies.

Another advantage of these approaches is that energy deposition within the treated area can be predicted using mathematical models [9–11]. These models have been able to accurately predict the size of the ablated volume using HIFU, not only ex vivo [9], but also in patients [12].

Nevertheless, several factors may impair the completeness of the destruction of the target volume. First, mis-targeting of the tumor volume may occur. This can be due to errors in treatment planning, inaccuracy of the placement of laser fibers, or patient motion during treatment. HIFU techniques that require the side-to-side placement of small focal lesions throughout the target volume [13], with relatively long treatment times, seem particularly sensitive to patient motion.

Second, local tissue perfusion may influence the extent of tissue destruction. Indeed, blood flow transports heat from the treated area, reducing temperature and treatment efficacy (heat sink effect) [14]. During HIFU treatment, the temperature can reach 80 °C at the focal site within a few seconds and the influence of blood flow on such important temperature increases over such short time periods has been questioned [14, 15]. Despite the high temperatures achieved with HIFU, experimental data suggested that the lesion size could be significantly influenced by local perfusion, probably because the latter impacts the extent of heat diffusion at the periphery of the treated volume [16, 17]. In a clinical evaluation of 48 patients treated with whole-gland transrectal HIFU ablation for prostate cancer, the regional prostate blood flow measured on preoperative magnetic resonance imaging (MRI) was significantly lower in patients who responded to the treatment (patients with a postoperative PSA nadir <0.2 ng/ml), than in nonresponders (PSA nadir >0.2 ng/ml) [18].

Third, complex interaction between successive HIFU shots (lesion-to-lesion interaction) or heat build-up phenomena may induce under- or overtreatment when firing parameters are suboptimal [19].

Finally, it has been suggested that some tumors could be more tolerant to heat than surrounding normal tissues. The history of neo-adjuvant androgen deprivation therapy (ADT) was found to negatively influence histological tissue destruction shown at postoperative biopsy in a cohort of 35 patients treated by whole-gland prostate HIFU ablation [14]. Recently, the history of pre-HIFU ADT was also found to be associated with a significantly worse outcome in 208 patients treated by salvage HIFU ablation for local recurrence after radiation therapy [20]. The latter result must be interpreted with care, since ADT was not standardized and was probably used in larger and more aggressive tumors. Nevertheless, it remains possible that some tumor cells may resist heat better than others, and this may be of therapeutic importance, especially in the areas located on the periphery of the ablated volume.

Taken together, all these data suggest that the final location, size, shape, and volume of tissue destruction due to thermal ablation techniques may differ from what is expected from preoperative mathematical modeling and treatment planning. Intraoperative monitoring of energy deposition and/or assessment of the tissue volume actually destroyed at the end of the treatment is therefore warranted.

9.2.2 Intraoperative Monitoring and Postoperative Evaluation of the Ablated Volume

MR-Guided Procedures

Intraoperative Monitoring of Temperature Changes
If the ablation is performed under MR guidance, intraoperative monitoring of the energy deposition is technically feasible and accurate. There are indeed several techniques for measuring temperature changes on MRI. Currently, the evaluation of

the proton resonance frequency shift (PRFS) due to temperature changes has achieved great acceptability in clinical settings. It makes it possible to monitor the temperature rise during HIFU or laser treatment, with an accuracy of approximately 1 °C, a spatial resolution on the order of 1 mm and a temporal resolution of a few seconds [10, 21–24]. Hence, MR thermometry allows (almost) real time monitoring of the temperature in the target volume. After integration of these data through time, cumulative thermal dose maps can be computed. It is even possible to use temperature feedback to actively control the treatment parameters to make sure that the prescribed thermal dose is actually obtained in the target volume [10, 23–25].

Although MR thermometry may seem ideal to avoid under- or overtreatments due to factors that are not taken into consideration during treatment planning (e.g., local blood perfusion), this approach still has some drawbacks and limitations. First, PRFS remains very sensitive to patient motion during treatment [21]. Second, its accuracy is limited in adipose tissue making it necessary to obtain efficient lipid suppression during MR thermometry. Any incomplete lipid suppression may induce inaccurate temperature readings. This may be problematic in subcapsular areas of the prostate because of their close vicinity with the periprostatic fat and in turn induce an overtreatment of the neurovascular bundles or an imperfect ablation of subcapsular tumors [21]. Third, the PRFS method relies on a relative change from a reference temperature obtained immediately before ablation. Any drop in core body temperature over the course of treatment could considerably influence the thermal dose [26]. Fourth, the presence of chelates of gadolinium in tissues will influence the local magnetic field and affect the proton resonance frequency. This will in turn affect temperature measurement. Thus, if an injection of chelates of gadolinium is performed before treatment (e.g., to localize the target tumor), subsequent MR thermometry may not be accurate [27]. Lastly, although ablated volumes measured by cumulative thermal dose positively correlate with histologically ablated volumes, they may slightly under- or overestimate them [26, 28].

Hence, even if MR thermometry increases the safety and precision of thermal ablation techniques, it remains necessary to evaluate at the end of the treatment the position and extent of the actual ablated tissue.

Postoperative Evaluation of the Ablated Volume

Since the 1990s it has been known that coagulation necrosis due to laser or HIFU ablation can be visible on gadolinium-enhanced T1-weighted MR images. Ablated areas appear as devascularized areas, sometimes surrounded by a rim of enhancement (Figs. 9.1, 9.2, and 9.3). Histological studies showed an excellent correlation between the volume of the devascularized area and the volume of the core of coagulation necrosis, the enhancement rim corresponding to the peripheral area of inflammation, edema, and partial necrosis [12, 26, 29–31]. This devascularized volume is visible within minutes following the end of the treatment. Thus, it seems easy to evaluate the position and volume of the tissue actually destroyed by obtaining gadolinium-enhanced imaging at the end of the procedure. Gadolinium-enhanced MRI may also show the extension of necrosis within periprostatic tissue or rectal wall (Fig. 9.4).

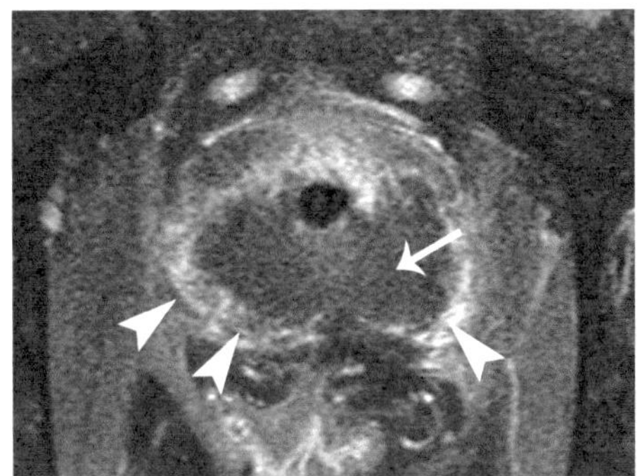

Fig. 9.1 Axial gadolinium-enhanced fat-saturated MR image obtained 2 days after HIFU ablation of the prostate. The HIFU-induced necrosis was visible as a devascularized area corresponding to homogeneous coagulation necrosis (*arrow*) surrounded by a peripheral rim of enhancement corresponding to edema inflammation and partial necrosis (*arrowheads*)

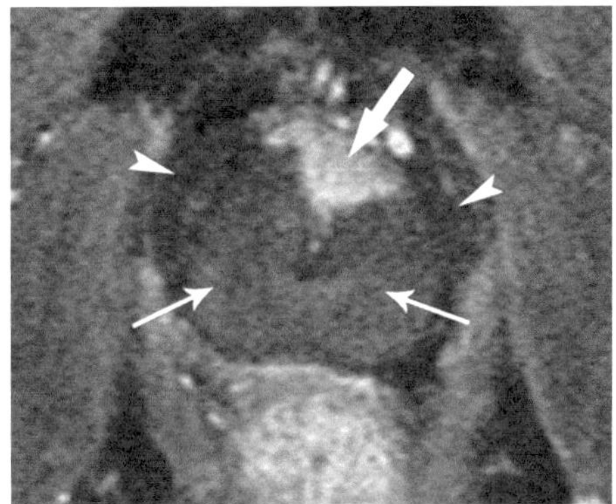

Fig. 9.2 Axial gadolinium-enhanced fat-saturated MR image obtained 2 days after HIFU ablation of the prostate. The HIFU-induced necrosis appeared as a devascularized area (*arrows*), but the rim of enhancement was not clearly visible. Note the extension of necrosis in the periprostatic tissues (*arrowheads*). Note also that an anterior strip of the left lobe remained untreated (*large arrow*)

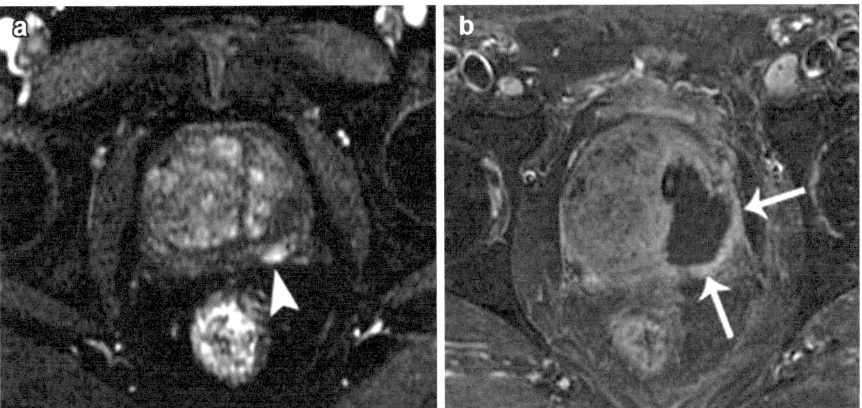

Fig. 9.3 Axial dynamic contrast-enhanced MR image showing a 7-mm Gleason 7 cancer in the left mid gland peripheral zone (**a**, *arrowhead*). Axial gadolinium-enhanced fat-saturated MR image obtained 3 days after focal HIFU ablation showing the position and extent of the ablated area (**b**, *arrows*)

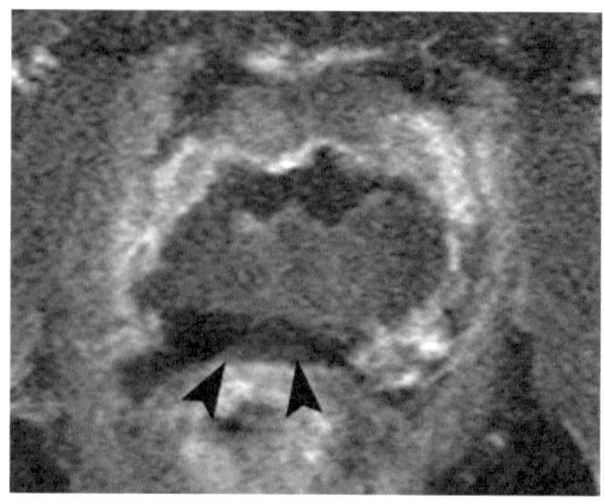

Fig. 9.4 Axial gadolinium-enhanced fat-saturated MR image obtained 2 days after HIFU ablation of the prostate and showing that the rectal wall had been partially included in the treated volume (*arrowheads*). Fortunately, only the most external part of the rectal wall was involved and the patient healed without any complication

Other MR sequences may be useful in the future. Ablated areas show a decreased diffusion of water molecules [32]. However, the incremental value of diffusion-weighted MRI as compared to gadolinium-enhanced T1-weighted imaging remains to be defined [26]. Dramatic increase in stiffness has been found in the ablated volume using MR elastography (MRE). This method seems particularly interesting because it can provide simultaneous measurement of temperature and tissue stiffness [33]. Thus, it may become feasible to monitor during the treatment – not only the temperature rise, but also the associated tissue changes. However, such monitoring remains technically challenging and is not used in daily practice.

Is Immediate Re-treatment Possible?

As seen above, it is possible to monitor the temperature during laser or HIFU ablation using MR thermometry and to assess whether the target volume has been correctly ablated using gadolinium-enhanced T1-weighted imaging.

This makes complete sense, however, only if it is possible to immediately re-treat the patient in case of unsatisfactory findings on gadolinium-enhanced imaging. There has been some concern that thermal ablation-induced mechanical and thermal stress may dissociate the gadolinium chelates used as contrast agents and lead to free Gd^{3+} ions. Free Gd^{3+} ions may be deposited as insoluble salts in bones, liver, and spleen, and their long-term retention has been strongly associated with the development of nephrogenic systemic fibrosis, a potentially fatal condition [34, 35]. A study was recently performed in vivo on rat muscle and subcutaneous tumors treated with HIFU after injection of gadopentetate dimeglumine (Gd-DTPA, Magnevist, Bayer-Schering, Berlin, Germany), a contrast medium widely used in human studies. The results showed a transient trapping of Gd-DTPA within the ablated volume, but no significant increase in gadolinium content in the principal target organs for translocated free Gd^{3+} ions (liver, spleen, and bone), as compared to sham-treated animals [27]. Thus, re-treating patients within minutes of the injection of chelates of gadolinium seems safe. It must be remembered, however, that the presence of gadolinium in tissues may alter MR thermometry performance and lead to inaccurate temperature readings.

US-Guided Procedures

Intraoperative Monitoring of Temperature Changes

Although some techniques based on changes in sound speed with temperature are under evaluation [36], there is currently no US-based method that can allow real time monitoring of temperature during US-guided procedures. On the Sonablate™ HIFU device (Focus Surgery, Indianapolis, IN, USA), it is possible to manually adjust the power to the B-mode US changes observed during the procedure [37]. However, this remains subjective, and whether such an approach induces more homogeneous necrosis remains to be proven in a large number of patients.

This lack of validated real time monitoring during treatment is a major limitation of US-guided procedures. On the other hand, US guidance has the advantage of being much cheaper than MR guidance that needs MR-compatible treatment systems and dedicated MR scanners. As a result, US guidance has been used much more for HIFU ablation of prostate cancers within the last 15 years [38, 39] and this may continue, given the current economic context. It should also be noted that despite the lack of real time temperature monitoring, whole-gland prostate cancer US-guided HIFU ablation yielded interesting clinical results [20, 38–40], suggesting that the treatment algorithms used provide an effective and safe tissue destruction.

Postoperative Evaluation of the Ablated Volume

Because there is no possibility of monitoring the temperature changes during US-guided thermal procedures, it is all the more important to assess the extent of tissue ablation at the end of US-guided procedures.

A contrast-enhanced power Doppler, using a galactose-based US microbubble contrast agent (SH U 508A, Levovist™, Schering, Berlin, Germany) was shown to reliably depict the position and volume of devascularized tissue in nine patients that underwent prostate cancer HIFU ablation 1 week before radical prostatectomy [41]. However, this technique was limited due to the short half-life of SH U 508A and the relatively low spatial resolution of the power Doppler. New US contrast agents, such as Sonovue™ (Bracco, Milan, Italy), a suspension of phospholipid stabilized sulfur hexafluoride microbubbles, can enhance the gray-scale echo pattern at specific imaging sequences, with excellent contrast-to-tissue ratio and spatial resolution, and prolonged half-life.

Contrast-enhanced US (CEUS) using Sonovue™ has been evaluated in a cohort of 34 patients treated with whole-gland prostate HIFU ablation and who underwent CEUS-guided biopsy 1 month after HIFU treatment [42]. CEUS showed the treated volume as a devascularized area that was visible immediately at the end of the treatment. This devascularized area was unchanged at 1-month CEUS control. CEUS findings were well correlated with the results of the gadolinium-enhanced MRI performed 1–3 days after treatment. CEUS-guided biopsy also showed good concordance between CEUS and biopsy results. Viable gland tissue was found in only 9 (6.2 %) of 140 biopsies performed in entirely devascularized parts of the prostate. In eight of these nine biopsies, viable tissue was found at one of the extremities of the biopsy cores, strongly suggesting that devascularized areas are made of homogeneous

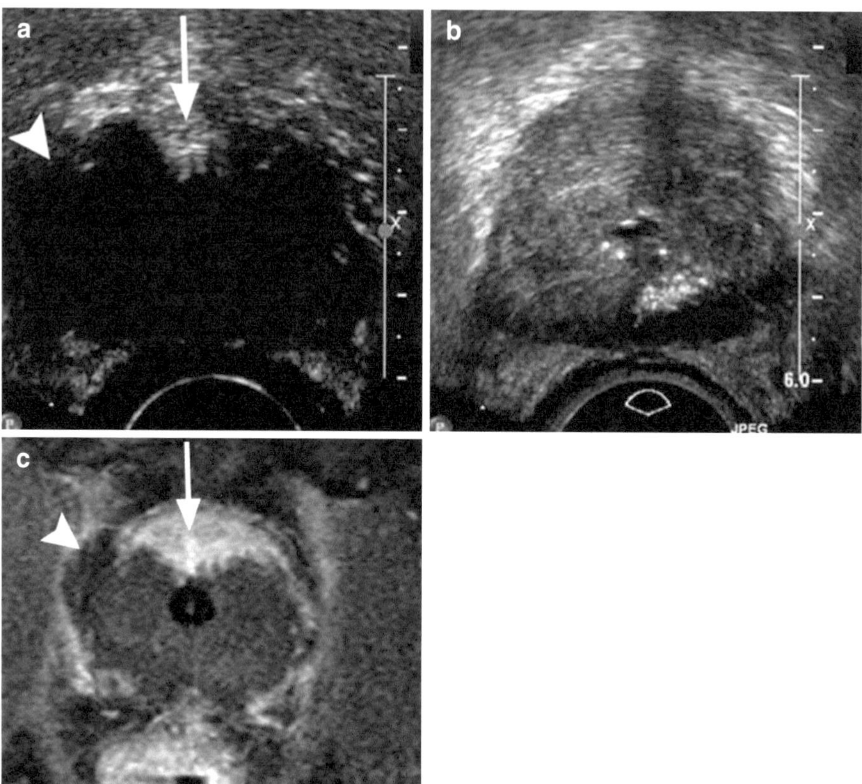

Fig. 9.5 Contrast-enhanced Ultrasound (CEUS) image (**a**) and corresponding gray-scale ultrasound image (**b**) obtained 1 day after HIFU ablation of the prostate. The ablated area appeared as a devascularized area on CEUS but was not visible on gray-scale imaging. The necrosis extended into the periprostatic tissues on the right (**a**, *arrowhead*) and an anterior and median strip of prostate parenchyma showed marked residual enhancement (**a**, *arrow*). A gadolinium-enhanced fat-saturated MRI performed 2 days later (**c**) confirmed the extension of the necrosis into the right periprostatic tissues (**c**, *arrowhead*) and the lack of destruction of an anterior and median strip of prostate tissue (**c**, *arrow*)

necrosis. In contrast, viable tissue was found in 10 (34 %) of 29 biopsies performed in prostate areas showing mild and/or patchy enhancement, and in 44 (60 %) of 72 biopsies performed in prostate areas showing marked enhancement. As compared to devascularized sites, the odds ratios for finding viable tissue at sites showing mild and/or patchy enhancement and at sites showing marked enhancement were 21 (95 % confidence interval: 6–71) and 73 (95 % confidence interval: 22–243) respectively ($p < 0.0001$). Residual cancer was found in only five biopsy cores in two patients, all in sites with marked enhancement. Thus, CEUS seems a promising tool for delineating ablated tissue in the operating room after US-guided thermal ablation (Figs. 9.5 and 9.6). One limitation of CEUS, however, is that it cannot clearly show the extension of necrosis to the rectal wall, at least with current US probes.

Quasi-static compression US elastography can show the treated volume as a stiff area and is feasible in the operating room [43]. However, the only clinical report,

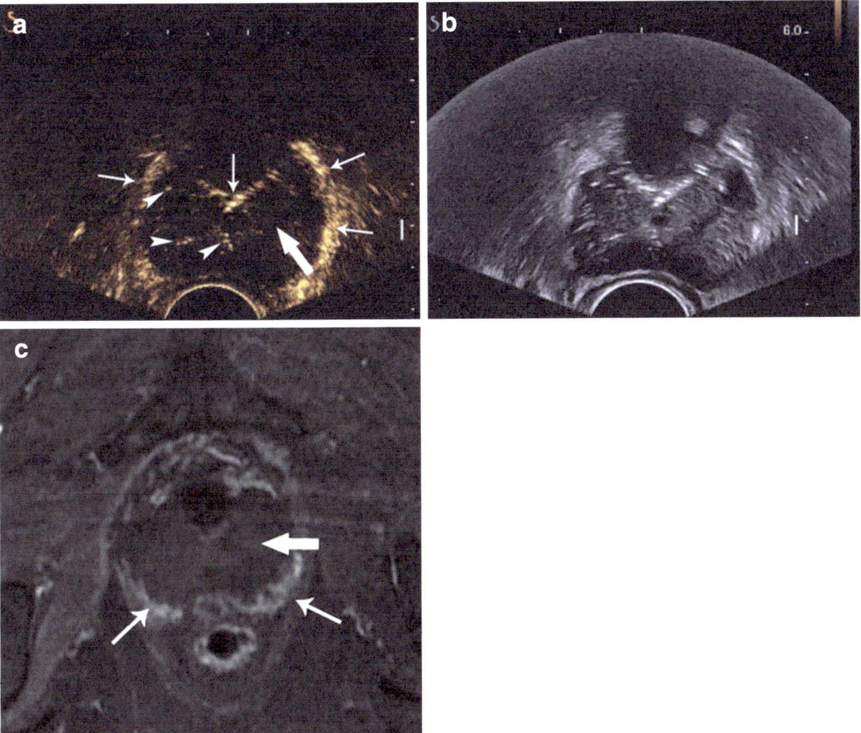

Fig. 9.6 Contrast-enhanced Ultrasound (CEUS) image (**a**) and corresponding gray-scale ultrasound image (**b**) obtained in the operating room, immediately after the end of HIFU ablation. CEUS image showed a complete devascularization of the prostate (**a**, *large arrow*), with a peripheral rim of enhancement (**a**, *small arrows*). The hyperechoic spots within the ablated area were visible at unenhanced imaging (not shown) and corresponded to residual cavitation bubbles. A gadolinium-enhanced fat-saturated MRI performed 2 days later (**c**) was confirmative and showed complete ablation of the gland (**c**, *large arrow*), with an incomplete peripheral rim of enhancement (**c**, *small arrows*)

featuring a prototype scanner, showed a mediocre correlation between the stiff volume shown at elastography and the devascularized volume shown at MRI [44]. We are currently evaluating US shear-wave elastography at our institution. This new technique allows the quantification of tissue stiffness and is, in theory, less operator-dependent than quasi-static compression US elastography. Preliminary results show that it can depict the treated area at the end of the treatment with reasonable accuracy (Fig. 9.7). It is, however, too soon to know whether it could challenge the results of CEUS.

Is Immediate Re-treatment Possible?

CEUS with injection of Sonovue™ is currently used at our institute on a routine basis to evaluate the ablated volume at the end of US-guided prostate cancer HIFU ablation. However, the contrast agent microbubbles may, at least in theory, interfere with subsequent repeat HIFU ablation. Because almost all microbubbles are eliminated from the blood within 20 min [45], repeat HIFU ablation is performed, when needed, more than 30 min after the end of the first HIFU ablation. Under these

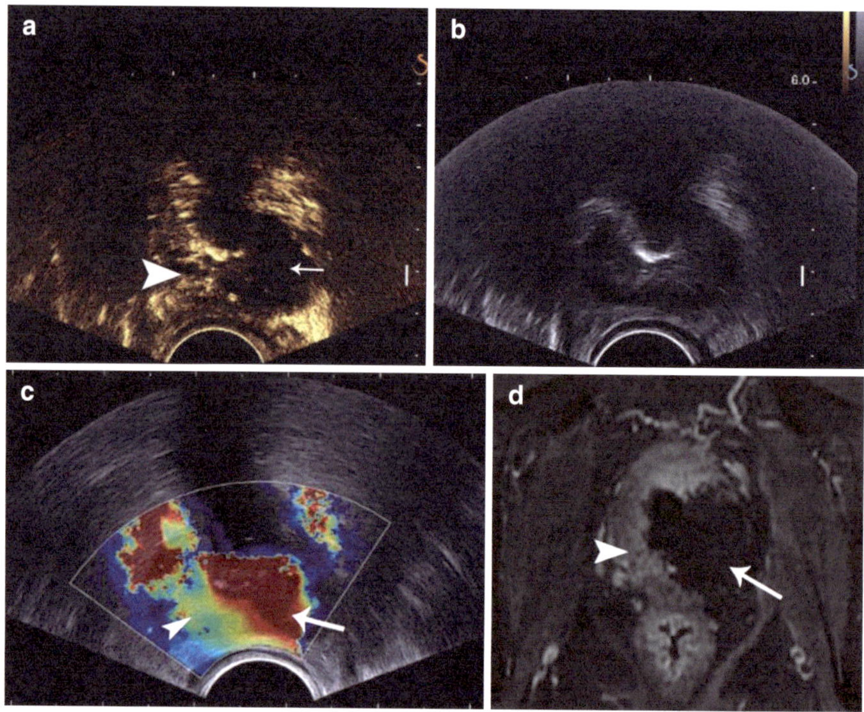

Fig. 9.7 Contrast-enhanced Ultrasound (CEUS) image (**a**) and corresponding gray-scale ultrasound image (**b**) obtained in the operating room, immediately after the end of HIFU ablation. CEUS image showed a complete ablation of the left lobe (**a**, *arrow*), with a right lobe remaining unaffected (**a**, *arrowhead*). Shear-wave ultrasound elastography, also performed at the end of the treatment, showed an increased stiffness within the left lobe (**c**, *arrow*) as compared to the right lobe (**c**, *arrowhead*). Gadolinium-enhanced fat-saturated MRI confirmed the ablation of the left lobe (**d**, *arrow*) and the preservation of the right lobe (**d**, *arrowhead*)

conditions, repeat HIFU treatment seems safe and so far we have not observed unexpected adverse events (Fig. 9.8).

9.3 Vascular-Targeted Photodynamic Therapy

Photodynamic therapy (PDT) involves the administration of a photosensitizing agent followed by the exposure of the target tissue to light of the appropriate wavelength, which stimulates the production of oxygen species that cause cell death. Palladium-bacteriopheophorbide (WST9, Tookad™, Steba-Biotech, The Hague, The Netherlands) is an intravascular photosensitizer with a short intravascular half-light and near-infrared (763-nm) absorption band that allows deep light penetration in tissues. Tookad-PDT induces tissue necrosis, but its mechanism is different from that of other thermal ablations techniques. Indeed, it induces rapid vascular occlusion which in turn creates necrosis in the target volume – hence the term "vascular targeted PDT" (VTP) proposed by some authors.

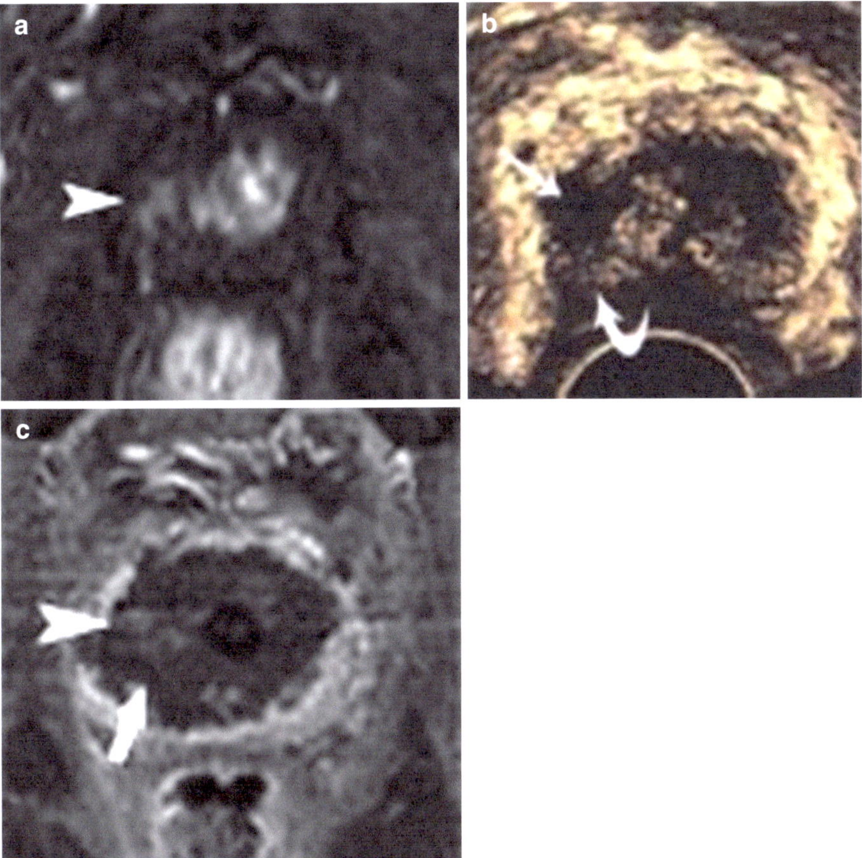

Fig. 9.8 Axial dynamic contrast-enhanced MR image (**a**) showing a prostate cancer focus in the right apex of the prostate (**a**, *arrowhead*) Contrast-enhanced Ultrasound image performed immediately after HIFU ablation showed partial destruction of the right apex (**b**, *arrow*), with a large amount of undestroyed posterior tissue (**b**, *curve arrow*). The right apex was immediately re-treated, within the same anesthesia. Gadolinium-enhanced fat-saturated MRI performed 2 days later showed an almost complete ablation of the prostate. The hyperintense area within the right apex (**c**, *arrowhead*) corresponds to interstitial hemorrhage already visible on unenhanced imaging (not shown), and not to enhancing tissue

9.3.1 Should We Assess Tissue Destruction Immediately After Treatment?

VTP-induced lesions are characterized by marked hemorrhagic and inflammatory necrosis [46–49]. The onset of necrosis and its extent depend on the drug-light dose administered. However, early histological studies showed that some tissues may be more sensitive to VTP than others [49]. In canine prostates, the induced lesion around the laser fiber was not always in a perfect spheral or oval shape as expected. Some lesions that were found to extend beyond the light-irradiated zone may be due to downstream vascular shutdown [48]. Clinical phase I/II studies on prostate cancer

VTP treatments also showed a wide variation in induced necrotic volumes between patients [50, 51]. The reasons for these large variations remain unclear. Prostate biopsies performed 6 months after VTP commonly show the presence of entrapped benign, atrophic-appearing prostate glands within the areas of VTP-induced fibrosis [50]. It is therefore possible, unlike what is observed after thermal ablation, that the VPT-induced necrosis is not homogeneous at the microscopic level. Even if there are some attempts at modeling the volume of necrosis [52], evaluating the amount of prostate destroyed at the end of the treatment seems to be warranted.

9.3.2 Intraoperative Treatment Monitoring and Postoperative Evaluation of the Ablated Volume

There is no intraoperative monitoring of the energy deposition within the prostate during VTP. A study on dogs showed a good spatial correlation between the histological necrotic areas of the prostate and the unenhancing zones found on gadolinium-enhanced T1-weighted MR images obtained 2 and 7 days after VTP. T2-weighted and diffusion-weighted imaging showed altered signals within the treated area but did not clearly define necrosis in all cases [53].

Gadolinium-enhanced T1-weighted MRIs performed 7 days after treatment also showed VTP-induced necrosis in humans (Fig. 9.9). It can also show the extension of necrosis to the rectum or the extraprostatic tissues [50, 51].

Even if it has not been tested so far, it would seem logical to think that CEUS using Sonovue™ as a contrast agent would show the necrotic areas at day seven, just as gadolinium-enhanced MRI does. However, it remains unclear whether the VTP-induced necrosis is entirely constituted (and thus potentially visible at imaging) immediately at the end of the treatment or not. In any such case, CEUS would probably be a convenient method to evaluate the treatment result in the operating room. Nevertheless, the safety and conditions (reinjection of the drug or not) of an immediate re-treatment have not been evaluated.

9.4 Cryotherapy

As for thermal ablation, the site treated by cryoablation is characterized by a central zone of coagulation necrosis, and a peripheral zone characterized by varying degrees of inflammation, hemorrhage, and cellular death [54–56]. There is little doubt that the central part of the target volume that is exposed to temperature below −40 °C, is homogeneously destroyed due to direct ice-related cell damage. In contrast, the periphery of the treated volume, exposed to a gradient of temperature from −40 to 0 °C is submitted to more complex injury mechanisms including direct ice-related cell damage and indirect injury due to ischemia and delayed apoptosis in which mitochondrial damage may play a role [54, 57, 58]. It is of course in this "gray area" that cells may survive and lead to cancer recurrence.

The progressive extension of the ice ball during cryotherapy is easy to monitor, whether one uses US or MR guidance [56]. Unfortunately, the ice ball only

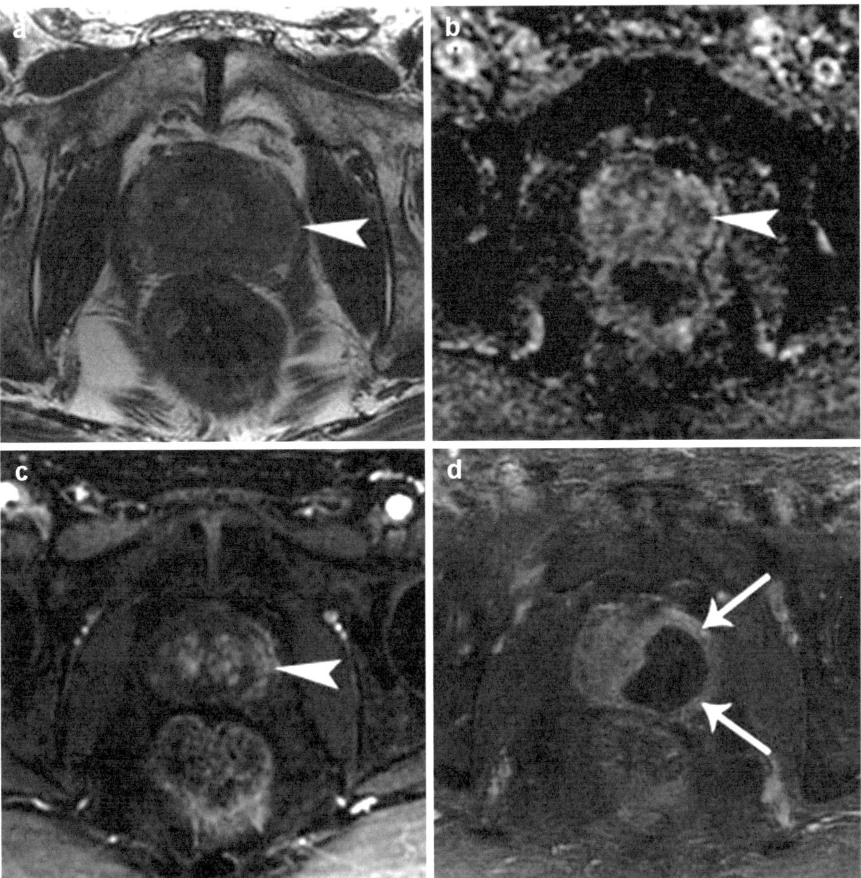

Fig. 9.9 Images obtained in a patient with Gleason 6 cancer of the left lobe. Multiparametric MRI shows the cancer that appears as an area with marked signal hypointensity at T2-weighted imaging (**a**, *arrowhead*) and on the Apparent Diffusion Coefficient map (**b**, *arrowhead*) and as an area with early enhancement at dynamiccontrast-enhanced imaging (**c**, *arrowhead*). Axial, gadolinium-enhanced fat-saturated MRI performed 7 days after focal VTP showed homogeneous devascularization of the left lobe (**d**, *arrows*)

indicates the amount of tissue exposed to temperatures below freezing. How exactly the position of the central core submitted to lethal temperature can be inferred from the position of the ice ball remains unclear. Furthermore, if transrectal US guidance is used, only the posterior part of the ice ball can be monitored, its anterior aspect being invisible due to the high attenuation of the US beam by the ice. Thus, the decision to further increase the size of the ice ball or to stop the freezing relies mostly on the experience of the operator.

As a result, it would be interesting to evaluate, at the end of the procedure, the size and position of the central core of necrosis actually obtained.

As for thermal ablation, the coagulation necrosis induced by cryotherapy appears as a devascularized volume at gadolinium-enhanced T1-weighted MRI [56]. It is likely that CEUS could provide the same information, even if, to our knowledge,

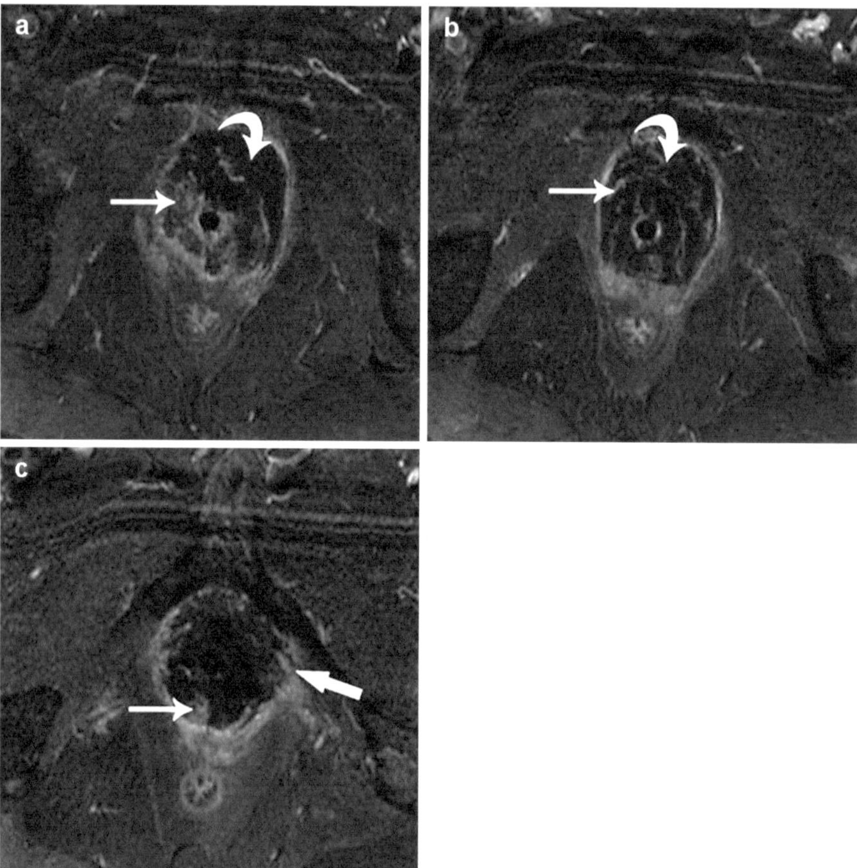

Fig. 9.10 Images obtained in a patient with history of radiation therapy, and treated by salvage cryotherapy for a cancer local recurrence. Axial gadolinium-enhanced fat-saturated MR images (**a–c**), performed 2 days after cryotherapy, showed a complete devascularization of the prostate. Note however that the devascularized area is not homogeneous, with persistence of areas of patchy enhancement (**a–c**, *arrows*). In our experience, these areas of patchy enhancement are replaced by homogeneous devascularization in the week following cryotherapy (not shown). Note the large extension of necrosis in the periprostatic tissues, anteriorly (**a**, **b**, *curve arrow*) and on the left (**c**, *large arrow*)

this has never been assessed. Unfortunately, this can be done only once the ice ball has totally disappeared, which may take several hours. Furthermore, in our experience, the central core of necrosis may take 1 or 2 weeks to become homogeneous at MRI. If the control imaging is performed too soon after the treatment, the ablated volume may show patchy residual enhancement that disappears within a week or two (Figs. 9.10 and 9.11). Hence, unlike what is observed after thermal ablation, contrast-enhanced imaging cannot provide an accurate evaluation of tissue destruction immediately at the end of the procedure.

One way to overcome this problem would be to use MR thermometry sequences to monitor the position of the −20 and −40 °C isotherms within the ice ball during cryotherapy. However, this is currently technically not possible [59].

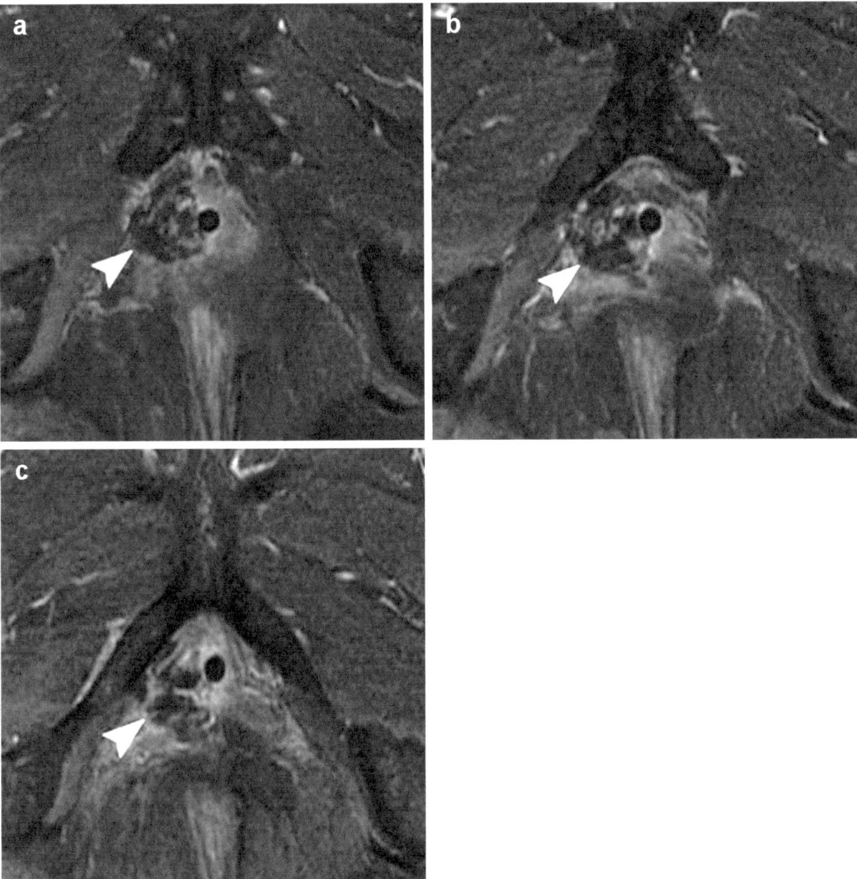

Fig. 9.11 Images obtained in a patient with history of radiation therapy, and treated by salvage hemi-cryotherapy for a cancer local recurrence within the right lobe. Axial gadolinium-enhanced fat-saturated MR images (**a–c**), performed 2 days after cryotherapy showed that the entire right lobe had been treated, with a typical patchy appearance of the devascularized area

Conclusion

Thermoablation procedures, using either HIFU or interstitial laser, induce tissue necrosis that is visible immediately at the end of the treatment on contrast-enhanced US or MR images. Immediate re-treatment is easily feasible and seems to be safe. Postoperative control of the correct destruction of the target volume is therefore highly recommended and possibilities of easy immediate re-treatment may appear in the near future as an important advantage of thermoablation procedures. Additionally, if the procedures are performed under MR guidance, real time monitoring of the temperature during treatment is possible.

It remains unknown whether the indirect necrosis induced by VTP is visible immediately at the end of the procedure. In such a case, the conditions for immediate re-treatment (need for a reinjection or not, safety and dose of the reinjection) still have to be determined.

Cryotherapy can provide a direct and real time monitoring of the ice ball size and position. However, the size of the ice ball indicates the amount of tissue submitted to freezing and not to lethal (below −40 °C) temperatures. Postoperative assessment of the volume of coagulation necrosis is difficult since it needs the complete disappearance of the ice ball. It remains to be determined whether in the future MR thermometry sequences will be able to monitor the position of the −20 and −40 °C isotherms within the ice ball during treatment.

References

1. Boyes A, Tang K, Yaffe M, Sugar L, Chopra R, Bronskill M. Prostate tissue analysis immediately following magnetic resonance imaging guided transurethral ultrasound thermal therapy. J Urol. 2007;178(3 Pt 1):1080–5.
2. Susani M, Madersbacher S, Kratzik C, Vingers L, Marberger M. Morphology of tissue destruction induced by focused ultrasound. Eur Urol. 1993;23 Suppl 1:34–8.
3. Beerlage HP, van Leenders GJ, Oosterhof GO, et al. High-intensity focused ultrasound (HIFU) followed after one to two weeks by radical retropubic prostatectomy: results of a prospective study. Prostate. 1999;39(1):41–6.
4. Chapelon JY, Margonari J, Theillere Y, et al. Effects of high-energy focused ultrasound on kidney tissue in the rat and the dog. Eur Urol. 1992;22(2):147–52.
5. Gelet A, Chapelon JY, Margonari J, et al. Prostatic tissue destruction by high-intensity focused ultrasound: experimentation on canine prostate. J Endourol. 1993;7(3):249–53.
6. Beerlage HP, Thuroff S, Debruyne FM, Chaussy C, de la Rosette JJ. Transrectal high-intensity focused ultrasound using the Ablatherm device in the treatment of localized prostate carcinoma. Urology. 1999;54(2):273–7.
7. Chen L, Rivens I, ter Haar G, Riddler S, Hill CR, Bensted JP. Histological changes in rat liver tumours treated with high-intensity focused ultrasound. Ultrasound Med Biol. 1993;19(1):67–74.
8. el-Ouahabi A, Guttmann CR, Hushek SG, et al. MRI guided interstitial laser therapy in a rat malignant glioma model. Lasers Surg Med. 1993;13(5):503–10.
9. Chavrier F, Chapelon JY, Gelet A, Cathignol D. Modeling of high-intensity focused ultrasound-induced lesions in the presence of cavitation bubbles. J Acoust Soc Am. 2000;108(1):432–40.
10. Feng Y, Fuentes D. Model-based planning and real-time predictive control for laser-induced thermal therapy. Int J Hyperthermia. 2011;27(8):751–61.
11. Prakash P, Diederich CJ. Considerations for theoretical modelling of thermal ablation with catheter-based ultrasonic sources: implications for treatment planning, monitoring and control. Int J Hyperthermia. 2012;28(1):69–86.
12. Rouviere O, Lyonnet D, Raudrant A, et al. MRI appearance of prostate following transrectal HIFU ablation of localized cancer. Eur Urol. 2001;40(3):265–74.
13. Rouviere O, Souchon R, Salomir R, Gelet A, Chapelon JY, Lyonnet D. Transrectal high-intensity focused ultrasound ablation of prostate cancer: effective treatment requiring accurate imaging. Eur J Radiol. 2007;63(3):317–27.
14. Rouviere O, Curiel L, Chapelon JY, et al. Can color doppler predict the uniformity of HIFU-induced prostate tissue destruction? Prostate. 2004;60(4):289–97.
15. Fry FJ. Intense focused ultrasound in medicine. Some practical guiding physical principles from sound source to focal site in tissue. Eur Urol. 1993;23 Suppl 1:2–7.

16. Zhou P, Zhou P, He W, et al. The influence of blood supply on high intensity focused ultrasound a preliminary study on rabbit hepatic VX2 tumors of different ages. Acad Radiol. 2012;19(1):40–7.
17. Chen L, ter Haar G, Hill CR, et al. Effect of blood perfusion on the ablation of liver parenchyma with high-intensity focused ultrasound. Phys Med Biol. 1993;38(11):1661–73.
18. Wiart M, Curiel L, Gelet A, Lyonnet D, Chapelon JY, Rouviere O. Influence of perfusion on high-intensity focused ultrasound prostate ablation: a first-pass MRI study. Magn Reson Med. 2007;58(1):119–27.
19. Chen L, ter Haar G, Hill CR. Influence of ablated tissue on the formation of high-intensity focused ultrasound lesions. Ultrasound Med Biol. 1997;23(6):921–31.
20. Crouzet S, Murat FJ, Pommier P, et al. Locally recurrent prostate cancer after initial radiation therapy: early salvage high-intensity focused ultrasound improves oncologic outcomes. Radiother Oncol. 2012;105(2):198–202.
21. Rieke V, Butts Pauly K. MR thermometry. J Magn Reson Imaging. 2008;27(2):376–90.
22. Chopra R, Wachsmuth J, Burtnyk M, Haider MA, Bronskill MJ. Analysis of factors important for transurethral ultrasound prostate heating using MR temperature feedback. Phys Med Biol. 2006;51(4):827–44.
23. Salomir R, Delemazure AS, Palussiere J, Rouviere O, Cotton F, Chapelon JY. Image-based control of the magnetic resonance imaging-guided focused ultrasound thermotherapy. Top Magn Reson Imaging. 2006;17(3):139–51.
24. Ramsay E, Mougenot C, Kohler M, et al. MR thermometry in the human prostate gland at 3.0T for transurethral ultrasound therapy. J Magn Reson Imaging. 2013. doi:10.1002/jmri.24063.
25. Goharrizi AY, N'Djin WA, Kwong R, Chopra R. Development of a new control strategy for 3D MRI-controlled interstitial ultrasound cancer therapy. Med Phys. 2013;40(3):033301.
26. Partanen A, Yerram NK, Trivedi H, et al. Magnetic resonance imaging (MRI)-guided transurethral ultrasound therapy of the prostate: a preclinical study with radiological and pathological correlation using customised MRI-based moulds. BJU Int. 2013. doi:10.1111/bju.12126.
27. Hijnen NM, Elevelt A, Grull H. Stability and trapping of magnetic resonance imaging contrast agents during high-intensity focused ultrasound ablation therapy. Invest Radiol. 2013;48(7):517–24.
28. Kickhefel A, Rosenberg C, Weiss CR, et al. Clinical evaluation of MR temperature monitoring of laser-induced thermotherapy in human liver using the proton-resonance-frequency method and predictive models of cell death. J Magn Reson Imaging. 2011;33(3):704–12.
29. Larson BT, Collins JM, Huidobro C, Corica A, Vallejo S, Bostwick DG. Gadolinium-enhanced MRI in the evaluation of minimally invasive treatments of the prostate: correlation with histopathologic findings. Urology. 2003;62(5):900–4.
30. Kirkham AP, Emberton M, Hoh IM, Illing RO, Freeman AA, Allen C. MR imaging of prostate after treatment with high-intensity focused ultrasound. Radiology. 2008;246(3):833–44.
31. Tazaki H, Nakashima J, Nakagawa K. MRI evaluation of cavitation induced by laser prostatectomy. J Endourol. 1995;9(2):171–3.
32. Chen J, Daniel BL, Diederich CJ, et al. Monitoring prostate thermal therapy with diffusion-weighted MRI. Magn Reson Med. 2008;59(6):1365–72.
33. Le Y, Glaser K, Rouviere O, Ehman R, Felmlee JP. Feasibility of simultaneous temperature and tissue stiffness detection by MRE. Magn Reson Med. 2006;55(3):700–5.
34. Laurent S, Elst LV, Copoix F, Muller RN. Stability of MRI paramagnetic contrast media: a proton relaxometric protocol for transmetallation assessment. Invest Radiol. 2001;36(2):115–22.
35. MacNeil S, Bains S, Johnson C, et al. Gadolinium contrast agent associated stimulation of human fibroblast collagen production. Invest Radiol. 2011;46(11):711–7.
36. Seo CH, Shi Y, Huang SW, Kim K, O'Donnell M. Thermal strain imaging: a review. Interface Focus. 2011;1(4):649–64.

37. Illing RO, Leslie TA, Kennedy JE, Calleary JG, Ogden CW, Emberton M. Visually directed high-intensity focused ultrasound for organ-confined prostate cancer: a proposed standard for the conduct of therapy. BJU Int. 2006;98(6):1187–92.
38. Murat FJ, Gelet A. Current status of high-intensity focused ultrasound for prostate cancer: technology, clinical outcomes, and future. Curr Urol Rep. 2008;9(2):113–21.
39. Zini C, Hipp E, Thomas S, Napoli A, Catalano C, Oto A. Ultrasound- and MR-guided focused ultrasound surgery for prostate cancer. World J Radiol. 2012;4(6):247–52.
40. Crouzet S, Rebillard X, Chevallier D, et al. Multicentric oncologic outcomes of high-intensity focused ultrasound for localized prostate cancer in 803 patients. Eur Urol. 2010;58(4): 559–66.
41. Sedelaar JP, Aarnink RG, van Leenders GJ, et al. The application of three-dimensional contrast-enhanced ultrasound to measure volume of affected tissue after HIFU treatment for localized prostate cancer. Eur Urol. 2000;37(5):559–68.
42. Rouvière O, Glas L, Girouin N, et al. Transrectal HIFU ablation of prostate cancer: assessment of tissue destruction with contrast-enhanced ultrasound. Radiology. 2011;259(2): 583–91.
43. Souchon R, Rouviere O, Gelet A, et al. Visualisation of HIFU lesions using elastography of the human prostate in vivo: preliminary results. Ultrasound Med Biol. 2003;29(7):1007–15.
44. Curiel L, Souchon R, Rouviere O, Gelet A, Chapelon JY. Elastography for the follow-up of high-intensity focused ultrasound prostate cancer treatment: initial comparison with MRI. Ultrasound Med Biol. 2005;31(11):1461–8.
45. Schneider M. SonoVue, a new ultrasound contrast agent. Eur Radiol. 1999;9 Suppl 3:S347–8.
46. Chevalier S, Anidjar M, Scarlata E, et al. Preclinical study of the novel vascular occluding agent, WST11, for photodynamic therapy of the canine prostate. J Urol. 2011;186(1):302–9.
47. Chevalier S, Cury FL, Scarlata E, et al. Endoscopic vascular targeted photodynamic therapy with the photosensitizer TOOKAD(R) soluble (WST11) for benign prostatic hyperplasia in the pre-clinical dog model. J Urol. 2013. doi:10.1016/j.juro.2013.05.014.
48. Huang Z, Chen Q, Dole KC, et al. The effect of Tookad-mediated photodynamic ablation of the prostate gland on adjacent tissues – in vivo study in a canine model. Photochem Photobiol Sci. 2007;6(12):1318–24.
49. Borle F, Radu A, Fontolliet C, van den Bergh H, Monnier P, Wagnieres G. Selectivity of the photosensitiser Tookad for photodynamic therapy evaluated in the Syrian golden hamster cheek pouch tumour model. Br J Cancer. 2003;89(12):2320–6.
50. Trachtenberg J, Weersink RA, Davidson SR, et al. Vascular-targeted photodynamic therapy (padoporfin, WST09) for recurrent prostate cancer after failure of external beam radiotherapy: a study of escalating light doses. BJU Int. 2008;102(5):556–62.
51. Haider MA, Davidson SR, Kale AV, et al. Prostate gland: MR imaging appearance after vascular targeted photodynamic therapy with palladium-bacteriopheophorbide. Radiology. 2007;244(1):196–204.
52. Betrouni N, Lopes R, Puech P, Colin P, Mordon S. A model to estimate the outcome of prostate cancer photodynamic therapy with TOOKAD Soluble WST11. Phys Med Biol. 2011;56(15): 4771–83.
53. Huang Z, Haider MA, Kraft S, et al. Magnetic resonance imaging correlated with the histopathological effect of Pd-bacteriopheophorbide (Tookad) photodynamic therapy on the normal canine prostate gland. Lasers Surg Med. 2006;38(7):672–81.
54. Maccini M, Sehrt D, Pompeo A, Chicoli FA, Molina WR, Kim FJ. Biophysiologic considerations in cryoablation: a practical mechanistic molecular review. Int Braz J Urol. 2011;37(6): 693–6.
55. Kimura M, Rabbani Z, Mouraviev V, et al. Morphology of hypoxia following cryoablation in a prostate cancer murine model: its relationship to necrosis, apoptosis and, microvessel density. Cryobiology. 2010;61(1):148–54.

56. van den Bosch MA, Josan S, Bouley DM, et al. MR imaging-guided percutaneous cryoablation of the prostate in an animal model: in vivo imaging of cryoablation-induced tissue necrosis with immediate histopathologic correlation. J Vasc Interv Radiol. 2009;20(2):252–8.
57. Yang WL, Addona T, Nair DG, Qi L, Ravikumar TS. Apoptosis induced by cryo-injury in human colorectal cancer cells is associated with mitochondrial dysfunction. Int J Cancer J Int Cancer. 2003;103(3):360–9.
58. Erinjeri JP, Clark TW. Cryoablation: mechanism of action and devices. J Vasc Interv Radiol. 2010;21(8 Suppl):S187–91.
59. Kickhefel A, Weiss C, Roland J, Gross P, Schick F, Salomir R. Correction of susceptibility-induced GRE phase shift for accurate PRFS thermometry proximal to cryoablation iceball. MAGMA. 2012;25(1):23–31.

Transperineal Template-guided Mapping Biopsy of the Prostate

Arjun Sivaraman and Rafael Sanchez-Salas

10.1 Definition

The Ginsburg study group defines transperineal template-guided mapping biopsy (TTMB) of the prostate as "exhaustive transperineal transrectal ultrasound (TRUS)-guided biopsies of the prostate performed with the patient in the lithotomy position using a 5-mm brachytherapy grid, with at least one biopsy from each hole" and transperineal template-guided saturation biopsy (TTSB) as "more than 20 transperineal TRUS-guided biopsies of the prostate performed with the intention of comprehensively sampling the prostate, according to a predefined core distribution pattern" [1]. Since different techniques are being adopted at various centers, these standard definitions will aid in uniform reporting and avoiding miscommunication and confusions.

10.2 Background

In developed countries, prostate cancer (PCa) is the most common solid organ tumor and third most common cause of cancer-related mortality [2]. Although prostate specific antigen (PSA) screening and testing has shown a reduction in PCa mortality, it detects both indolent and aggressive tumors [3]. Contemporary TRUS-guided biopsy (TRUS-B) used for the diagnosis of PCa has been shown to miss 25–30 % of cancers [4–7]. On the other hand, long-term follow-up studies on PCa have shown that the number of patients needed to be screened and treated to avert

A. Sivaraman
Department of Urology, St. John's Medical College, Bangalore, India

R. Sanchez-Salas (⊠)
Department of Urology, Institut Montsouris, Paris, France
e-mail: rafael.sanchez-salas@imm.fr

© Springer-Verlag France 2015
E. Barret, M. Durand (eds.), *Technical Aspects of Focal Therapy in Localized Prostate Cancer*, DOI 10.1007/978-2-8178-0484-2_10

one PCa-related death is as high as 1,055 and 37 patients respectively [3]. Hence we face the dual challenge of false negative biopsies, and among the patients with cancer, possible overdiagnosis and overtreatment.

Extended and saturation biopsies can reduce the false negative rate, and the incorporation of image-guided biopsies can possibly reduce overdiagnosis [8]. But reduction of overtreatment requires active surveillance protocols/focal therapy to treat low-risk prostate cancers. To safely assign patients to active surveillance (AS)/focal therapy, we need a reliable biopsy technique that can precisely characterize the lesion in terms of grade, volume, location and organ-confined stage. Clinical studies have shown that although saturation biopsy increases the diagnostic yield, its accuracy in characterizing the lesion is similar to standard 10-, 12-core biopsies [9].

Transperineal biopsy (TPB) techniques are safe and efficacious alternatives to transrectal biopsies. Different techniques of TBP have been reported in the literature, varying in number and distribution of cores, showing results better than TRUS-B. Barzell et al. introduced the transperineal template-guided saturation biopsy (TTSB) scheme, using a brachytherapy grid and dividing the prostate into 24 zones [10]. Later, Crawford et al. proposed a unique technique of TBP, a 3-dimensional (D) transperineal template-guided mapping biopsy (TTMB) of the prostate, using computer simulations on autopsy and radical prostatectomy (RP) specimens [11]. In this technique, multiple transperineal biopsies were performed, spaced at 5 mm intervals throughout the volume of the prostate; a high degree of accuracy and sensitivity for detecting cancer were demonstrated. Onik et al. reported their 4-year experience of this volume-based technique in clinical practice and showed superior sensitivity and staging information as compared to TRUS-B [12]. In the review, we focus on the present technique, indications, and outcomes of TTMB. Future studies will provide better evidence on optimal techniques, their positions in the algorithm of PCa diagnoses and follow-up, and their use in image fusion studies.

10.3 Rationale

TRUS-guided 10- or 12-core biopsy is the standard diagnostic modality for men with suspected prostate cancer. Saturation biopsy is used in the setting of negative initial sextant biopsy and a high index of suspicion of cancer. These procedures are performed at outpatient clinics with local anesthesia with prophylactic antibiotics. The procedure is generally well tolerated by the patients with decreasing toleration noted in younger patients and on repeat biopsies. The major limitations of TRUS-B include infection, false negativity and inability to precisely characterize the cancer. These limitations may be inherent to the transrectal approach of prostate biopsy and may not be reduced by increasing the number or changing the distribution of cores taken during the biopsy.

Urosepsis is a notable complication of TRUS-B, with 1.3 % of patients requiring hospitalization [13]. Adoption of saturation techniques correlates to more cores and higher bacterial translocation. Increasing reports of quinolone- resistant intestinal flora and inadequate prostatic tissue penetration by antibiotics are issues of concern in the prophylaxis and treatment of these patients [14]. Logically, the infection rates of TPB should be less than TRUS-B, as the needle passes through the cleaned perineal skin rather than the bowel or feces. However, Shen et al., in their systematic review, reported a similar incidence of infection in TRUS-B and TPB [15].

The cancer detection rate of 10-, 12-core TRUS-B from contemporary series is 20–35 % and it increases to 30–40 % with saturation biopsies [15]. The TTSB and TTMB performed after initial negative TRUS-B that detects cancer is 35–68 % [16] and 68.8 % [17] of patients respectively. Bittner et al. reported a high cancer detection rate of 73.3 % when TTMB was used as the initial biopsy to establish the diagnosis [18]. The possible rationale for the superior results of TPB are that TRUS-B has an inherent physical and technical limitation to the biopsy transition zone and anterior regions of the prostate, whereas TBP can sample these regions in a way similar to those of other regions; the needle in TPB is parallel to the prostate rather than perpendicular – as in TRUS-B – and therefore more tissue is sampled in every core; TRUS-B is more prone to inaccuracies in mapping and sampling when using unstabilized manual positioning of the guide needle and relying on the 3-D visual recall for guidance; and finally, exhaustive biopsy protocols, such as TTMB, which involve multiple biopsies, if performed transrectally, will cause extensive rectal injury and bleeding.

The accuracy of TRUS-B in characterizing the lesion is disappointing. Past studies with large series of patients have shown that Gleason upgrading from TRUS-B to RP specimens is 29 % and it improved to 20 % when 10-core biopsy was performed [19, 20]. Onik et al. reported a Gleason upgrade of 23 % from TRUS-B to TTMB, which is similar to the upgrading noted in RP specimens [12]. Bittner et al. used TTMB to map the approximate location of cancer within the prostate and proposed that theoretically, a 12-core TRUS-B scheme would have missed 23.7 % of these cancers and 18 % of the cancers would have been wrongly reported as low Gleason [18]. Crawford et al. studied the clinical-pathological correlation of TTMB with 3-D reconstruction of RP specimens and demonstrated that 72 % of the TTMB cores were identical in grade to RP specimens, with 80 % accuracy in predicting laterality [11]. These data indicate that TTMB is more accurate in predicting the tumor characteristics than TRUS-B. This accuracy is very important in the present, when much emphasis is on AS/focal therapy to avoid overtreatment. More prospective studies comparing TTMB with RP specimens will further validate the accuracy of TTMB.

Another advantage of TTMB is in post-radiotherapy biopsy, where the incidence of rectal complications are high, with TRUS-B and in patients at high risk of infection (such as diabetes mellitus, an immunocompromised state, recent overseas travel and prior antibiotic use) [16]. The downside of TTMB, as compared to TRUS-B, is the need for general anesthesia, the large number of cores to be examined, and the possible increased complication associated with a higher number of cores.

10.4 Indication

TTMB is an elaborate procedure with superior results compared to the other diagnostic techniques. The current indications for performing TTMB are:

Prior negative TRUS-B: Patients with a previous transrectal negative biopsy and with risk factors such as rising total PSA, falling free PSA, strong family history, and previous prostate biopsy showing cellular atypia or high grade risk of harboring cancer. The cancer detection rate of TTSB and TTMB after initial negative TRUS-B is shown in Table 10.1 is much better than the detection rate of saturation with TRUS-B. One of the concerns in this group of patients is that cancer in the antero-apical region of the prostate is being missed by transrectal biopsy. The combination of an aggressive and anterior tumor – known as prostatic evasive anterior tumor syndrome (PEATS) – manifests as a rising PSA in the setting of a prior negative TRUS-B [40]. Greshman et al. have reported that 94.1 % of the cancers detected by TTSB after a prior negative TRUS-B are in the apical and anterior regions of the prostate [24].

Active Surveillance (AS): Prostate cancer is a multifocal disease. Patients with minimal low-grade cancers as met by Epstein criteria can be managed with AS. We need a reliable biopsy technique that can accurately exclude high- grade cancer in other regions of the prostate. The present evidence has shown that when patients with prostate cancer on AS based on TRUS-B findings underwent TTSB/TTMB, upstaging (Gleason/volume upgrade) was noted in up to 30 % of the patients (Table 10.1). At our institute, we noticed that TMMB upstaged 30.6 % of patients with TRUS-B diagnosed low-risk prostate cancer. TTMB is the best available biopsy technique to precisely characterize the cancer within the prostate.

Focal therapy: Pathological studies of RP specimens have revealed that 20–25 % of patients had single-index cancer only, and 40–60 % had single-index cancer with an additional small (less than 0.5 ml) clinically insignificant cancer [41, 42]. Based on this data, focal therapy can be tried for low-grade single-index tumors to avoid the overtreatment of RP. The success of focal therapy depends on proper patient selection in whom the clinically significant cancer is confined to a single location. Standard/sextant TRUS-B or MRI with or without spectroscopy failed to adequately stage the patients for focal therapy [43, 44]. TTMB has shown superior staging information for focal therapy, as demonstrated by Onik et al. and Barzell et al. [12, 38, 39]. Further research on the balance of cost, complications and the diagnostic yield will define the future indications of TTMB in the primary biopsy setting and image fusion studies.

Table 10.1 Outcomes and complications of transperineal template-guided biopsy of prostate in the initial and repeat biopsy setting

Study	No. of patients	Design	Mean age	Mean PSA	Indication	Mean no. of cores	Technique of TPB	Cancer detection rate	Gleason upgrade	Additional points
Klatte et al. (2013) [21]	50	Prospective	57.5	7.3	Prior negative TRUS-B	24	Template-guided saturation	48 %	–	Insignificant cancer – 25 %
Vyas et al. (2013) [22]	634	Retrospective	63	7.66	Prior negative TRUS-B – 174	31	Template-guided saturation	Prior negative TRUS-B – 36 %	29 %	17 % had cancer in anterior sectors
					Primary – 153			Primary – 54 %		
					Active surveillance – 307					
Symons et al. (2013) [23]	409	Prospective	63	9.69	Primary – 273	19	Template-guided saturation	Primary – 64.4 %	–	Significantly higher detection rates were found in prostates <50 mL
					Repeat – 136			Repeat – 35.6 %		
Greshman et al. (2013) [24]	34	Retrospective	66.2	23.6	Prior negative TRUS-B	24.8	Template-guided saturation	50 %	–	94.1 % had cancer in either apical or anterior zone
Ekwueme et al. (2013) [25]	270	Prospective	64	10	Prior negative TRUS-B	28	Template-guided saturation	55 %	–	21 % had cancer in anterior sectors
Crawford et al. (2013) [26]	25	Retrospective	56	5	Correlation of TTMB and RP specimen	49	Template-guided mapping	–	–	TTMB accurately detected gleason in 72 % cores and over all laterality 80 %

(continued)

Table 10.1 (continued)

Study	No. of patients	Design	Mean age	Mean PSA	Indication	Mean no. of cores	Technique of TPB	Cancer detection rate	Gleason upgrade	Additional points
Bittner et al. (2013) [27]	485	Retrospective	64.8	8.7	Prior negative TRUS-B	59	Template-guided saturation	46.60 %	–	Most common cancer location is apex Insignificant cancer – 13.3 %
Losa et al. (2013) [28]	87	Prospective	63.9	6.9	Focal therapy	42.3	Template-guided saturation	–	29.60 %	
Bittner et al. (2013) [18]	191	Prospective	64.6	5.2	Primary	54	Template-guided saturation	73.30 %	–	11.4 % insignificant cancer
OUR EXPERIENCE (2013)	98	Retrospective	63	6.3	Active surveillance	24	Template-guided mapping	–	16.30 %	9.1 % had bilateral disease, 5 % had both gleason and volume upgrade
Huo et al. (2012) [29]	414	Retrospective	60.9	7.7	–	23.5	Template-guided saturation	–	25.60 %	Sensitivity – 48 % and specificity – 84.1 % for TTSB in this accuracy study
Mabjeesh et al. (2012) [30]	92	Prospective	63.8	14.1	Prior negative TRUS-B	33.3	Template-guided saturation	26 %	–	83.3 % cancers in the anterior zones
HU et al. (2012) [31]	107	Computer simulation of RP specimen	61	8.5	–	55	Template-guided mapping	–	–	TTMB had accuracy of 0.9

Dimmen et al. (2012) [32]	69	Prospective	64.5	25.2	Prior negative TRUS-B	18.4	Template-guided saturation	55 %	–	Final RP specimen showed majority anterior tumors
Pal et al. (2012) [33]	40	Prospective	63	21.9	Prior negative TRUS-B	36	Template-guided saturation	68 %	–	
Ayres et al. (2012) [34]	101	Prospective	68	5.4	Active surveillance	47	Template-guided saturation	–	34 %	The upgrade includes both gleason and volume upgrade
Lecornet et al. (2012) [35]	96	Computer simulation of RP specimen		2.1	–		Template-guided mapping	100 % (for lesions > 0.5 ml)	–	7 % of lesions 0.2–0.5 ml were missed by TTMB
Barqawi et al. (2011) [17]	215	Prospective	60.5	4.8	Active surveillance – 180; Prior negative TRUS – 35	56	Template-guided mapping	68.80 %	27.20 %	Upstaging noted in 45.6 % patients
Abdollah et al. (2011) [36]	140	Prospective	66.4	10	Prior negative TrUS	24	Template-guided saturation	25.70 %	–	
Taira et al. (2010) [37]	373	Prospective	63.8	8.3	Primary – 79; Prior negative TRUS-B – 294	54	Template-guided saturation	Primary – 75.9 %; Prior negative TRUS-B – 43.7 %	–	

(continued)

Table 10.1 (continued)

Study	No. of patients	Design	Mean age	Mean PSA	Indication	Mean no. of cores	Technique of TPB	Cancer detection rate	Gleason upgrade	Additional points
Onik et al. (2009) [38]	180	Prospective			Active surveillance	50	Template-guided mapping	–	22.70 %	Upstaging noted in 61.1 % patients
Barzel et al. (2007) [39]	80	Prospective	68.2	16.5	Focal therapy/ active surveillance	66.3	Template-guided saturation	–	16 %	TTSB detected cancer in 47 % patients with negative repeat TRUS-B
Onik et al. (2008) [12]	110	Retrospective	–	7.4	Focal therapy	50.2	Template-guided mapping	–	23 %	Bilateral disease found in 55 % patients who had unilateral disease in TRUS-B
Crawford et al. (2005) [11]	106	Computer simulation of autopsy and RP specimen	63.1		Autopsy – 86, RP specimen – 20	–	Template-guided mapping	Autopsy – 86 %, RP specimen – 100 %	–	

10.5 Technique

Several techniques of TTMB have been described; they vary in the number and distribution of cores. All patients are ensured of sterile urine prior to the procedure. The routine use of Tamsulosin in the periprocedure period can prevent acute urinary retention [45], and prophylactic antibiotics are used to prevent infection. Logically, antibiotics should be aimed at both bowel and skin pathogens. Biopsies are performed by a single operator in the dorsal lithotomy position under general anesthesia (Figs. 10.1 and 10.2). A Foley catheter might be placed to identify the location of the urethra and also to assess hematuria. A standard brachytherapy grid with holes 5 mm apart as demonstrated by Barzell is used as a template [10]. The rationale of using a 5 mm grid is that any cancer less than 5 mm may not be clinically significant. To accurately mark the location of each core, grid coordinates A-M are placed in the x axis and 1–12 in the y axis, and the coordinate D2 is positioned at the

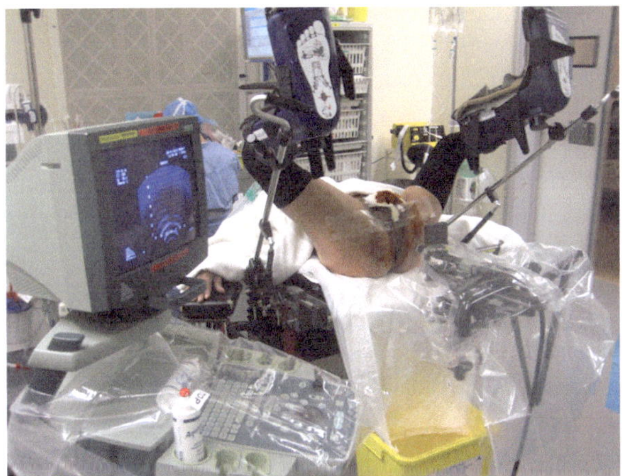

Fig. 10.1 Patient positioning for prostatic TTMB

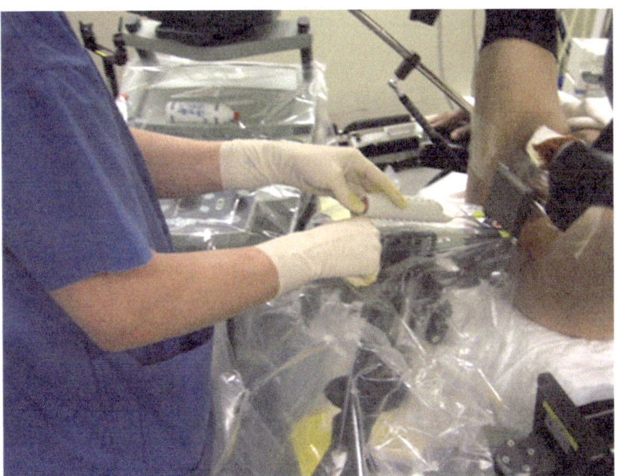

Fig. 10.2 TTMB procedure

Fig. 10.3 Grid with urethra in the midline

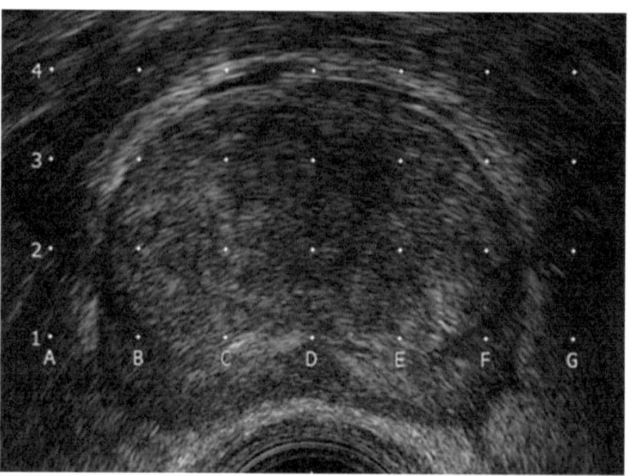

midline corresponding to the urethra (Fig. 10.3). All the biopsy cores are named according to the coordinates and if more than one core is taken from a single hole, an additional tag as a proximal (apex) or distal (base) is used (Fig. 10.3a, b). The grid is attached to a cradle and firmly positioned against the perineum. A standard transrectal probe with 5–7.5 MHz transducer is introduced, the prostate is scanned from base to apex, and the volume is calculated by prostate ellipsoid formula (height × length × width × pi/6). Biopsies are performed with an 18G automated biopsy gun. The position of the biopsy gun during the biopsy is tracked through the TRUS probe and the whole length of the prostate is biopsied. Care should be taken to avoid injury to the urethra and the bladder neck region. Biopsies in the midline are taken only posterior to the urethra to avoid injury. All the biopsy containers are appropriately tagged and each core should be reported for core length, presence of cancer, Gleason grade, cancer length and ratio of cancer to core length. Patients are discharged from the hospital on the same day unless there are complications.

10.6   Total Number of Cores

Barzell et al. originally proposed the biopsy technique for TTMP in which the prostate is divided into the proximal and distal halves. Each half is again divided into four parts: anterior/posterior and right/left. In addition, each octant is divided into three zones: medial, intermediate and lateral, resulting in 24 zones and 1 – 3 biopsies are taken from each zone [10]. Later, Onik et al. in their PCa mapping study, followed a different technique in which at least one biopsy was taken in each aperture of the template throughout the volume of the prostate and hence the number of biopsies is directly proportional to the volume of the gland [12]. Recently, the Ginsburg study has standardized the definition that TTMB should have at least one biopsy through each hole of the 5 mm brachytherapy grip throughout the volume of the prostate [1]. This model will be ideal to map the morphometric location of the cancer within the prostate. At our institute, we aim for a volume-adjusted saturation biopsy, meaning that a higher number of cores are taken for prostates with more volume.

10.7 Complications

The complications of TTMB are not studied as extensively as those of TRUS-B. From the available literature, the overall incidence of complications in TTMB is comparable to TRUS-B with a similar incidence of urosepsis [46]. Acute urinary retention is the primary complication following TTMB. Merrick et al. showed in their series that 39.4, 7.1 and 1.6 % patients were catheter-dependent following TTMB on days 0, 3 and 6. All the patients were catheter-free after the 12th day and the median catheter dependency for the entire group was 1 day [46]. The incidence of acute urinary retention is substantially higher than TRUS-B and it is strongly related to the size of the gland. The exact mechanism of this voiding difficulty is not clear. Bozlu et al. have shown that the routine use of Tamsulosin in the periprocedure period decreases the incidence of AUR. Contrary to the presumption, the incidence of urinary tract infection is similar in TPB and TRUS-B [15, 46]. Other reported complications include hematuria, hematospermia, mild transient erectile dysfunction, perineal discomfort, and transient worsening of urinary symptoms [28, 46, 47]. Most of the symptoms after TTMB appear to be secondary to prostatic edema and usually resolve within 30 days. Although rare, there is a small chance of malignant seeding of the biopsy tract and it carries a poor prognosis [48].

10.8 State of the Art: Outcomes

The technique of TTMB is evolving to improve the outcomes of its diagnostic accuracy. Barzell et al. assessed 80 patients who were due to undergo focal cryoablation, with both TTMB and TRUS-B. In their study, 47 % of patients found suitable for focal therapy by TRUS-B actually had high-risk cancer in TTMB [39]. However, the technique used in this study is different from the present definition for mapping biopsies, and according to the Ginsburg study group, Barzell's technique may be termed "transperineal template-guided saturation biopsy." Onik et al. used the Crawford model of TTMB to perform mapping biopsies in 110 patients with TRUS-B proven unilateral disease. He demonstrated that TTMB found bilateral disease in 55 % and Gleason upgrading in 25 % of these patients [12]. Intraprostatic mapping of cancer by TTMB was tested by Crawford, using 3-D reconstruction of RP specimens. The laterality was accurate in 80 % of the specimens, with 72 % of the cores precisely diagnosing the Gleason score [26]. At our institute, we performed volume-based TTMB in 98 patients with low-risk prostate cancer diagnosed by TRUS-B, and we found that 30.6 % of the patients were upstaged (9.2 % had bilateral disease, 16.3 % had Gleason upgrade and 5.1 % had both). According to present evidence, the cancer detection rate of TTSB/TTMB after initial negative TRUS-B is 46–68 % (Table 10.1). The diagnostic performance of TTMB in the initial biopsy setting is 73–76 %, which is superior to all the diagnostic modalities used for PCa until now [18, 37]. These data reflect the superior results of TTMB in the detecting, grading and mapping of PCa as compared to TRUS-B.

10.9 The Future

The results of TTMB are very encouraging and it has the potential to become an essential tool in the management of PCa. Future studies will broaden the indications of this excellent technique and define the limitations. Considering the exceptional cancer detection rate of TTMB, its use in the primary biopsy setting needs to be debated. However, the cost – benefit ratio of the procedure in this setting – will determine the utility. Recent advances in image-guided – histoscanning/multiparametric magnetic resonance imaging (MRI) – biopsies have enhanced the TRUS-B cancer detection. The fusion of this image guidance with TTMB will be an interesting advance in prostate cancer diagnosis and can potentially overcome most of the shortcomings of present biopsy techniques.

References

1. Kuru T, Wadhwa K, Chang RTM, et al. Definitions of terms, processes and a minimum dataset for transperineal prostate biopsies: a standardization approach of the Ginsburg Study Group for Enhanced Prostate Diagnostics. BJU Int. 2013;112:568–77.
2. Jemal A, Bray F, Center MM, Ferlay J, Ward E, Forman D. Global cancer statistics. CA Cancer J Clin. 2011;61:69–90.
3. Schröder FH, Hugosson J, Roobol MJ, et al. Prostate-cancer mortality at 11 years of follow-up. N Engl J Med. 2012;15:981–90.
4. Eskew LA, Bare RL, McCullough DL. Systematic 5 region prostate biopsy is superior to sextant method for diagnosing carcinoma of the prostate. J Urol. 1997;157:199–202; discussion 202–3.
5. Presti JC, Chang JJ, Bhargava V, Shinohara K. The optimal systematic prostate biopsy scheme should include 8 rather than 6 biopsies: results of a prospective clinical trial. J Urol. 2000;163:163–6; discussion 166–7.
6. Rabbani F, Stroumbakis N, Kava BR, Cookson MS, Fair WR. Incidence and clinical significance of false-negative sextant prostate biopsies. J Urol. 1998;159:1247–50.
7. Babaian RJ, Toi A, Kamoi K, et al. A comparative analysis of sextant and an extended 11-core multisite directed biopsy strategy. J Urol. 2000;163:152–7.
8. Moore CM, Robertson NL, Arsanious N, et al. Image-guided prostate biopsy using magnetic resonance imaging-derived targets: a systematic review. Eur Urol. 2013;63:125–40.
9. Abouassaly R, Lane B, Jones J. Staging saturation biopsy in patients with prostate cancer on active surveillance protocol. Urology. 2008;71:573–7.
10. Barzell WE, Whitmore WF. Transperineal template guided saturation biopsy of the prostate: Rationale, indications, and technique. Urology Times. 2003;31(5):41–2.
11. Crawford ED, Wilson SS, Torkko KC, et al. Clinical staging of prostate cancer: a computer-simulated study of transperineal prostate biopsy. BJU Int. 2005;96(7):999–1004.

12. Onik G, Barzell W. Transperineal 3D mapping biopsy of the prostate: an essential tool in selecting patients for focal prostate cancer therapy. Urol Oncol. 2008;26:506–10.
13. Rosario DJ, Lane JA, Metcalfe C, et al. Short term outcomes of prostate biopsy in men tested for cancer by prostate specific antigen: prospective evaluation within ProtecT study. BMJ. 2012;344:d7894. doi:10.1136/bmj.d7894.
14. Loeb S, van der Heuvel S, Zhu X, Bangma CH, Schroder FH, Roobol MJ. Infectious complications and hospital admissions after prostate biopsy in a European randomized trial. Eur Urol. 2012;61:1110–4.
15. Shen PF, et al. The results of transperineal versus transrectal prostate biopsy: a systematic review and meta-analysis. Asian J Androl. 2012;14:310–5.
16. Chang DT, Challacombe B, Lawrentschuk N. Transperineal biopsy of the prostate-is this the future? Nat Rev Urol. 2013. doi:10.1038/nrurol.2013.195.
17. Barqawi AB, et al. The role of 3-dimensional mapping biopsy in decision making for treatment of apparent early stage prostate cancer. J Urol. 2011;186:80–5.
18. Bittner N, Merrick GS, Abbey Bennett BS, Wayne M, Butler, Hugo J, Andreini W, Taubenslag EA. Diagnostic performance of initial transperineal template guided mapping biopsy of the prostate gland. Am J Clin Oncol. 2013. doi:10.1097/coc.0b013e31829a2954.
19. Pinkstaff DM, Igel TC, Petrou SP, et al. Systematic transperineal ultrasound guided template biopsy of the prostate: three year experience. Urology. 2005;65(4):735–9.
20. Chuu FK, Steuber T, Erbersdobler A, et al. Development and internal validation of a nomogram predicting the probability of prostate cancer Gleason sum upgrading between biopsy and radical prostatectomy pathology. Eur Urol. 2006;49(5):820–6.
21. Klatte T, Swietek N, Schatzl G, Waldert M. Transperineal template-guided biopsy for diagnosis of prostate cancer in patients with at least two prior negative biopsies. Wien Klin Wochenschr. 2013;125(21–22):669–73.
22. Vyas L, et al. Indications, results and safety profile of transperineal sector biopsies of the prostate: a single centre experience of 634 cases. BJU Int. 2014;114:32–7. http://dx.doi.org/10.1111/bju.12282.
23. Symons JL, Huo A, Yuen CL, Haynes AM, Matthews J, Sutherland RL, Brenner P, Stricker PD. Outcomes of transperineal template-guided prostate biopsy in 409 patients. BJU Int. 2013;112(5):585–93. doi:10.1111/j.1464-410X.2012.11657.x.
24. Gershman B, Zietman AL, Feldman AS, McDougal WS. Transperineal template-guided prostate biopsy for patients with persistently elevated PSA and multiple prior negative biopsies. Urol Oncol. 2013;31(7):1093–7. doi:10.1016/j.urolonc.2012.01.001.
25. Ekwueme K, Simpson H, Zakhour H, Parr NJ. Transperineal template-guided saturation biopsy using a modified technique: outcome of 270 cases requiring repeat prostate biopsy. BJU Int. 2013;111(8):E365–73. doi:10.1111/bju.12134.
26. Crawford ED, Rove KO, Barqawi AB, Maroni PD, Werahera PN, Baer CA, Koul HK, Rove CA, Lucia MS, La Rosa FG. Clinical-pathologic correlation between transperineal mapping biopsies of the prostate and three-dimensional reconstruction of prostatectomy specimens. Prostate. 2013;73(7):778–87.
27. Bittner N, Merrick GS, Butler WM, Bennett A, Galbreath RW. Incidence and pathological features of prostate cancer detected on transperineal template guided mapping biopsy after negative transrectal ultrasound guided biopsy. J Urol. 2013;190(2):509–14. doi:10.1016/j.juro.2013.02.021.
28. Losa A, et al. Complications and quality of life after template-assisted transperineal prostate biopsy in patients eligible for focal therapy. Urology. 2013;81:1291–6.
29. Huo AS, Hossack T, Symons JL, PeBenito R, Delprado WJ, Brenner P, Stricker PD. Accuracy of primary systematic template guided transperineal biopsy of the prostate for locating prostate cancer: a comparison with radical prostatectomy specimens. J Urol. 2012;187(6):2044–9. doi:10.1016/j.juro.2012.01.066.
30. Mabjeesh NJ, Lidawi G, Chen J, German L, Matzkin H. High detection rate of significant prostate tumours in anterior zones using transperineal ultrasound-guided template saturation biopsy. BJU Int. 2012;110:993–7.

31. Hu Y, et al. A biopsy simulation study to assess the accuracy of several transrectal ultrasonography (TRUS)-biopsy strategies compared with template prostate mapping biopsies in patients who have undergone radical prostatectomy. BJU Int. 2012;110:812–20.
32. Dimmen M, et al. Transperineal prostate biopsy detects significant cancer in patients with elevated prostate-specific antigen (PSA) levels and previous negative transrectal biopsies. BJU Int. 2012;110:E69–75.
33. Pal RP, Elmussareh M, Chanawani M, Khan MA. The role of a standardized 36 core template-assisted transperineal prostate biopsy technique in patients with previously negative transrectal ultrasonography-guided prostate biopsies. BJU Int. 2012;109:367–71.
34. Ayres BE, et al. The role of transperineal template prostate biopsies in restaging men with prostate cancer managed by active surveillance. BJU Int. 2012;109:1170–6.
35. Lecornet E, Ahmed HU, Hu Y, Moore CM, Nevoux P, Barratt D, Hawkes D, Villers A, Emberton M. The accuracy of different biopsy strategies for the detection of clinically important prostate cancer: a computer simulation. J Urol. 2012;188(3):974–80. doi:10.1016/j.juro.2012.04.104.
36. Abdollah F, et al. Trans-rectal versus trans-perineal saturation rebiopsy of the prostate: is there a difference in cancer detection rate? Urology. 2011;77:921–5.
37. Taira AV, et al. Transperineal template-guided mapping biopsy as a staging procedure to select patients best suited for active surveillance. Am J Clin Oncol. 2013;36:116–20.
38. Onik G, Miessau M, Bostwick DG. Three-dimensional prostate mapping biopsy has a potentially significant impact on prostate cancer management. J Clin Oncol. 2009;27:4321–6.
39. Barzell WE, Melamed MR. Appropriate patient selection in the focal treatment of prostate cancer: the role of transperineal 3-dimensional pathologic mapping of the prostate—a 4-year experience. Urology. 2007;70 Suppl 6:27–35.
40. Lawrentschuk N, et al. 'Prostatic evasive anterior tumours': the role of magnetic resonance imaging. BJU Int. 2010;105:1231–6.
41. Rukstalis DB, Goldknopf JL, Crowley EM, et al. Prostate cryoablation: a scientific rationale for future modifications. Urology. 2002;60(2A):19–25.
42. Noguchi M, Stamey TA, McNeal JE, et al. Prognostic factors for multifocal prostate cancer in radical prostatectomy specimens: lack of significance of secondary cancers. J Urol. 2003;170(2 Pt 1):459–63.
43. Dhingsa R, Qayyum A, Coakley FV, et al. MR imaging and MR spectroscopic imaging: effect of clinical data on reader accuracy. Radiology. 2004;230(1):215–22.
44. Sved PD, Gomez P, Manoharan M. Limitations of biopsy Gleason grade: implications for counseling patients with biopsy Gleason score 6 prostate cancer. J Urol. 2004;172(1):98–102.
45. Bozlu M, Ulusoy E, Doruk E, Cayan S, Canpolat B, Schellhammer PF, Akbay E. Voiding impairment after prostate biopsy: does tamsulosin treatment before biopsy decrease this morbidity? Urology. 2003;62(6):1050–3.
46. Merrick GS, et al. The morbidity of transperineal template-guided prostate mapping biopsy. BJU Int. 2008;101:1524–9.
47. Tsivian M, Abern MR, Qi P, Polascik TJ. Short-term functional outcomes and complications associated with transperineal template prostate mapping biopsy. Urology. 2013;82:166–70.
48. Moul JW, et al. Risk factors for perineal seeding of prostate cancer after needle biopsy. J Urol. 1989;142:86–8.

Focal Cryotherapy

Matthieu Durand, Zeinab Mahate, and Victoria Wijeratne

Abbreviations

ASTRO	American Society for Therapeutic Radiology and Oncology
BPH	Benign prostate hyperplasia
DRE	Digital rectal examination
EBRT	External beam radiation therapy
ED	Erectile dysfunction
HIFU	High-intensity focused ultrasonography
IQR	Interquartile range
PCa	Prostate cancer
TRUS	Transrectal ultrasound
US	Ultrasound
VTP	Vascular-targeted photodynamic therapy

With acknowledgments to Romain Haider, Damien Ambrosetti, Lisa Camus (photography credits)
Romain Haider, MD, Department of Urology, Hôpital Pasteur 2 – Centre Hospitalier Universitaire de Nice, University of Nice-Sophia-Anitpolis, 3à voie Romaine, 06000, Nice, France
Damien Ambrosetti, MD, PhD, Department of Pathology, Hôpital Pasteur 2 – Centre Hospitalier Universitaire de Nice, University of Nice-Sophia Antipolis, France

M. Durand, MD (✉)
Department of Urology, Hôpital Pasteur 2 – Centre Hospitalier Universitaire de Nice,
University of Nice-Sophia-Antipolis, 30 voie Romaine,
06000, Nice, France
e-mail: durand.m@chu-nice.fr

Z. Mahate • V. Wijeratne
Department of Urology, Hôpital Pasteur 2 – Centre Hospitalier Universitaire
de Nice, University of Nice-Sophia-Antipolis, 30 voie Romaine,
06000, Nice , France

MbChb Medicine with European Studies, University of Manchester, Manchester, UK

© Springer-Verlag France 2015
E. Barret, M. Durand (eds.), *Technical Aspects of Focal Therapy in Localized Prostate Cancer*, DOI 10.1007/978-2-8178-0484-2_11

11.1 Introduction

Cryotherapy has been used for years. The prospect of its use in focal therapy has spurred renewed interest in it, which in its recent evolutions enhance both the accuracy and reliability that are especially needed for focal ablation while preserving adjacent tissue. Improvements in thermoimaging monitoring and new percutaneous cryoprobes have resulted in lowering technical limitations and make cryotherapy fit for both primary localized prostate cancer treatment with intention to treat and salvage therapy for locally recurrent prostate cancer following radiation therapy.

11.2 The History of Cryotherapy: The Renaissance

Before being applied to the prostate, cryotherapy was used for various other medical reasons, such as lung and cervical cancer treatment. The initial methods of cryotherapy involved using a combination of ice and salt to reduce the size of tumors; however, various improvements in the materials available have led to further developments in cryotherapy techniques. The history of cryotherapy can be best categorized into four different generations.

In the first generation of cryotherapy, Cooper and Lee [1] made the first catheter (1961) with still liquid nitrogen inside and it was used to treat neuromuscular disease. This catheter was first used in urology by Gonder et al. (1964) [30] as a transurethral treatment for prostate cancer or benign prostate hyperplasia. In 1972, Flocks et al. proposed a transperitoneal incision to open up Denonvillier's space, allowing direct contact with the posterior face of the prostate; however, this technique also caused a high mortality rate. That same year, Reuter recommended using rigid cystoscopy alongside digital rectal examination to improve procedural monitoring. Following this, Megalli et al. then described the first transperineal technique using cryotherapy needles, with a median line incision (1974). This procedure involved controlling the placement and temperature of needles with digital rectal examination and perirectal thermometers along with repositioning the needles throughout the procedure. However, during the 1980s, the above method was abandoned because of inadequate procedural surveillance, thus ending the first generation of cryotherapy and somehow slowing down the evolution of cryotherapy.

The second generation began in 1984 with the introduction of endorectal echography and urethral reheating to the cryotherapy procedure, which lowered the risk of complications. In the same year, Onik also demonstrated how to visualize frozen tissue using echography. In 1988 Onik further developed cryotherapy imaging by showing how to visualize the volume of prostatic tissue in real tissue. 1994 Saw the evolution of percutaneous transperineal cryotherapy with multiple needles by Chang et al., and from then until 1999, urethral reheating was continuously improved to reduce complications. This transperineal approach by means of cryoprobes associated with both the thermal monitoring and visual control mark a turning point for cryotherapy.

In the following third generation of cryotherapy, argon gas began to be used instead of liquid nitrogen. This idea involved using high-pressure argon gas to freeze the tissue and helium to reheat it via the Joule-Thompson effect (described later in detail). Smaller caliber needles were also developed, thereby eliminating the need for incisions, and template grids were introduced to optimize needle positioning, leading to the ability to perform real minimally invasive cryosurgery.

Finally, during the last decade (the fourth generation of cryotherapy), improved thermoimaging technology and better needles, coupled with real-time monitoring of the constants, continued to enhance and to ease the process, resulting in more safety, reliability, and less postoperative complications. Various needle lengths produced an improved quality of ablation while preserving adjacent tissue with regard to both the rectum and urethra. During this time, software was also developed for procedural control. Nowadays, various cryotherapy systems are designed to freeze and ablate prostate tissue by the application of extreme cold based on these similar and competing technologies.

11.3 Principles of Cryotherapy

11.3.1 The Physiology of Cryotherapy

The Cellular Physiology of Cryotherapy
The cellular damage caused by cryotherapy [2] is varied and includes direct damage through rupturing membranes and indirect vascular damage due to ischemia and coagulative necrosis leading to tissue destruction based on the freezing. The cellular physiology of cryotherapy by type is summarized in Table 11.1.

At $-7\ ^{\circ}$C, ice is formed in the extracellular compartment which, in turn, leads to an osmotic imbalance. This then causes water to be drawn out of the intracellular space and into the extracellular compartment, leading to intracellular dehydration. The main consequence of this is a disrupted intracellular pH that causes protein denaturation [3].

Table 11.1 Cellular physiology effects of the cryotherapy sorted out by physiological phenomenon

Mechanical	Extracellular ice crystals, followed by intracellular crystals, exert shearing forces on cell membranes
Necrotic and apoptotic	Necrosis, in the central zone ($-40\ ^{\circ}$C) circumscribed by a sublethal apoptotic peripheral tissue (cf. Fig 11.1)
Biochemical	pH modification, osmotic modification, concentration of toxins
Ischemic	Disseminated vascular thrombosis lead to ischemic necrosis
Immunological	Hypothesis of immune stimulation originating from the antigenic antitumoral response [3]

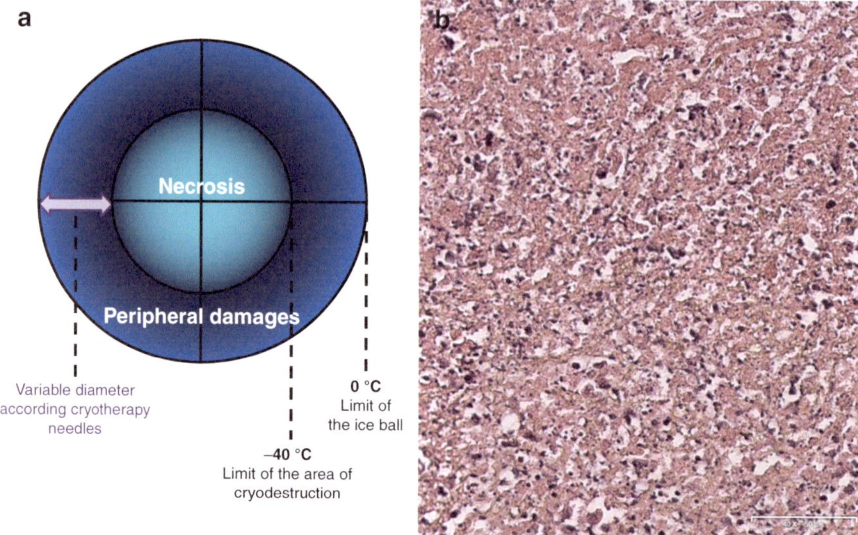

Fig. 11.1 Tissue damage of cryotherapy. (**a**) Schematic representation of necrosis coagulation in the central zone to −40 °C surrounded by a peripheral tissue damage induced by temperature between −40 and 0 °C, the width of which is directly dependent on the type and number of cryotherapy needles used. (**b**) Histological section of cryotherapy's effects on the tissue. Necrosis (*top left*) is circumscribed by a sublethal apoptotic peripheral zone tissue (hematoxylin and eosin staining, ×400)

Once a temperature of −15 °C has been reached, ice is formed inside the cell. The shearing forces exerted by the ice crystals both intracellularly and extracellularly induce the rupture of cell membranes.

Beyond these temperatures, blood clots form in the vessels of the tissue being targeted and this provokes a local reactional edema. Furthermore, a cascade of inflammatory agents is then activated which causes damage to the endothelium. These two factors combined lead to disseminated microthrombi formation and the cells become hypoxic and die. This phenomenon initiates ischemic necrosis.

The Tissular Effect

In tissue ablation, cryotherapy consists of freezing by means of percutaneous cryoprobes placed directly into the prostate tissue within the target zone, including the suspected index lesion. The cryolesion consists of both central necrosis and a peripheral edema reaction (Fig. 11.1). The lesion sizes vary, depending on the technical features of cryotherapy including the type and the number of needles (described in further detail in materials for cryotherapy procedures) the duration of the process, the number of freeze-thaw cycles, and the distance between the needles and their placement within the prostatic tissue target. Apoptosis has still been reported roughly 8 h following the cryoablation. It is important to note that the cryotherapy-induced lesion extends to the edge of the ice ball used during the process.

After therapy, the onset of cryolesion scarring starts from the peripheral ring, in contact with safe tissue, healing step by step to the central necrosis. Inflammatory cells are involved in wound healing by progressive infiltration leading to a tissue fibrosis reaction. If the transrectal route offers an excellent acoustic window to monitor the ice ball during the procedure to focally ablate the target, the cryotherapy-induced lesions are not visible by standard US after treatment. Magnetic resonance imaging (MRI) remains the gold standard technique for efficacy assessment. But because of this fibrosis reaction, neither diffusion-weighted nor T2-weighted imaging enables assessment of the cryolesion; only gadolinium-enhanced T1-weighted images can assess the extent of this devascularized tissue.

The Joule-Thompson Effect

The Joule-Thompson effect is a physiological principle that forms the basis of modern cryotherapy. According to this principle, various gases undergo unique temperature changes when depressurized, according to unique gas coefficients [4]. Argon gas, used in cryotherapy, has a constant enthalpy expansion that causes it to cool rapidly to its boiling point −185.7 °C – i.e., to gas.

For the purposes of cryotherapy, high-pressure (3,000 psi) ambient temperature argon is circulated to the probe tip, where it expands rapidly and its pressure then decreases to room pressure (15 psi). According to the Joule-Thompson effect, this decrease in the argon pressure also leads to a sharply decreased temperature of the gas, which can then be used to achieve the low temperatures desired for tissue freezing in cryotherapy, resulting in an ice ball at the tip of the needle.

When expanded, helium gas heats up rather than cools, and so expansion of helium gas at the needle tip provides an increased temperature that can be used to reheat the urethra. In general, this means that by altering the pressures of the different gases used, the various temperatures needed for active freezing and reheating in the cryotherapy process can be achieved (Fig. 11.2).

11.3.2 Factors Influencing Cryoablation

Many factors can affect the outcome of cryotherapy treatment. Their efficacy is directly linked to the speed and temperature of freezing and reheating [5]. At temperatures greater than −20 °C, cell death is not likely to be achieved, whereas −40 °C achieves systematic cell death. Therefore, the nadir temperature range is between −40 and −50 °C. A rapid freezing rate followed by a more progressive reheating period provides the best results to induce cell death.

Other factors influencing cryotherapy include the duration of the freezing portion of the cycle and the number of freeze-thaw cycles carried out [6]. The optimum duration of freezing is not clearly defined and may, in fact, be tissue-dependent, and the freeze-thaw cycle needs to be repeated in order to achieve the best results. The first cycle increases the thermal conductivity of the tissue due to cellular damage and the second cycle can then induce the same cellular stress but on a more conductive target tissue.

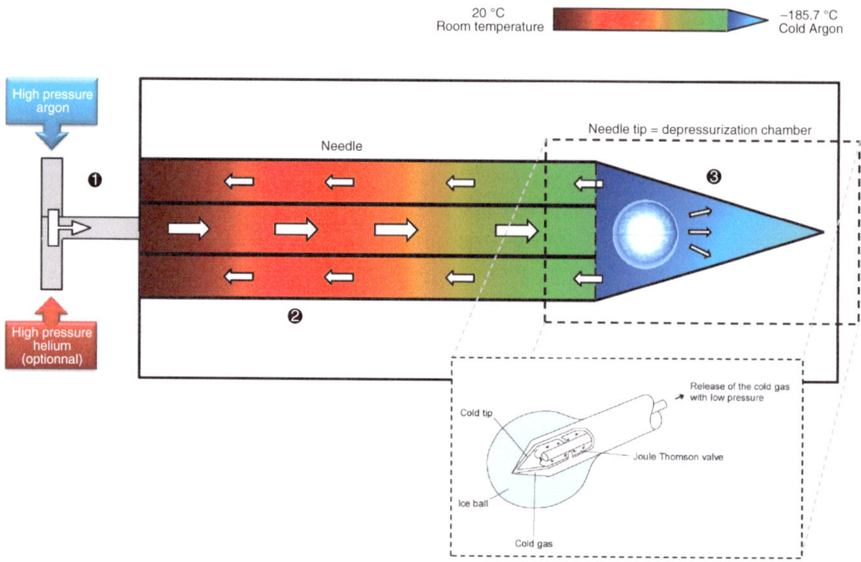

Fig. 11.2 The Joule-Thompson effect. • Gas inlet, previously packaged in high-pressure cylinders. • Gas flow in the tubing of the needle. • Sudden depressurization of gas – argon temperature drop – cryotherapy by diffusion in tissues

11.4 Specific Indications and Limitations

11.4.1 Indications for Focal Cryotherapy

The indications for focal cryotherapy depend on the context in which it is being used, i.e., whether as a primary therapy or a salvage therapy after external beam radiation therapy (EBRT) or brachytherapy.

Focal Primary Treatment for Unilateral Prostate Cancer with Curative Intent

Recent reports suggest that focal cryotherapy may be considered a management option for selected cases of clinically localized prostate cancer with a biochemical disease-free survival of 5 years, similar to whole-gland treatment modalities [7]. Many protocols have already been published to carefully select the patients in focal cryotherapy with comparable oncological and functional outcomes [8, 9].

For some, the selection criteria are similar to those of active surveillance, provided that the tumor is unilateral. In such cases, focal cryotherapy may be an attractive option for men who fit active surveillance criteria but do not want to consider this option or any type of invasive or radical treatment. This focal cryotherapy may also improve failure rates in men who initially pursue active surveillance protocols. For others, patient selection has been expanded to those of intermediate d'Amico risk of prostate cancer including maximum PSA value up to 15 ng/ml and higher, up to the Gleason score of 7 (3+4) [9]. At this point, based on short-term published outcomes, no difference has been reported between the two options regarding the two main selection criteria options.

Whatever the patient selection, patients are being treated with a curative intent that consists of a hemi-cryoablation of one prostatic lobe in which the index lesion of prostate cancer has been established after a combination of both, mostly with repeated biopsy and multiparametric MRI. Inclusion criteria include the clinical stages of T1c to T2a, PSA value <10 ng/ml or <15 ng/ml, low volume index lesion (i.e., less than 30 % of positive biopsies with the extent of prostate cancer less than 50 % of any positive core), Gleason score ≤6 (3+3) or ≤7 (3+4).

Prostate volume is not restricted with focal cryotherapy because needle placement and the number of needles are not also limited. The main selection criteria for primary treatment for unilateral prostate cancer with curative intent are shown in Table 11.2.

Focal Salvage Therapy for Locally Recurrent Prostate Cancer Following Organ-Sparing Treatment of Unilateral Prostate Cancer

The main goal is to locally control the prostate cancer by ablating the local-recurrent lesion with the highest possible oncological efficiency and the lowest possible risk of side effects. The indications for focal salvage cryotherapy are a unilateral recurrent disease of low-intermediate risk that has failed to respond to primary radiotherapy or brachytherapy. Local radio-recurrent prostate cancer has to be confirmed by a biopsy-proven unilateral recurrent prostate cancer and/or rising PSA level after therapy (ASTRO or Nadir +2 ng/ml according to the Phoenix criteria) with a corresponding local recurrence imaging as well as a negative metastatic extension [14].

For carefully selected patients, focal salvage therapy is an option that could be associated with lower treatment-related morbidity compared with total focal therapy without being life threatening and leading to mid-term oncological outcomes similar to other treatment options [15]; in most cases, recurrent prostate cancer is located at the same area within the lobe where it had been primarily treated. Focal salvage therapy has to consider the primary treatment using radiation leading to minimize the intensity of salvage cryotherapy and to limit the number of needles. Indeed, the shorter the time from primary radiation therapy to salvage cryotherapy, the higher the likelihood of successful curative-intent treatment.

11.4.2 Limitations of Focal Cryotherapy

The limitations for focal cryotherapy can be classified into two main groups: relative and absolute. The relative limitations include any previous history of transurethral prostate resection (TURP), as this increases the risk of sloughing and urinary retention. A significant urinary obstruction symptom before treatment would also be seen as a limitation, as would any pubic arch interference because this would affect needle placement.

The absolute limitations are an advanced local cancer of T3b and above, or a history of abdo-perineal resection for rectal pathology. A urinary fistula and any form of prostate distortion due to previous surgery or trauma are also included as absolute limitations.

Table 11.2 Inclusion criteria in primary focal cryotherapy protocols

	Onik et al. [10]	Ellis et al. [11]	Lambert et al. [12]	Bahn et al. [8]	Ward et al. [13]	Durand et al. [9]
Clinical study design	Retrospective	Retrospective	Retrospective	Prospective	Retrospective	Prospective
Adjuvant PCa treatment	NHT[a]	NR	None	None	None	None
Clinical stage	NR	T1 to T3, N0, M0	T1, N0, M0	T2	cT1, T2	T1, T2, N0, M0
PSA (ng/ml)	NR	NR	<15		NR	<10
Gleason score	NR	$\leq$6/7/$\geq$8	<6/7 (3+4)	6/7	$\leq$6/7/$\geq$8	6
D'Amico risk	Low/high	Low to high	Low/Int	Low/Int	Low/Int/High	Low
Number of core biopsy	Every 5 mm throughout the prostate volume	NR	12	NC	NR	$\geq$12
Biopsy approach	Transperineal[b]	Transrectal/sextant	Transrectal/sextant	Transrectal/ sextant + targeted	NR	Tansrectal/sextant/ 2 series
Number of positive cores (%)	NR	NR	$\leq$2 contiguous biopsy	NC	NR	<33
Tumor volume	NR	NR	<10 %	NC	NR	Not used
Core involvement of a single core (%)	NR	NR	<50	NC	NR	<50
Gland involvement	Unilateral	NR	Unilateral	Unilateral[d]	NR	Unilateral
Extraprostatic extension on multiparametric-MRI (T2W-DCE-DW)	Not applied	Not applied	Not applied	NC	NR	No EPE on mpMRI
Biochemical follow-up	PSA/3 months at 2 first year	PSA/3 months at first year	PSA/3 months at first year	PSA/3 months at first year	NR	PSA/3 months at first year
	PSA/6 months thereafter	PSA/6 months thereafter	PSA/6 months thereafter	PSA/6 months thereafter		PSA/6 months thereafter
Rebiopsy follow-up	Yearly	Not in routine	Not in routine (if suspicion of BCR)	Yearly	Not in routine	Yearly

Table 11.2 (continued)

BCR	ASTRO	ASTRO	Nadir <50 % iPSA OR		NR	ASTRO	Nadir + 2 ng/ml
			Nadir + 2 ng/+ml				
Standardized questionnaires	Not applied	Not applied	Morbidity		IPSS	Not applied	IPSS
					IIEF-5		IIEF-5
Penile rehabilitation protocol	With or without oral	With or without oral Vacuum[c]	With or without oral		With or without oral	NR	With or without oral

Int intermediate, *FC* focal cryotherapy, *NHT* neoadjuvant hormonal therapy, *NC* not considered, *NR* not reported, *PSA* prostate-specific antigen, *yr* year
[a]6-month NHT were given in Gleason score 7 and greater patients prior to FC
[b]Not carried out in beginning original series
[c]Using of vacuum on regular basis
[d]pT3a at entry biopsy were not included

11.5 Cryotherapy Technique

11.5.1 Official Guidelines for Cryosurgery

Guidelines on the practice of cryosurgery have been written by both the American Urological Association (AUA) [16] and National Institute for Health and Clinical Excellence (NICE). The AUA recommends that diseased tissue should be frozen rapidly and the temperatures adequately monitored; this monitoring should be carried out using thermometric catheters in the target zone and close to the rectum through the Denonvilliers fascia in order to optimize the desired temperature of the target tissue and to reduce freezing of the rectum, thereby reducing the risk of a fistula forming.

The nadir temperature must be achieved at least down to $-40°$ at the heart of the tumor. The AUA also recommends that the speed of reheating should be controlled and progressive – as opposed to aggressive. Based on clinical studies, two freeze-thaw cycles are advised, since the first cycle induces cellular distress but the second is more lethal to the cell, providing optimal tissue destruction. NICE sets out general guidelines [17] on focal cryotherapy that recommend that the patient have a thorough understanding of the risks and uncertainty of the treatment, and this should be also be given in written form. The selection and treatment of patients should be done by a multidisciplinary urology and cancer team. Furthermore, in the U.K., all patient data needs to be collected and entered into EuCAP to review the outcomes.

NICE recommends using specific guidelines regarding the procedure. The size and suitability of the tumor should be confirmed by imaging and biopsy-mapping studies. Catheterization should be carried out under local or general anesthesia. Additionally, it should be ensured that transrectal ultrasonography is performed and a template grid placed on the perineum to guide the placement of the transperineal needles. Pressurized argon gas should then be passed through the cryotherapy needles. Appropriate measures should be taken to prevent surrounding tissues from the effects of freezing. Postoperatively, regular patient follow-up should include the monitoring of PSA levels, biopsies, and the appropriate imaging.

11.5.2 Materials for Cryotherapy Procedure

The materials needed for focal cryotherapy include the following:

Gas
Argon gas and helium gas (optional; not necessarily needed for some needles, e.g., IceRod (Galil Medical Inc.))
Cryotherapy System
Various systems are designed for cryosurgery and some are dedicated to urologist care. The systems manage gas flow and allow the control of the development of the ice ball during the procedure. Real-time temperature could be monitored by tuning the power of the cold production; some devices may also incorporate the view of transrectal ultrasound.

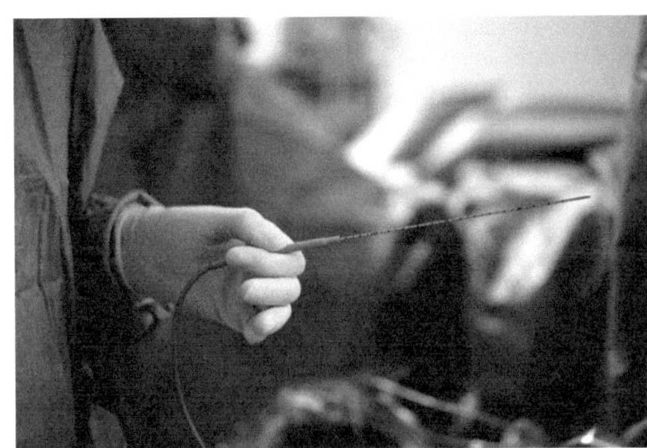

Fig. 11.3 Cryoneedle for prostate cryotherapy. Ultra-thin 17-gauge needles are used for cryotherapy and are connected to the cryosystem using flexible gas tubing. Gas flows through the cryo-system from the gas cylinder into needle, producing a cold temperature at the tip of the needle. Many needles could be provided (e.g., IceRod, IceSeed, IceBulb (Galil Medical Inc.))

Cryoneedles

Ultra-thin 17-gauge needles are used for cryotherapy and are connected to the cryosystem using flexible gas tubing (Fig. 11.3). Gas flows through the cryosystem from the gas cylinder into the needle, producing a cold temperature at the tip of the needle. Many needles could be provided (e.g., IceRod, IceSeed, IceBulb (Galil Medical Inc.)). For each needle there is a specific volume of ice ball. Based on the choice of the type of the needle, the ice ball encompasses the index lesion and destroys the targeted tissue. Needles are shaped to be used percutaneously.

A prostate procedure template is required to enable the surgeon to insert the needle through it within the targeted prostate. Either a single-use plastic version or a multiuse metal version is available, and the template is attached to the ultrasound stand.

Ultrasound System

A 7.5-MHz-endocavity biplane ultrasound probe is required for real-time imaging and controlling the development of the ice ball.

The TRUS is attached to an ultrasound probe stand secured to the surgical table, usually named "stepper."

A standoff or a brachy-balloon filled in water is necessary to cover the TRUS probe enabling contact with the posterior face of the prostate through the rectal wall.

Thermometer and Warming System

Thermocouples are essential for real-time monitoring of the temperature. One of the probes is placed directly within the targeted tissue to achieve the nadir temperature and another probe is positioned into the Denonvilliers space to protect the rectum from temperatures under 0 °C.

A warming catheter is inserted into the bladder through the urethra to keep it warm and protect it from a freezing injury.

11.5.3 Focal Cryotherapy Procedure

The surgical technique advised for focal cryotherapy can be divided into three main categories – patient preparation, operative, and postoperative.

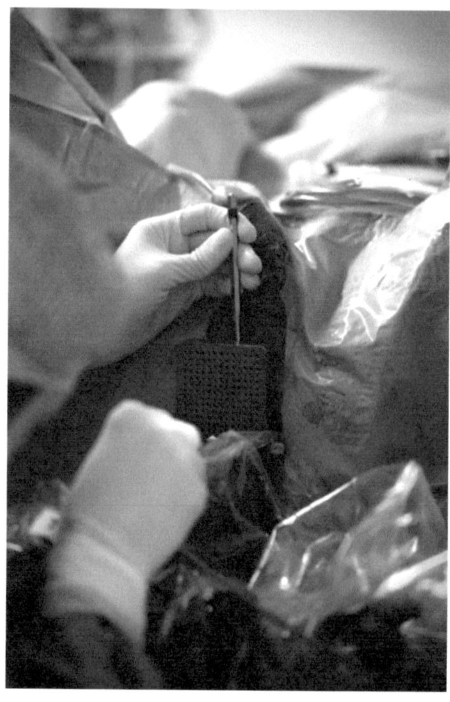

Fig. 11.4 Prostate cryotherapy by transperineal approach throughout a mapping template. The mapping template attached to the ultrasound is placed close to the perineum. The ultrasound stand is set correctly by real-time visualizing the urethral opening at the level of D2 as mentioned on the grid of the template

Patient Preparation and Positioning

Before the operation, a laxative must be used to empty the rectum. Antibiotic prophylaxis (gentamicin 3 mg/kg aminoglycoside) should also be given before the procedure.

Cryotherapy is performed under general anesthesia. The patient should be appropriately placed in the lithotomy position. Once anesthetized, anogenital and perineal scrubbing are to be done and an Ch.18–Ch.20 Foley catheter is inserted and left at beginning for TRUS setting and needle placement.

Sterile drapes have to be placed over the patient, with open access to the perineum. TRUS is prepared with ultrasound gel; the probe is covered by the standoffs filled in gel or using the brachy-balloon. The ultrasound stand is set correctly by real-time visualizing the urethral opening at the level of D2 as mentioned on the grid of the template. The mapping template attached to the ultrasound is placed close to the perineum (Fig. 11.4). Prostate volume is performed by appropriate biplanar measurements in both sagittal and transversal views.

Surgical Technique

Cryotherapy is performed through a transperineal percutaneous approach. Needle placement is done under TRUS imaging guidance. The 17-gauge cryoneedles are inserted percutaneously, through the template, into the area to be treated within the prostate parenchyma (Fig. 11.5). The cryoneedles should be placed in two groups [14]: group 1 should be placed away from the posterior surface of the prostate, within the central and anterior zone, and group 2 should be placed near the posterior lateral surface within the peripheral zone. In total, from 2 to 5 or more needles can

Fig. 11.5 Cryoneedle placement for focal therapy. Cryotherapy is performed through a transperineal percutaneous approach. Needle placement is done under TRUS imaging guidance. The 17-gauge cryoneedles are inserted percutaneously, through the template, into the area to be treated within the prostate parenchyma

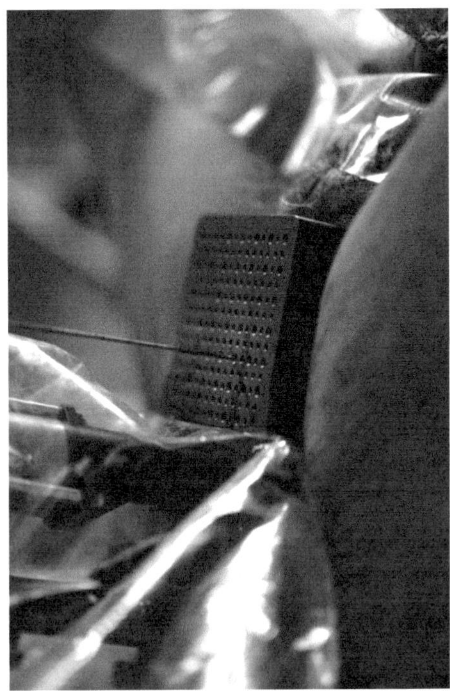

be placed, based on the targeted volume of the diseased prostate. Placement complies with safety distance recommendations. All the needles should be equidistant and a maximum of 1.8 cm apart from each other. They should also be a minimum of 1 cm away from the prostate capsule, and a minimum of 0.8 cm away from the urethra.

After needle placement, two thermocouples have to be inserted for temperature monitoring. One probe is placed centrally to the needles to check the nadir temperature of less than −40 °C during the procedure, and one placed rectally to prevent rectal freezing at >0 °C – within the Denonvilliers' fascia, on the ipsilateral side to needles.

Once the needle and thermocouple placement is completed, a flexible cystoscopy is performed to check no needle tip into the urethra or bladder wall. One 0.035 semirigid guidewire is inserted through the cystoscope before its removal in to place over this guide the warming catheter

The procedure can then begin by delivering argon gas that flows through the cryosystem into the needles to freeze the targeted prostate gland under ultrasound imaging and temperature control monitoring. First, initiate active freezing involving needles of group 1 followed by group 2, with a 1-min interval between the two groups; the freezing will be going on for 10 min. Once adequate freezing is achieved, the thawing part of the procedure is then conducted, using either hydrogen gas for 10 min if necessary or passive thawing for 5 min and then 5 min more of active thawing if applicable (based on the type of needle). The process is repeated one more time because, in total, two consecutive freeze-thaw cycles should be carried out. Once completed, the end of the cycles are marked by normal prostate echogenicity and the needles, thermocouples, warming catheter, and TRUS are removed and an Ch.18–Ch.20 Foley catheter is inserted and left in place to prevent acute postoperative urinary retention.

Postoperative

The urinary catheter is removed 1–2 days after the procedure and the patient's urine output may be checked. Some physicians also advise performing an early post-procedure multiparametric MRI to check that all intended areas have been successfully treated.

After all this has been done, the patient should be discharged with directions for the oral administration of a mild analgesic when pain occurs, starting (if the patient is not in severe pain) with non-opioid drugs such as paracetamol. Low-molecular-weight heparin (LMWH) daily injections for 10 days, and an alpha-blocker for at least15 days are also recommended. Note that the patient can also be discharged on the day of the procedure, and the catheter can be removed later at home.

11.6 Outcomes and Complications

11.6.1 Outcomes on Prostate Cancer Control

A few series have not reported on robust mid-, long-term outcomes, especially in the context of controlled clinical trials comparing their use with established interventions that have so far never been achieved. Overall, nevertheless, the biochemical disease-free survival at 5 years is likely to be similar to whole-gland treatment modalities. Onik et al. who first reported on focal cryotherapy outcomes in 2002 [18], published results from 48 patients with at least a two-year follow-up [10]; of them, 45 had a stable PSA according to the ASTRO definition [19]. Moreover, to date the largest data sets ever issued about cryotherapy have been provided from the Cryo On-Line Database (COLD). This registry has included 1,160 patients treated with focal cryotherapy. Ward et al. [13] have stratified patients into low-, intermediate-, and high-risk groups with 47, 41 and 12 %, respectively. The overall biochemical-free survival was 74, 7 % at a 3-year follow-up, similar to those patients in the COLD database treated with global cryotherapy. Likewise, Bahn et al. [8] wrote about 73 patients treated with focal cryotherapy, with a mean follow-up of 3.7 years, 75 % of biochemical-free survival rate based on ASTRO definition. Oncological outcomes are summarized in Table 11.3.

Based on Durand et al. [9], the oncological follow-up was recently carried out by monitoring PSA levels and doing mandatory12-transrectal biopsies between 6 months and a year after focal cryotherapy as recommended by Pister [20]. The primary endpoint for oncological assessment was no cancer in the ipsilateral prostatic lobe at this 12-month rebiopsy. This was a prospective, single-arm cohort study that included 48 consecutive patients with a mean age of 67 and a median follow-up of 13.2 months (IQR: 7.4–26.5) from January 2009 to March 2012. Eligibility criteria were patients with localized low-risk prostate cancer who refused active surveillance protocols and PCa treatment prior to inclusion. For the first time, this study used mandatory follow-up biopsy for oncological assessment and reported that FC could eradicate PCa in 86 % of rebiopsied patients confirmed with negative mandatory follow-up biopsy at 1 year. In addition, the mean PSA value dropped significantly, by 55 % at 3 months (Fig. 11.6).

Biological assessment remains a concern. The nadir value for PSA after cryotherapy has not yet been defined. For some, this should be approximately +2 ng/ml [21]. However, a reassuring fall in PSA levels does not necessarily mean a completely successful treatment and failure could only be definitively identified by positive rebiopsies in the treated area. Given that, Durand et al. assumed that unique PSA monitoring was not accurate enough to follow up patients treated with FC since their biological outcomes did not match well with their proven-cancer 1-year rebiopsy rate. Due to the multifocality of prostate cancer [22], the initial risk of underdetection, and imperfect PSA monitoring, the standardization of follow-up protocols including mandatory biopsies of both lobes at some point should be rethought. Also, it is likely that the routine sextant prostate biopsy lacked accuracy in detecting multiple locations of localized PCa [23] at entry, thereby misleading to the eligibility of inappropriate patients in FC. In the FC cohort from the COLD Registry, Ward reported on 73.8 % of negative follow-up biopsies that had been performed only in cases of biochemical recurrence. For instance, this rate is comparable to Durand et al outcomes even though mandatory 1-year rebiopsies were not standardized in the follow-up protocols, showing that how we follow up patients for FC still needs to be agreed upon.

While positive rebiopsies have detected localized PCa in cases of failure, re-treatment using FC was achieved successfully [9]. By the time the rebiopsy had detected larger PCa ineligible for any focal treatment, overall treatments such as radical prostatectomy, radiation therapy, or global cryotherapy were carried out and they were associated with low morbidity [12].

11.6.2 Functional Assessment

FC is a procedure done without major surgery or radiation exposure, something that seems particularly attractive to patients who aim for disease control and low comorbidity. The maintenance of potency and rate of continence are strongly encouraging after FC; functional outcomes are presented in Table 11.3.

Erectile dysfunction (ED) is uncommon after FC; its outcomes are homogeneous and encouraging, regardless of age and even among elderly patients [Pister LL]. Potency assessment using the IIEF-5 (International Index of Erectile Function-5) questionnaire [24] and the ability to maintain sexual activity ranged from 70 to 90 % after FC, except for the COLD registry, which has reported on 58 %. This high ED in Ward's study is likely to be due to the length of the cohort of the registry, associating multiple devices of FC treatment, various medical experiences in FC, and unstandardized criteria at entry or for follow-up assessment. Apart from the Ward's outcomes, the high rate of potency maintained makes CF compelling and

Table 11.3 Oncological and functional outcomes of focal cryotherapy

	Onik et al. [10]	Ellis et al. [11]	Lambert et al. [12]	Bahn et al. [8]	Ward et al. [13]	Durand et al. [9]
Study period	Jun 1995–Dec 2004	Dec 2000–Dec 2005	June 2002–Dec 2005	Sept 2002–Mar 2011	1997–2007	Jan 2009–Mar 2012
No. of pts. (with F/U)	48 (46)	60 (51)	25	73	1,160	48
Mean age, years	NR	69	68	64	68	67
Median follow-up, yrs	4.5	1.3	2.3	3.7	1.8	1.1
Clinical stage, n (%)	NR	$\leq$T2a: 55 (92) $\geq$T2b: 5 (8)	T1c: 25 (100)	T1c: 41 (56) T2a: 31 (43) T2b: 1 (1)	$\leq$T2a: 1,013 (87) $\geq$T2b: 147 (13)	T1c: 42 (88) T2a: 6 (12)
Gleason score, n (%)	NR	$\leq$6: 47 (78) =7: 12 (20) $\geq$8: 1 (1.7)	=6: 13 (52) =7: 12 (48)	=6: 30 (41) =7: 43 (59)	$\leq$6: 844 (74) =7: 240 (21) $\geq$8: 64 (6)	=5 (2) =6: 47 (98)
D'Amico risk, n (%)	NR[d]	Low: 40 (67) Int: 14 (23) High: 6 (10)	NR	Low: 24 (33) Int: 49 (67)	Low: 541 (47) Int: 473 (41) High: 143 (12)	Low: 48 (100)
Preop PSA, mean, ng/ml	7.8	7.2	6.0	5.9	7.2	6.1
Post PSA, mean, ng/ml	2.2	2.2	2.4	1.6	2.2	2.8
Biochemical recurrence-free survival, %	94	80	84	75	76	NA
Repeat biopsy, n (%)	NR	NR	7 (28)	48 (66)	164 (14)	42 (88)

(continued)

Biopsy-proven recurrence-free prostate cancer, %	Treat.100[a]	Treat. 98[a]	Treat 85[a]	Treat 98[a]	Treat NR	Treat 89[a]
	Both 92[b]	Both 77[b]	Both 57[b]	Both 75[b]	Both 74[c]	Both 74[b]
Continence, n (%)[e]	48 (100)	58 (96)	25 (100)	70 (100)	(98.4)	48 (100)
Potency, n (%)[f]	Pre 40	Pre 40	Pre 24	Pre 42	Pre NR	Pre 39
	Post 36/40 (90)	Post 24/34 (71)	Post 17/24 (71)	Post 31/42 (86)	Post NR (58.1)	Post NR

Int intermediate, *F/U* follow-up, *NA* not available, *PSA* prostate-specific antigen, *Treat* Treated

[a]Biopsy-proven recurrence-free prostate cancer based on negative biopsy in treated prostatic lobe

[b]Biopsy-proven recurrence-free prostate cancer based on negative biopsy in both treated and unfrozen prostatic lobe

[c]Biopsy-proven recurrence-free prostate cancer were based on both lobes negative biopsy, in only 14.1 % of the cohort of those suspected of PCa recurrence

[d]$n = 25$ (52 %) patients were intermediate to high-risk

[e]Continence is defined as no use of any pads

[f]Potency percentage was calculated out of patients who were preoperatively potent

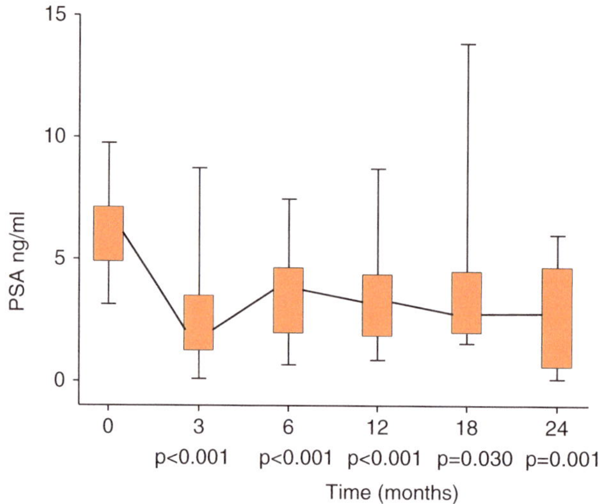

Fig. 11.6 PSA monitoring after focal cryotherapy. The mean PSA value dropped by 55 % to 2.8 ng/ml at 3 months ($p < 0.001$) and the decline persisted throughout the follow-up period. No undetectable PSA was reported (Courtesy of Durand et al. [9])

among the best focal devices to preserve erections while controlling PCa [8–13]. Few studies have reported prospective standardized functional questionnaires. Durand et al. [9] reported a slight decrease in the IIEF-5 score present at 3 months, but that it was not significantly different from the baseline at a 6-month follow-up. These superior functional outcomes for FC, compared with an equivalent unilateral nerve-sparing radical prostatectomy, could be explained by less invasive vascular disruption and the absence of any manipulation of the contralateral neurovascular bundle. Regarding ED outcomes, the majority of protocols allowed patients to take on-demand PDEi therapy if needed. No systematic regimen was recommended and again, to allow better data from functional outcomes of assessment after FC in the future, agreement and standardization remain eagerly awaited for reliable comparison.

Outcomes of FC series show a very high rate of urinary continence after treatment, ranging around 100 % [8–10, 12]. Incontinence assessment is established on the absence of pads at the FC follow-up as well as using the scoring system IPSS (International Prostate Symptoms Score) [25]. At the worst, very low rates of incontinence have been reported in Ward's and Ellis's cohorts, with 1.6 %, 3.6 % respectively, making FC a very safe technique in terms of the preservation of functional postoperative urinary quality.

11.6.3 Focal Cryotherapy-Related Complications

Complications are minimal and comparable with other local treatment modalities.

Durand et al. have applied Clavien-Dindo [26] scoring for surgical complication assessment during follow-up. Close attention was paid to previous types of complications reported from prior studies on both focal and global cryotherapy treatment [27]. There were 15 % grade 1 and 4 % grade 2 complications including mainly short-term complications as such acute urinary retention, genito-scrotal inflammation, and urinary tract infection. It has been found that the more long-term complications include urethral stenosis, and an uncommon case of Urinary rectal fistulae, and the above-described erectile dysfunction and urinary incontinence [28]. With a longer cohort, Ward reported mainly the same level of overall complications with no more risk of rectourethral fistulae (0, 1 %).

Although many measures are taken to avoid complications from the procedure, both patient and practitioner should be aware of the possibility of the low-rate complications of FC.

To compare it with other focal therapies, Barret et al. [29] have assessed the morbidity of their initial experience, regardless of the technique performed at their tertiary referral center for PCa management from 2009 until 2011 that included 1,213 patients with clinically localized PCa. Of these, 106 of the patients met with focal therapy criteria at entry and underwent either FC, high-intensity focused ultrasonography (HIFU), brachytherapy, or vascular-targeted photodynamic therapy (VTP). Of these 106 patients, 50 underwent FC. Overall, less than 2 % of grade 3 Clavien-Dindo complications have been reported, and only 13 % of the patients experienced focal treatment-related complications regardless of the techniques and there was no significant difference reported between them.

Conclusions

FC can eradicate cancer in 80 % of rebiopsied low-risk unilateral PCa patients with an acceptable morbidity with <2 % major complications in a highly selected population. Agreement and commitment to standardized inclusion criteria and follow-up are needed. Surgeons offering FC should agree with other groups to share and collect data for purposes of a standardization process. To this end, FC should still be considered as a part of controlled clinical trials.

References

1. In the first generation of cryotherapy, Cooper and Lee made the first catheter (1961).
2. Robilotto AT, et al. Development of a tissue engineered human prostate tumor equivalent for use in the evaluation of cryoablative techniques. Technol Cancer Res Treat. 2007;6(2):81–9.
3. Hoffmann NE, Bischof JC. The cryobiology of cryosurgical injury. Urology. 2002;60(2 Suppl 1):40–9.
4. http://www.cryogenicsociety.org/resources/defining_cryogenics/joule-thomson_effect/.
5. Tatsutani K, et al. Effect of thermal variables on frozen human primary prostatic adenocarcinoma cells. Urology. 1996;48(3):441–7.
6. Babaian RJ, et al. Best practice statement on cryosurgery for the treatment of localized prostate cancer. J Urol. 2008;180(5):1993–2004.

7. Nguyen HD, Allen BJ, Pow-Sang JM. Focal cryotherapy in the treatment of localized prostate cancer. Cancer Control Juill. 2013;20(3):177–80.

8. Bahn D, de Castro Abreu AL, Gill IS, et al. Focal cryotherapy for clinically unilateral, low-intermediate risk prostate cancer in 73 men with a median follow-up of 3.7 years. Eur Urol. 2012;62(1):55–63.

9. Durand M, Barret E, Galiano M, Rozet F, Sanchez-Salas R, Ahallal Y, et al. Focal cryoablation: a treatment option for unilateral low-risk prostate cancer. BJU Int. 2014;113(1):56–64.

10. Onik G, Vaughan D, Lotenfoe R, et al. The "male lumpectomy": focal therapy for prostate cancer using cryoablation results in 48 patients with at least 2-year follow-up. Urol Oncol. 2008;26(5):500–5.

11. Ellis DS, Manny Jr TB, Rewcastle JC. Focal cryosurgery followed by penile rehabilitation as primary treatment for localized prostate cancer: initial results. Urology. 2007;70(6 Suppl 1):S9–15.

12. Lambert EH, Bolte K, Masson P, Katz AE. Focal cryosurgery: encouraging health outcomes for unifocal prostate cancer. Urology. 2007;69:1117–20.

13. Ward JF, Jones JS. Focal cryotherapy for localized prostate cancer: a report from the national Cryo On-Line Database (COLD) Registry. BJU Int. 2012;109(11):1648–54.

14. Ellis DS, Manny Jr TB, Rewcastle JC. Cryoablation as primary treatment for localized prostate cancer followed by penile rehabilitation. Urology. 2007;69(2):306–10.

15. De Castro Abreu AL, Bahn D, Leslie S, Shoji S, Silverman P, Desai MM, et al. Salvage focal and salvage total cryoablation for locally recurrent prostate cancer after primary radiation therapy. BJU Int. 2013;112(3):298–307.

16. Babaian RJ, Donnelly B, Bahn D, Baust JG, Dineen M, Ellis D, et al. Best practice statement on cryosurgery for the treatment of localized prostate cancer. J Urol. 2008;180(5): 1993–2004.

17. http://www.nice.org.uk/.

18. Onik G, Narayan P, Vaughan D, et al. Focal "nerve-sparing" cryosurgery for treatment of primary prostate cancer: a new approach to preserving potency. Urology. 2002;60(1):109–14.

19. Consensus statement: guidelines for PSA following radiation therapy. American society for therapeutic radiology and oncology consensus panel. Int J Radiat Oncol Biol Phys. 1997;37(5):1035–41.

20. Pisters LL. Cryotherapy for prostate cancer: ready for prime time? Curr Opin Urol. 2010;20(3):218–22.

21. Williams SG, et al. An international multicenter study evaluating the impact of an alternative biochemical failure definition on the judgment of prostate cancer risk. Int J Radiat Oncol Biol Phys. 2006;65(2):351–7.

22. Villers A, McNeal JE, Freiha FS, Stamey TA. Multiple cancers in the prostate. Morphologic features of clinically recognized versus incidental tumors. Cancer. 1992;70(9):2313–8.

23. Mayes JM, Mouraviev V, Sun L, Tsivian M, Madden JF, Polascik TJ. Can the conventional sextant prostate biopsy accurately predict unilateral prostate cancer in low-risk, localized, prostate cancer? Urol Oncol. 2011;29(2):166–70.

24. Rosen RC, et al. Development and evaluation of an abridged, 5-item version of the International Index of Erectile Function (IIEF-5) as a diagnostic tool for erectile dysfunction. Int J Impot Res. 1999;11(6):319–26.

25. Barry MJ, et al. The American Urological Association symptom index for benign prostatic hyperplasia. The Measurement Committee of the American Urological Association. J Urol. 1992;148(5):1549–57. discussion 1564.

26. Clavien PA, Barkun J, de Oliveira ML, Vauthey JN, Dindo D, Schulick RD, et al. The Clavien-Dindo classification of surgical complications: five-year experience. Ann Surg. 2009;250(2):187–96.

27. Caso JR, et al. Complications and postoperative events after cryosurgery for prostate cancer. BJU Int. 2012;109:840–5. http://www.ncbi.nlm.nih.gov/pubmed/21883827.

28. Eggener SE, Scardino PT, Carroll PR. Focal therapy for localized prostate cancer: a critical appraisal of rationale and modalities. J Urol. 2007;178(6):2260–7.
29. Barret E, Ahallal Y, Sanchez-Salas R, Galiano M, Cosset JM, Validire P, et al. Morbidity of focal therapy in the treatment of localized prostate cancer. Eur Urol. 2013;63:618–22.
30. Gonder MJ, Soanes WA, Smith V. Experimental prostate cryosurgery. Invest Urol. mai 1964;1:610–9.

Focal High-Intensity Focused Ultrasound (HIFU)

12

Sebastien Crouzet, Olivier Rouvière, Cyril Lafond, Jean-Yves Chapelon, and Albert Gelet

12.1 Introduction

Transrectal high-intensity focused ultrasound (HIFU) is highly suitable for focal therapy of localized prostate cancer (PCa) for several reasons. HIFU induces immediate and irreversible coagulative necrosis with sharply delineated boundaries. The treatment can be accurately targeted to a portion of the prostate gland. Unlike radiation, there is no lifetime dose limit, allowing HIFU to be repeated if necessary.

S. Crouzet, MD (✉)
Department of Urology, Edouard Herriot Hospital, Lyon, France

Therapeutic Ultrasound Research Laboratory, Inserm, U1032, Lyon F-69003, France

Université de Lyon, Lyon F-69003, France

Urology and Transplantation Department, Edouard Herriot Hospital,
5 place d'Arsonval, Lyon 69437, France
e-mail: sebastien.crouzet@chu-lyon.fr

O. Rouvière
Therapeutic Ultrasound Research Laboratory, Inserm, U1032, Lyon F-69003, France

Department of Urology, Université de Lyon, Université Lyon 1, Lyon F-69003, France

Department of Radiology, Edouard Herriot Hospital, Lyon, France

C. Lafond • J.-Y. Chapelon
Department of Urology, Inserm, U1032, Lyon F-69003, France

Université de Lyon, Lyon F-69003, France

A. Gelet
Department of Urology, Edouard Herriot Hospital, Lyon, France

Therapeutic Ultrasound Research Laboratory, Inserm, U1032, Lyon F-69003, France

Université de Lyon, Lyon F-69003, France

© Springer-Verlag France 2015
E. Barret, M. Durand (eds.), *Technical Aspects of Focal Therapy in Localized Prostate Cancer*, DOI 10.1007/978-2-8178-0484-2_12

HIFU does not create a potential therapeutic impasse, and additional radical therapy can be performed involving radical surgery [1], external beam radiation therapy [2], and cryotherapy [3]. Moreover, HIFU is a minimally invasive therapy that can be performed under spinal anesthesia on an outpatient basis.

12.2   Principles of HIFU

Spherical ultrasound (US) sources can generate high focal intensity. The first prostate investigations were performed on dogs [4], and subsequent human trials were performed on men with either benign prostate hypertrophy (BPH) [5] or localized PCa [6]. US waves deposit energy in the media through which they pass. For imaging purposes, pulses of nonfocused ultrasound (US) waves travel through tissue, resulting in an insignificant deposit of energy. Increasing the intensity of the waves increases the amount of energy deposit, and tissue temperatures can rise substantially. Further, focusing the waves enables temperatures to be reached that result in tissue destruction through cellular disruption and coagulative necrosis [7] in the focal volume while preserving adjacent tissues. The focal volume need not include tissue adjacent to the piezoelectric crystal, and, if required, the tissue between the crystal and the focal volume is preserved as well by using a distal focal point. The two mechanisms involved in the destruction of tissue are the thermal effect and cavitation [8]. Thermal effects rely on the absorption of US energy by the tissue and its conversion into heat. Under the right conditions, the temperature within sonicated tissue will rise to a level sufficient to induce irreversible damage. Cavitation is the result of the interaction between US and microbubbles in the sonicated tissue, an interaction that may lead to enhanced heating through nonlinear oscillation of these microbubbles and mechanical disruption of tissue through the violent collapse of the bubbles. HIFU is a technique for thermal ablation based on the combination of absorption and cavitation, while lithotripsy uses cavitational mechanisms to produce nonthermal tissue destruction [9].

The deposit of energy during HIFU can be mathematically modeled using the bioheat transfer equation. This allows determination of the optimal acoustic intensity necessary to achieve irreversible tissue destruction in a variety of clinical situations, particularly with previously irradiated prostate tissue [10]. The aim of focal HIFU is to treat the cancer foci inside the prostate gland by juxtaposition of elementary lesions. The exposure conditions are defined by the time-averaged acoustic intensity, duration of sonication, on/off ratio, distance between the two elementary lesions, and displacement path when multiple lesions are made. The transrectal route offers an excellent acoustic window to ablate the prostate. The combination of focused US sources and active cooling of rectal mucosa minimizes the risk of rectal injury. HIFU-induced lesions are visible with standard US as hyperechoic areas, but their extent is not always accurately defined visually. Magnetic resonance imaging (MRI) is the gold standard technique for assessing HIFU treatment efficacy, and gadolinium-enhanced T1-weighted images can effectively reveal the extent of necrosis [11]. MRI has also been used to guide and monitor temperature changes during HIFU treatment, but it should be noted that this technology remains in the early preclinical stage of evaluation for use in transrectal PCa treatment. More recently, contrast-enhanced ultrasound (CEUS) demonstrated that ablated (devascularized) and viable (enhancing) tissue can be distinguished immediately after HIFU treatment [12]. Pulse-echo US backscattered signals have also been used to estimate changes in tissue properties induced by HIFU [13]. These less expensive US-based techniques are now incorporated into routine clinical use with various devices for assessing post-HIFU thermal injury to prostatic targets.

Following HIFU treatment, the absence of a prostate-specific antigen (PSA) bounce allows greater convenience and less anxiety during follow-up for both the urologist and the patient.

Unlike radiotherapy, late-onset bladder or rectal toxicities have not been reported with HIFU, and radiotherapy has the potential to induce malignant tissue transformation, leading to an increased risk in development of secondary malignancies [14]. Also unlike radiation therapy, there is no dose limitation and no limited number of sessions with HIFU.

12.3 Specific Indication and Limitations

HIFU can be used either as primary cancer therapy or salvage therapy in patients with local recurrence following primary treatment with external beam radiation therapy (EBRT), brachytherapy, or surgery.

12.3.1 Focal HIFU as Primary PCa Treatment

Various treatment protocols are used in the primary treatment of PCa. In the PSA era, unilateral tumor is identified in roughly 20 % of patients [15]. With unilateral tumor, hemi-ablation is applied with or without adjunctive transurethral resection of the prostate (TURP).

Strategies used in the treatment of bilateral tumor include treatment of the index lesion or treatment of all identified tumor foci including the index lesion.

The limitations are similar to other focal therapy approaches:

- The ability to identify the tumor foci in 3D.
- The optimal margin around the region of interest (ROI) to ensure oncological safety is not yet defined.
- Real-time control of the treated area.

Prostate size is a limitation with HIFU technologies (Ablatherm Integrated Imaging® and Sonablate 500®). This is due to limits of the focal depth of therapy transducers that result in incomplete prostate gland penetration in prostate volumes >35 cc.

Most HIFU limitations have been overcome with the latest-generation HIFU device (Focal One®, EDAP TMS, Vaulx en Velin, France), which features a dynamic focusing transducer. This allows the treatment of large prostates (up to 60 cc) by moving the focal point of the transducer and it can create up to eight different focal points that lie 32–67 mm from the transducer. This system offers the possibility of image fusion between preoperative MRI and the live US prostate image in order to precisely target the identified ROI. The imaging transducer can perform contrast-enhanced US imaging for precise localization of the treated volume. Treatment can be completed in the same session if necessary, taking into account preoperative MR tumor mapping with use of US/MRI fusion software.

Bowel pathology, such as inflammatory disease, is a contraindication because treatment is applied using a transrectal approach. Anatomical conditions that interfere with probe introduction or placement within the rectum are a potential contraindication, and unless removed with TURP, significant prostatic calcifications are a contraindication because they can impair ultrasonic wave transmission.

12.3.2 Focal HIFU for Locally Recurrent PCa

In patients with locally recurrent tumor following radiation therapy, the primary objective of focal HIFU is to eradicate recurrent tumor foci using the lowest thermal dose delivered inside the whole gland. Side effect rates following whole-prostate salvage HIFU are high [16]; the rates of grade 2/3 incontinence, urethral stricture, and rectal injury have been 19, 16.9, and 0.4 %, respectively. Most recurrence has occurred in the lobe where the tumor was identified before radiation therapy. In post-EBRT recurrence, early detection is important when the malignancy is still small and amenable to focal therapy. The parameter for treating radiorecurrence with Ablatherm devices incorporates the specific characteristics of irradiated tissue such as reduced vascularization induced by radiation fibrosis [17], and salvage HIFU hemi-ablation must be performed with a dedicated strategy that includes the urethra. In 50 salvage prostatectomies, Leibovici et al. found that 66 % of patients had a solitary tumor focus, with tumor invasion of the median line in 74 % of cases [18]. It is therefore important to perform an "extended" hemi-ablation involving the contralateral lobe without the intention of urethral preservation. Rectal stricture is the primary contraindication for post-EBRT salvage HIFU; MRI performed with a rectal balloon filled with 100 ml saline solution can be used to predict HIFU feasibility in more difficult cases. Patient selection is essential to optimize oncological outcomes with focal salvage therapy; the process for accurate patient selection should first exclude patients with infra-clinical metastases and then consider for focal treatment only patients with small unilateral local recurrence.

12.4 Materials and Technique

Three HIFU devices are currently available for the treatment of PCa. They include the Sonablate 500® (Sonacare, Charlotte, NC, USA), the Ablatherm Integrated Imaging® (EDAP-TMS SA, Vaulx en Velin, France), and the Focal One® (EDAP-TMS SA, Vaulx en Velin, France) (Fig. 12.1). Experimental MRI-guided HIFU devices remain in the development stage (ExAblate, InSightec, Tirat Carmel, Israel, and Profound Medical Inc., Toronto, Canada).

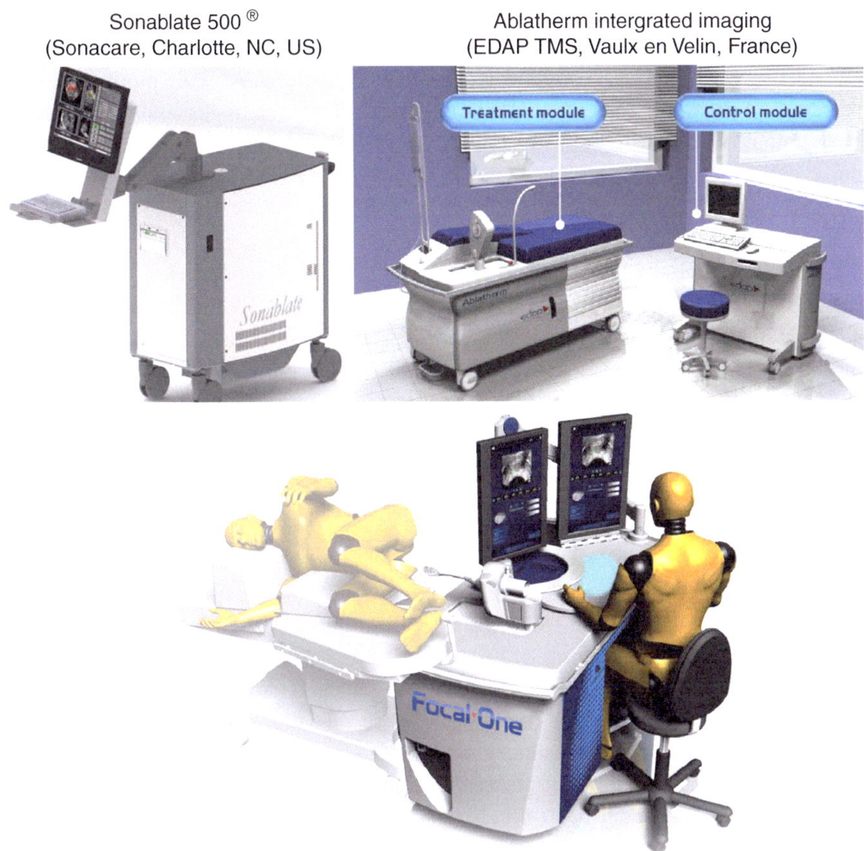

Focal One (EDAP TMS, Vaulx en Velin, France)

Fig. 12.1 Commercially available HIFU devices

12.4.1 Sonablate 500

The Sonablate 500® uses a single transducer (4 MHz) for imaging and treatment (Fig. 12.1). Several probes are available with focal lengths from 25 to 45 mm. The size of the elementary lesion is 10 mm in length and 2 mm in diameter. The Sonablate procedure is conducted in a dorsal position with the patient lying on a conventional operating table. Sonablate uses a single treatment protocol, and the power must be manually adapted by the operator. The treatment is usually made in three consecutive coronal layers that starts from the anterior prostate area and moves to the posterior area, and at least one probe switch is made during the procedure [19]. The probe is chosen to match the prostate size, with larger glands requiring longer focal length probes.

The latest generation of Sonablate (Sonablate 500®) used a tissue change monitoring (TCM®) system that allows visual confirmation of the treated prostate. The TCM's color-coding feature highlights tissue that had not been adequately "heated," alerting the operator of the need to retreat that section of the prostate in real-time for confirmation of adequate treatment of the entire prostate. A radiofrequency (RF) signal is sent to the treated prostate site before HIFU delivery, with another RF signal sent to the same site after HIFU delivery. TCM calculates and displays the change that occurred, with tissue change quantified through comparison of RF US pulse-echo signals at each treatment site.

12.4.2 Ablatherm Integrated Imaging

The Ablatherm Integrated Imaging® incorporates both the imaging (7.5 MHz) and therapeutic (3 MHz) transducers into a single endorectal probe focused at 40 mm. A custom bed is required with the Ablatherm device, where the patient lies in a lateral position (Fig. 12.1). The lateral treatment position permits gas bubbles produced through the heating of prostatic tissue to rise with gravity to a position lateral to the prostate, thus reducing the risk of acoustic interference with the HIFU waves. The Ablatherm device includes four treatment protocols specifically designed for the treatment parameters required in different clinical indications. These include standard, HIFU re-treatment, post-EBRT, and post-brachytherapy. Size of the elementary lesion varies from 19 to 26 mm in length and is 1.7 mm in diameter. Ablatherm Integrated Imaging offers real-time US monitoring of treatment. The HIFU probe is robotically adjusted, with a permanent control of the distance between the transducer and the rectal wall. A precise volume is treated by repeating the shots and moving the transducer, which is defined by the operator in the planning phase. Treatment is made in transversal layers. The device has many safety features, including a control of the distance between the transducer and the rectal wall, a urethral cooling system, and a patient motion detector.

12.4.3 Focal One

The Focal One® is the latest and most advanced HIFU device for the treatment of PCa (Fig. 12.1). With this device, the procedure is performed using a conventional operating table with the patient in the lateral position. Included in this device is the new dynamic focusing transducer, made of 16 isocentric rings (Fig. 12.2). Each ring is driven by a dedicated electronic system comprised of 16 different power lines. Adjustment of the respective phases of the 16 electrical signals supplying the transducer allows the operator to electronically steer the US beam and move the focal point of the transducer to a maximum of eight different points that are 32–67 mm from the transducer (Fig. 12.2). Treatment with dynamic focusing involves unitary HIFU lesion stacking within the prostate along the transducer US beam axis. Each lesion size is as small as 5 mm, and by stacking 2–8 unitary lesions, it is possible to extend the necrotic lesion 5–40 mm to adequately target either small or large prostate glands. Each US pulse lasts 1 s, and there is no interruption time between the different US pulses. Compared to HIFU treatment using fixed focusing, dynamic

Fig. 12.2 Dynamic focusing probe principles (Focal One®)

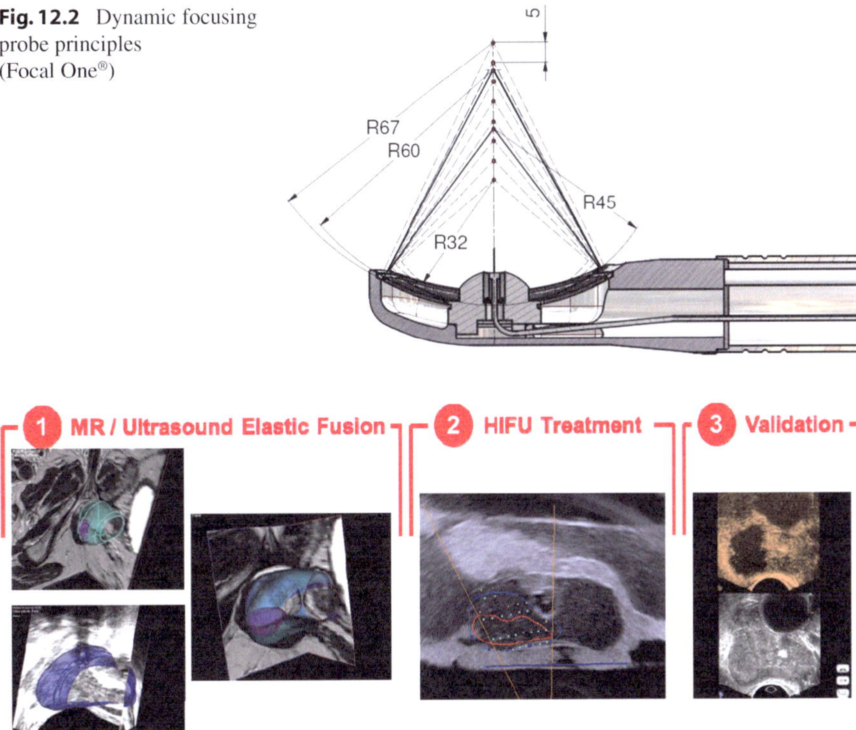

Fig. 12.3 Main steps of focal treatment with the Focal One®

focusing allows the treatment of larger prostates because the maximum lesion height is 40 mm instead of 26 mm with previous-generation devices. The wide range in lesion height (5–40 mm) enables highly precise contouring of the prostate, and treatment duration of PCa is shortened with the continuous shooting process and lack of interruption between firings. Finally, HIFU using dynamic focusing is anticipated to provide a more homogeneous necrotic zone due to improved energy distribution within the prostate.

Focal One® is the first HIFU device specifically designed for focal therapy of PCa and combines all the necessary tools to visualize, target, treat, and confirm the focal treatment (Fig. 12.3). The process is divided into four logical steps: treatment preparation using imported MRI images and fusion with real-time US volume, focal target definition, application of precise destructive energy, and confirmation of the devascularized target area.

MR/US Image Elastic Fusion

Focal One is capable of importing standard DICOM MR images either from a removable storage device (CD, DVD, USB key, etc.) or directly from the PACS through a hospital local network. Using this MR volume image, the operator can define the contours of the prostate and one or several ROIs that have been confirmed as prostate tumors. These contours can be performed on a desktop computer or on Focal One just before beginning the treatment. The same prostate contouring is executed by the operator on the live US volume feature of the Focal One transrectal probe. The software automatically registers the two volumes and proceeds to an "elastic fusion": the live US volume is used as the reference volume, and the MR volume is smoothly deformed to every dimension, so the 3-D contour of the prostate on the MR volume matches perfectly in three dimensions the contours of the prostate on the US volume. The same 3-D elastic transformation is applied to the ROI initially indicated in the MR image, so they appear at the appropriate position on the live US image.

Treatment Planning and HIFU Energy Delivery

The application of HIFU energy is planned for transversal slices. On each slice, the operator defines the contour of the area to be treated. The section of the ROI initially defined on MR image and transformed in the previous "elastic fusion" step automatically appears on the live US image of the transversal view being planned, serving to guide the planning process by surrounding the tumor focus with the appropriate margin. The Focal One software automatically directs the focus of the HIFU shot to entirely destroy the defined area. Delivery of HIFU energy begins when all slices within the block are defined. Focal One is equipped with the latest generation of HIFU probe (dynamic focusing) and is able to electronically vary the focal point along the acoustic axis using a HIFU-phased array transducer. The focal point can be steered from 32 to 67 mm from the probe without any mechanical movement. A longer lesion is achieved by stacking unitary 5 mm HIFU lesions. At any point during the HIFU energy delivery process, the operator can observe a live US image of the treated area and if necessary can pause the treatment to readjust the treatment planning in cases such as a shifting prostate or change in some other aspect (such as swelling).

Treatment Validation

At the end of the treatment process, while the probe remains in the patient's rectum, the integrated US probe is able to acquire a CEUS volume after intravenous injection of microbubbles (Sonovue®, Braco, Switzerland). The acquired volume clearly shows the devascularized area. This image volume can be superimposed with the treatment planning and the initial MR image showing the targeted lesions. The physician can choose to complete treatment by planning additional HIFU energy spots.

12.4.4 Experimental MRI-Guided Devices

Several devices have been developed based on the principle of combining HIFU and MRI. The manufacturers have developed treatment probes compatible with commercially available MRI devices such the ExAblate (endorectal probe) and Profound (endourethral applicator). With MRI, an alternative method involves use of thermometry to control the power during the sonication [20], so that the desired exposure is induced without wasting energy. Feedback control may reduce the treatment time for thermal coagulation of the prostate with intraurethral applicators that slowly rotate to sweep the whole gland [21]. These closed-loop feedback systems can optimize the energy delivery. However, MRI-guided devices are in use only with preclinical trials.

12.5 Postoperative Evaluation of the Ablated Area and Detection of Post-HIFU Local Recurrences

12.5.1 Postoperative Evaluation of the Ablated Area

Ideally, imaging should indicate the extent of prostate volume destroyed after an HIFU ablation session so that another HIFU ablation can be immediately performed in the event of unsatisfactory results. Unfortunately, the transrectal US that guides HIFU treatment cannot show the ablated area with the necessary accuracy [11].

Gadolinium-enhanced (non-dynamic) MRI clearly displays the treated volume as a devascularized zone corresponding to the central core of the coagulation necrosis, surrounded by a peripheral rim of enhancement that corresponds with edema; however, MRI images cannot be obtained in the operating room [22, 23].

We have recently shown that CEUS, using Sonovue™ as a contrast agent, displayed the ablated volume immediately following treatment, with excellent correlation between the MRI and biopsy findings. All prostate sectors not showing enhancement with CEUS following a HIFU ablation can be safely determined as entirely destroyed. On the other hand, any prostate sector that shows a degree of enhancement can be considered as harboring living benign or malignant tissue [24]. These results should allow immediate re-treatment of the gland areas showing residual enhancement that are within the range of the transducer.

12.5.2 Detection of Post-HIFU Local Recurrences

After HIFU ablation, the residual prostate is composed of fibrotic scarring and BPH tissue that, because of its anterior position, has not been destroyed. With the ability to treat local recurrence or residual cancer following HIFU ablation with a second session of HIFU ablation or by radiation therapy [25], early detection is imperative. The precise location of recurrence can also assist in selection of the salvage modality.

Even if TRUS is sensitized with color Doppler [26], US-based techniques lack the accuracy to detect early local recurrence and guide the biopsy.

MRI, and particularly DCE MRI, seems effective in the early detection and accurate localization of recurrent cancer, which produce an earlier and more pronounced enhancement than post-HIFU fibrosis [27, 28]. However, DCE MRI lacks specificity, making it difficult to differentiate recurrent cancer from residual BPH tissue. In a retrospective study at our institute of 65 patients with biochemical recurrence following HIFU ablation, neither the enhancement pattern nor the apparent diffusion coefficient (ADC) was able to significantly differentiate BPH nodules from recurrent malignancy, even when the latter had, on average, higher wash-in rates, lower wash-out rates, and lower ADCs (unpublished results). Thus, to date, all patients with rising PSA after HIFU ablation should undergo MRI of the whole prostate, and early intense enhancement should be biopsied to distinguish cancer from BPH residual tissue.

12.6 Review of Literature: Oncological Side Effects and Functional Outcomes

12.6.1 Focal HIFU as Primary Care Treatment

In 2008, Muto et al. reported the outcomes of 29 patients treated with the Sonablate™ device [29]. In selected patients with cancer confined to a single lobe based on multiregional biopsy, the total peripheral zone and a half portion of the transitional zone were ablated. The average prostate volume decreased from 35.8 to 30.3 cc, and the mean PSA level decreased from 5.36 ± 5.89 ng/ml to 1.52 ± 0.92 at 36 months. Of the 29 patients, 28 underwent control biopsy 6 months after the procedure. Residual cancer foci were found in three patients (10.7 %). At 12 months post-HIFU, 17 patients underwent control biopsy. Residual cancer foci were found in four patients (23.5 %); only one patient had a urethral stricture. No significant differences were found in 2-year disease-free survival rates between low- and intermediate-risk patients treated with whole prostate (90.9 % vs. 49.9 %, respectively) and focal therapy (83.3 % vs. 53.6 %, respectively). Indwelling urethral catheter following HIFU remained in place a mean 15 ± 4 days; the frequency of urethral stricture and urinary tract infection was 4 % for both. No significant changes were found in IPSS score and maximal flow rate pre-HIFU and 12 months post-HIFU. No information was provided regarding erectile function.

Ahmed et al. presented the first published series of prostate hemi-ablation with HIFU [30]. Patients with low-moderate risk (Gleason ≤ 7, PSA ≤ 15 µg/ml), unilateral ($\leq$T2bN0M0) PCa on TRUS biopsy underwent multi-sequence MRI (T2, DCE, diffusion) and 5 mm-spaced transperineal template biopsy for disease localization. All patients received transrectal HIFU that involves ablation of the entire positive hemi-prostate up to the urethra. Of the 20 patients (mean age 60.4 years), 25 % had low-risk and 75 % intermediate-risk PCa. Before HIFU, the mean PSA was 7.3 ng/ml, 95 % were pad free, and 95 % could achieve an erection sufficient for penetrative sex. At the 12-month follow-up, the mean PSA decreased to 1.5 ng/ml ± 1.3, and 89 % had no histological evidence of cancer. Two patients (11.1 %) had a positive protocol biopsy at 6 months with residual 1 mm Gleason $3 + 3$; one elected to have HIFU re-treatment and the other active surveillance. Trifecta status was achieved by 89 %.

The French Urological Association (AFU) initiated a multi-institutional study to evaluate HIFU hemi-ablation as a primary treatment in patients >50 years, T1C or

T2A, PSA <10 ng/ml, Gleason ≤7 (3+4), and with ≤2 contiguous positive biopsies in no more than one lobe after MRI and random and targeted biopsy. Additional inclusion criteria were that the tumor had to be >6 mm from the apex and >5 mm from the midline. Only one prostatic lobe was treated.

To date, the 87 treated patients (Gleason ≤6 in 77 %, Gleason 7 in 23 %) have shown a negative biopsy rate in the treated lobe of 90.6 % and a mean PSA that decreased from a baseline 5.35 ng/ml ±3.3 to 2.07/ml ± 1.75 at 6-month follow-up. No significant changes have been observed before and after HIFU in the scores on any standardized measure of urinary or sexual function (IPSS, ICS, IIEF 5, EORTC-QLC30) [31].

In 2012, Ahmed et al. published a prospective trial of focal therapy for localized unifocal and multifocal PCa [32]. Included were 42 patients with localized PCa (stage T1/T2, PSA ≤15 ng/ml, Gleason score ≤4+3:7) of whom 27 % had low-risk, 63 % intermediate-risk, and 10 % had high-risk PCa. Patients received HIFU focal therapy using the Sonablate 500® device, delivered to all suspected tumor lesions that were localized using multiparametric MRI and transperineal template mapping biopsy. A maximum 60 % of the prostate was ablated. The edge of the ablation zone was ≥10 mm from a neurovascular bundle in unilateral disease and ≥5 mm from the neurovascular bundles in bilateral disease. Of 41 treated patients, 49 % received unilateral single-area ablation, 37 % received bilateral two-area ablation, and 15 % received a midline one-area ablation. All patients were able to void through the urethra on the first postoperative day. A significant decrease in PSA was reported at 12 months, with median baseline PSA of 6.6 and 1.9 ng/ml at 12 months ($p=0.0001$). Histological evidence of tumor was negative in 30 of 39 (77 %) patients biopsied at 6 months. Of the 39 men biopsied (transrectal route) at 6 months, 9 (23 %) had evidence of tumor, and 3 (8 %) had evidence of clinically significant tumor (Epstein criteria: Gleason >3+3, > 2 cores positives, >2 mm involvement). Of those with positive biopsy, five were placed on active surveillance and four received a second HIFU session. None of the four that underwent a repeat focal therapy consented to further biopsies, but all received control MRI. After re-treatment in four patients, 39 of 41 (95 %) had no evidence of disease on multiparametric MRI at 12 months. All 38 men were pad-free at baseline and remained pad-free at 12 months. IPSS score improved, with a decrease between baseline and 12 months ($p=0.026$). Of the 35 men with good baseline erectile function, 31 (89 %) had erection sufficient for penetration 12 months after focal therapy. Finally, of the 31 men with good baseline erectile function, 26 (84 %) achieved the trifecta status of being leak-free and pad-free, with erections sufficient for intercourse, and no evidence of clinically significant disease on multiparametric MRI at 12 months. One patient experienced acute urinary retention requiring a urethral catheter for 5 days. One patient received a partial rectal wall injury with extravasation of urine outside the prostate. The patient was successfully managed with suprapubic catheter and quinolone antibiotics. This patient required an endoscopic dilatation for a delayed urethral stricture. Two patients with large prostate size required a limited TURP because voiding did not return to normal. This study supports the proposition that tissue preservation leads to functional preservation. The histological outcomes were slightly less than those achieved after hemi-ablation, likely due to reduction in margin around the tumor.

12.6.2 Focal HIFU as Salvage Treatment

Focal salvage HIFU (FSH) represents a new therapeutic option. The aim of FSH is to destroy the recurrent tumor with minimal risk of severe side effects. The initial results of this new treatment approach were recently published [33]. In this trial, 39 patients received focal salvage HIFU therapy for localized recurrence after EBRT (hemi-ablation, $n=16$; quadrant ablation, $n=23$). Patients with multifocal tumor foci underwent index lesion ablation if the untreated areas had ≤ 1 core with ≤ 3 mm $3+3$ Gleason score. A PSA response was observed in 87 % of patients; 44 % of treated patients achieved a PSA nadir <0.5 ng/ml. Of those who achieved a nadir <0.5, the 3-year biochemical-free survival rate (BFSR) (Phoenix criteria) was 63 %. Of those who achieved a nadir >0.5, the 3-year BFSR was 0 %. Two patients developed metastasis, and 40 % required salvage androgen deprivation therapy. Twenty-five patients (64 %) were continent (pad-free, leak-free) at last follow-up. The mean pre-salvage IIEF-15 score decreased from 18 ± 16 to 13 ± 21 after FSH.

More recently, Baco et al. [34] (*BJUI* 2013, in press) reported the short-term results of hemi-salvage HIFU ablation (HSH) for unilateral recurrent PCa following radiation therapy. Between 2009 and 2012, 48 patients were prospectively enrolled from two European centers. Inclusion criteria were positive MRI and at least one positive biopsy in one lobe after primary radiation therapy; mean age was 68.8 ± 6 years and the mean pre-HIFU PSA was 5.2 ± 5.2 ng/ml. With a median follow-up of 16.3 months, the mean PSA nadir after HSH was 0.69 ± 0.83 ng/ml. Disease progression occurred in 16 patients (35.5 %). Local recurrence was found in the untreated lobe in four patients and bilaterally in four patients. Six patients developed metastases, and two had rising PSA without local recurrence or radiologically proven metastasis. Progression-free survival (Phoenix criteria) rates at 12, 18, and 24 months were 83, 64, and 52, respectively. No rectal fistula were observed. There were no significant changes in EORTC-QLC30 and IPSS scores. Pad-free, leak-free urinary continence status after HSH was attained in 36 of 48 patients (75 %). Four patients (8.3 %) experienced severe post-HSH incontinence; all four had a post-EBRT local recurrence involving the apex, and HSH was voluntarily performed without a sphincter safety margin. Three of the four did not show disease progression; their PSA values at last follow-up were 0.12, 0.05, and 0.07 ng/ml. No rectourethral fistulas were observed. Two patients (4 %) experienced a delayed pubic osteitis that was conservatively managed. There were no statistically significant differences in IPSS and QoL (EORTC-QLQ C30) scores before between baseline and follow-up. A significant decrease in erectile function score was observed (IIEF-5 score), with a median of 7.5 to 5 at the 24-month follow-up. One rectourethral fistula occurred and was resolved with urinary and bowel diversion. Sloughing occurred in 18 % of patients and urinary tract infection or epididymitis in 8 %; no osteitis was observed.

Conclusions

The results of preliminary studies demonstrated that HIFU is an effective focal therapy option for localized PCa, either as primary therapy or as salvage therapy in patients with radiorecurrent PCa. Hemi-ablation is an option for patients with low-intermediate risk unilateral localized PCa, which characterizes 10–20 % of patients diagnosed following a PSA test. The efficacy of HIFU hemi-ablation must be demonstrated in randomized trials using active surveillance as the control condition. Focal HIFU treatment of the index tumor is a minimally invasive option for patients with small tumors involving a limited portion of the prostate gland, but studies with long-term follow-up, including randomized trials comparing focal HIFU with radical therapies, are needed. Focal salvage HIFU appears to be the best option for treating limited recurrence after EBRT that offers good cancer control efficacy and minimal risk of significant side effects. The technical development of devices that are guided with new US technologies or MRI will increase the role of this strategy in the near future.

References

1. Lawrentschuk N, Finelli A, Van der Kwast TH, Ryan P, Bolton DM, Fleshner NE, et al. Salvage radical prostatectomy following primary high intensity focused ultrasound for treatment of prostate cancer. J Urol. 2011;185(3):862–8.
2. Riviere J, Bernhard JC, Robert G, Wallerand H, Deti E, Maurice-Tison S, et al. Salvage radiotherapy after high-intensity focussed ultrasound for recurrent localised prostate cancer. Eur Urol. 2010;58(4):567–73.
3. Matillon X, Crouzet S, Murat FJ, Cherasse A, Gelet A, Martin X. Cryothérapie de rattrapage pour récidive de cancer de prostate après radiothérapie externe. 106ème Congrès Français d'Urologie; 2012; Paris 2012.
4. Gelet A, Chapelon JY, Margonari J, Theillere Y, Gorry F, Cathignol D, et al. Prostatic tissue destruction by high-intensity focused ultrasound: experimentation on canine prostate. J Endourol. 1993;7(3):249–53.
5. Gelet A, Chapelon JY, Margonari J, Theillere Y, Gorry F, Souchon R, et al. High-intensity focused ultrasound experimentation on human benign prostatic hypertrophy. Eur Urol. 1993;23 Suppl 1:44–7.
6. Beerlage HP, Thuroff S, Debruyne FM, Chaussy C, de la Rosette JJ. Transrectal high-intensity focused ultrasound using the Ablatherm device in the treatment of localized prostate carcinoma. Urology. 1999;54(2):273–7.
7. Beerlage HP, van Leenders GJ, Oosterhof GO, Witjes JA, Ruijter ET, van de Kaa CA, et al. High-intensity focused ultrasound (HIFU) followed after one to two weeks by radical retropubic prostatectomy: results of a prospective study. Prostate. 1999;39(1):41–6.
8. Kennedy JE, Ter Haar GR, Cranston D. High intensity focused ultrasound: surgery of the future? Br J Radiol. 2003;76(909):590–9.
9. Styn N, Hall TL, Fowlkes JB, Cain CA, Roberts WW. Histotripsy homogenization of the prostate: thresholds for cavitation damage of periprostatic structures. J Endourol. 2011;25(9):1531–5.
10. Chavrier F, Chapelon JY, Gelet A, Cathignol D. Modeling of high-intensity focused ultrasound-induced lesions in the presence of cavitation bubbles. J Acoust Soc Am. 2000;108(1):432–40.
11. Rouviere O, Souchon R, Salomir R, Gelet A, Chapelon JY, Lyonnet D. Transrectal high-intensity focused ultrasound ablation of prostate cancer: effective treatment requiring accurate imaging. Eur J Radiol. 2007;63(3):317–27.
12. Rouviere O, Glas L, Girouin N, Mege-Lechevallier F, Gelet A, Dantony E, et al. Prostate cancer ablation with transrectal high-intensity focused ultrasound: assessment of tissue destruction with contrast-enhanced US. Radiology. 2011;259(2):583–91.

13. Chen WH, Sanghvi NT, Carlson R, Uchida T. Real-time tissue change monitoring on the Sonablate 500 during high intensity focused ultrasound (HIFU) treatment of prostate cancer. AIP Conf Proc. 2001;391–6.

14. Bostrom PJ, Soloway MS. Secondary cancer after radiotherapy for prostate cancer: should we be more aware of the risk? Eur Urol. 2007;52(4):973–82.

15. Mouraviev V, Mayes JM, Polascik TJ. Pathologic basis of focal therapy for early-stage prostate cancer. Nat Rev Urol. 2009;6(4):205–15.

16. Crouzet S, Murat FJ, Pommier P, Poissonnier L, Pasticier G, Rouviere O, et al. Locally recurrent prostate cancer after initial radiation therapy: early salvage high-intensity focused ultrasound improves oncologic outcomes. Radiother Oncol. 2012;105(2):198–202.

17. Murat FJ, Poissonnier L, Rabilloud M, Belot A, Bouvier R, Rouviere O, et al. Mid-term results demonstrate salvage high-intensity focused ultrasound (HIFU) as an effective and acceptably morbid salvage treatment option for locally radiorecurrent prostate cancer. Eur Urol. 2009;55(3):640–7.

18. Leibovici D, Spiess PE, Heller L, Rodriguez-Bigas M, Chang G, Pisters LL. Salvage surgery for locally recurrent prostate cancer after radiation therapy: tricks of the trade. Urol Oncol. 2008;26(1):9–16.

19. Uchida T, Ohkusa H, Nagata Y, Hyodo T, Satoh T, Irie A. Treatment of localized prostate cancer using high-intensity focused ultrasound. BJU Int. 2006;97(1):56–61.

20. Salomir R, Vimeux FC, de Zwart JA, Grenier N, Moonen CT. Hyperthermia by MR-guided focused ultrasound: accurate temperature control based on fast MRI and a physical model of local energy deposition and heat conduction. Magn Reson Med. 2000;43(3):342–7.

21. Chopra R, Burtnyk M, Haider MA, Bronskill MJ. Method for MRI-guided conformal thermal therapy of prostate with planar transurethral ultrasound heating applicators. Phys Med Biol. 2005;50(21):4957–75.

22. Rouviere O, Lyonnet D, Raudrant A, Colin-Pangaud C, Chapelon JY, Bouvier R, et al. MRI appearance of prostate following transrectal HIFU ablation of localized cancer. Eur Urol. 2001;40(3):265–74.

23. Kirkham AP, Emberton M, Hoh IM, Illing RO, Freeman AA, Allen C. MR imaging of prostate after treatment with high-intensity focused ultrasound. Radiology. 2008;246(3):833–44.

24. Rouvière O, Glas L, Girouin N, Mège-Lechevallier F, Gelet A, Dantony E, et al. Prostate cancer ablation with transrectal high-intensity focused ultrasound: assessment of tissue destruction with contrast-enhanced US. Radiology. 2011;259(2):583–91.

25. Pasticier G, Chapet O, Badet L, Ardiet JM, Poissonnier L, Murat FJ, et al. Salvage radiotherapy after high-intensity focused ultrasound for localized prostate cancer: early clinical results. Urology. 2008;72(6):1305–9.

26. Rouviere O, Mege-Lechevallier F, Chapelon JY, Gelet A, Bouvier R, Boutitie F, et al. Evaluation of Color Doppler in guiding prostate biopsy after HIFU ablation. Eur Urol. 2006;50(3):490–7.

27. Ben Cheikh A, Girouin N, Ryon-Taponnier P, Mege-Lechevallier F, Gelet A, Chapelon JY, et al. MR detection of local prostate cancer recurrence after transrectal high-intensity focused US treatment: preliminary results. J Radiol. 2008;89(5 Pt 1):571–7.

28. Rouviere O, Girouin N, Glas L, Ben Cheikh A, Gelet A, Mege-Lechevallier F, et al. Prostate cancer transrectal HIFU ablation: detection of local recurrences using T2-weighted and dynamic contrast-enhanced MRI. Eur Radiol. 2010;20(1):48–55.

29. Muto S, Yoshii T, Saito K, Kamiyama Y, Ide H, Horie S. Focal therapy with high-intensity-focused ultrasound in the treatment of localized prostate cancer. Jpn J Clin Oncol. 2008;38(3):192–9.

30. Ahmed HU, Freeman A, Kirkham A, Sahu M, Scott R, Allen C, et al. Focal therapy for localized prostate cancer: a phase I/II trial. J Urol. 2011;185(4):1246–54.

31. Crouzet S, Villers A, Rischmann P, Pasticier G, Chevallier D, Rouviere O, et al. Focal treatment of prostate cancer with HIFU. 5th International symposium on focal therapy and imaging in prostate & kidney cancer, Duke, 2012.

32. Ahmed HU, Hindley RG, Dickinson L, Freeman A, Kirkham AP, Sahu M, et al. Focal therapy for localised unifocal and multifocal prostate cancer: a prospective development study. Lancet Oncol. 2012;13(6):622–32.
33. Ahmed HU, Cathcart P, McCartan N, Kirkham A, Allen C, Freeman A, et al. Focal salvage therapy for localized prostate cancer recurrence after external beam radiotherapy: a pilot study. Cancer. 2012;118(17):4148–55.
34. Baco E, Gelet A, Crouzet S, Rud E, Rouvière O, Tonoli-Catez H, et al. Hemi salvage high-intensity focused ultrasound (HIFU) in unilateral radiorecurrent prostate cancer: a prospective two-centre study. BJU Int. 2014;114(4):532–40.

Jean-Marc Cosset and Noelle Pierrat

13.1   Introduction

Recent data have triggered a worldwide interest in new techniques of "limited" prostate cancer treatment: "focal" techniques that would be able to selectively treat (and eradicate) a well-defined tumoral area of the prostate. It is hoped that in addition to leading to the same cure rate as the "classic" therapies, those focal prostate therapies could reasonably be expected to lead to a number of advantages: (1) They will overcome the limitations and the doubts about "active surveillance," which is sometimes poorly accepted psychologically by some patients (and in some countries). (2) They may provide a reasonable answer to accusations of "overtreatment," more and more often addressed to the clinicians' aggressively treating the whole prostate when the tumor involvement is limited. (3) The expected toxicity of the "focal" therapies can reasonably be anticipated to be low, and, it is hoped, lower than the treatment of a whole prostate. (4) The possibilities of a "salvage treatment" after such focal therapies would most probably be easier than after the conventional treatment of the whole prostate.

Among the techniques that can be proposed to focally treat the prostate, brachytherapy stands as an interesting competitor. In this chapter, after a rapid reminder of the principles of prostate brachytherapy, we concentrate on the selection of patients, on the various techniques that can be proposed to patients, and on the still limited data dealing with the preliminary results of such a prostate focal brachytherapy

J.-M. Cosset (✉)
Department of Urology, Institut Mutualiste Montsouris,
Paris 75014, France

Department of Oncology/Radiotherapy, Institut Curie,
Paris 75005, France
e-mail: jeanmarc.cosset@gmail.com

N. Pierrat
Department of Oncology/Radiotherapy, Institut Curie,
Paris 75005, France

© Springer-Verlag France 2015
E. Barret, M. Durand (eds.), *Technical Aspects of Focal Therapy
in Localized Prostate Cancer*, DOI 10.1007/978-2-8178-0484-2_13

procedure, in terms of biochemical control, side effects, and complications, available in the literature.

13.2   Principles of Prostate Brachytherapy

Born in the very first decades of the twentieth century, brachytherapy is defined as the technique of radiotherapy that uses radioactive sources located at contact of the tumors, or directly implanted in these tumors. Actually, the term *brachytherapy* derives from the Greek word for "short" – *brachy* (βραχμζ), referring to the distance between the therapeutic agent and the target lesion. In France, the technique is named "Curiethérapie," in honor of Pierre and Marie Curie.

Brachytherapy started essentially with radium tubes and needles, and as early as 1913 a few authors proposed using radium to treat prostate cancers. In the first decades of the twentieth century, various brachytherapy techniques were proposed, and actually performed, using the insertion of radium tubes in the urethra, or the implantation of radium needles directly into the prostate. Mostly because of radioprotection problems, the use of radium was abandoned in most countries in the 1970s–1980s. and gold seeds (Au198) were then proposed to replace radium as the radioactive sources to be used for prostate implantation. But the real step forward was the introduction of iodine 125 seeds (and later on of the palladium 103 seeds), together with the introduction of endorectal echography, which allowed the brachytherapists to master a precise positioning of their seeds in the prostate. Of note is that all the above mentioned seeds are low-dose rate (LDR) sources, used for permanent implants.

With the experience of more than 25 years for the pioneers, permanent implant brachytherapy using (essentially) iodine 125 seeds is now recognized as a valuable alternative therapy for localized low-risk prostate cancer patients [1, 2]. The possible extension of the indications of exclusive brachytherapy toward selected patients in the intermediate-risk group has now been confirmed by several studies [3]. Moreover, for other patients in the intermediate-risk group and for patients of the high-risk group, brachytherapy, as an addition to external radiotherapy, could represent one of the best ways to escalate the dose for selected patients [3].

Various permanent implant brachytherapy techniques have been proposed: preplanning or real-time procedures, with loose or stranded seeds (or a combination of both), manual or automatic injection of the seeds. The main point here is the ability to master the procedure and to comply with the dosimetric constraints that have been defined by the international societies [4, 5]. Mid- and long-term results that are now available in the literature indicate relapse-free survival rates of about 90 % at 5–10 years, the best results being obtained with satisfactory dosimetric data [3, 2]. Comparative data have shown that the incontinence and impotence rates after brachytherapy seemed to be significantly lower than those currently observed after surgery. However, a risk of urinary retention up to 5–10 % is often reported after brachytherapy, as well as an irritative urinary syndrome that may significantly alter the quality of life of the patients and last for several months.

More recently, high-dose rate (HDR) sources have been introduced for prostate brachytherapy, first to "boost" an external irradiation [6], and more and more as monotherapy [7, 8].

13.3   Selection of Patients

The selection of patients for focal treatment of prostate cancer is obviously of paramount importance.

Most authors advise only offering this treatment to a carefully selected subpopulation among "low-risk" localized prostate cancer patients, and a number of the authors have devoted specific papers to this topic [9–14]. Two authors [15, 16], among others, insisted on the importance of performing transperineal template-guided mapping biopsy (TTMB) in the initial and repeat biopsy setting. As a whole, most authors presently base their patients' selection for focal therapy on more than 20 transperineal biopsies (often in two series) thus allowing a real prostate "cartography" as well as on the more sophisticated imaging techniques available, such as multiparametric MRI [17, 18] and choline PET-CT scans [14].

Overall, a recently published consensus [14] defined as selection criteria for focal low-dose rate brachytherapy: 1) a life expectancy of more than 10 years; 2) a PSA less than or equal to 15 ng/mL; 3) the use of a multiparametric (T1W/T2W, diffusion-weighting, dynamic contrast enhancement ± spectroscopy) magnetic resonance imaging prior to biopsy (in order to avoid the false images linked to the biopsies); 4) bilateral template-guided prostate mapping biopsy with 5 mm sampling frame; 5) unilateral disease, lesion size ≤0.5 mL (approximately equates to maximum cancer length of 10 mm) with or without clinically insignificant disease on the contralateral side (cancer core length ≤3 mm); 6) Gleason score of index lesion 6–7 (3+4), (7) tumor stage ≤T2b (clinical); and 8) prostate size ≤60 mL.

In one of the rare published series on focal brachytherapy [19], patients among the low-risk disease group were selected as follows: life expectancy of more than 10 years, clinical stage T1c or T2a, MRI (multiparametric MRI, most often with an endorectal probe) stage T1c or T2a, prostate-specific antigen (PSA) less than 10 ng/mL, Gleason score less than or equal to 7 (3+4), unilateral disease, no individual biopsy core with more than 50 % involvement, no more than 25 % of cores involved, a total number of biopsies exceeding 20 (with a minimum of two series performed a few months apart, the second series being usually for "saturation": a minimum of 20 biopsies systematically involving all quadrants, realizing a prostate "cartography"), a total prostate volume no greater than 60 cubic centimeters (cc) on the pre-implantation endorectal ultrasound or MRI, and an IPSS score equal to or less than 15. Although established 2 years prior to the publication by the panel of experts on patient selection for focal therapy in 2012 [14], those selection criteria were actually very close to their consensus.

13.4   Types of Focal Brachytherapy

It is currently accepted that the clinical target volume (CTV) for prostate brachytherapy should be the whole prostate gland plus a 3 mm margin, possibly reduced to 1–2 mm, in particular posteriorly, to better spare the anterior rectal wall [4, 5]. When dealing with a focal brachytherapy, new terminology should be proposed. The abovementioned consensus paper [14] proposed F (for focal) Gross Target

Volume (F-GTV) for the gross visible or clinically demonstrable location and extent of the targeted cancer. Focal Clinical Target Volume (F-CTV) corresponds to the F-GTV plus the area of clinically insignificant disease. Focal Planned Target Volume (F-PTV) corresponds to the F-CTV plus a margin to compensate for uncertainties in image registration and treatment delivery. The authors of the consensus wrote that 'the actual margin size is undetermined at the present time.'

Moreover, the consensus paper describes three types of focal brachytherapy: "ultrafocal" brachytherapy, covering the gross lesion (GTV) with a margin (to be determined – see above); "focal" brachytherapy, for the authors, corresponding to a hemi-gland; and "focused" brachytherapy, an option that might be considered with 145 Gy given to the side of the prostate with the index lesion plus a lower dose applied to the contralateral side. Of note, this last proposal is close to the procedure already applied by a number of groups, delivering 145 Gy to the entire prostate, with a focal "boost" for the index lesion.

13.5　Techniques

A number of techniques have been proposed for focal treatments of prostate cancers (reviews by [20–22]): cryotherapy [23], HIFU-High Intensity Focused Ultrasounds [24, 25], photodynamic therapy, and laser-activated nanoparticles.

Brachytherapy can offer two techniques, using either low-dose rate (LDR) sources (essentially using iodine-125 and palladium-103 seeds,) or high-dose rate (HDR) sources (iridium 192 or cobalt 60).

In contrast with some of the techniques mentioned above, brachytherapy (LDR and HDR) benefits from an accurate dosimetry, being able to deliver a very precise dose in a very precise volume of the prostate. Moreover, a focal implantation (in the same way as the conventional "whole-prostate" implantation) is able to "cover" 3–5 mm *outside* the prostate, thus efficiently treating possible limited extracapsular extensions, which could have been left undetected by the pretreatment workup.

For an "ultrafocal" volume, due to the limited number of seeds to be implanted, the precise positioning of each seed is more important than for a whole-prostate implantation. One of the simplest techniques to be used (for ultrafocal brachytherapy) can be directly derived from a "real-time total prostate" procedure [26, 27], with the implantation of "free" iodine-125 seeds and with dynamic dose calculations (continuous feedback as per the actual position of each seed). The consensus paper [14] indicates that for the ultrafocal protocol, the use of loose seeds "might be preferable."

A double contour is usually performed; the whole prostate first, then the chosen volume to be treated. The drawing of the latter volume should be based on the site of the positive biopsies and on the MRI images. A rather large safety margin should probably be planned around the gross lesion (at least 1 cm). For what is defined in the consensus report [14] as the F-PTV for an "ultrafocal" treatment, the treated volume could represent about one-third of the total prostatic volume (Figs. 13.1 and 13.2) [19].

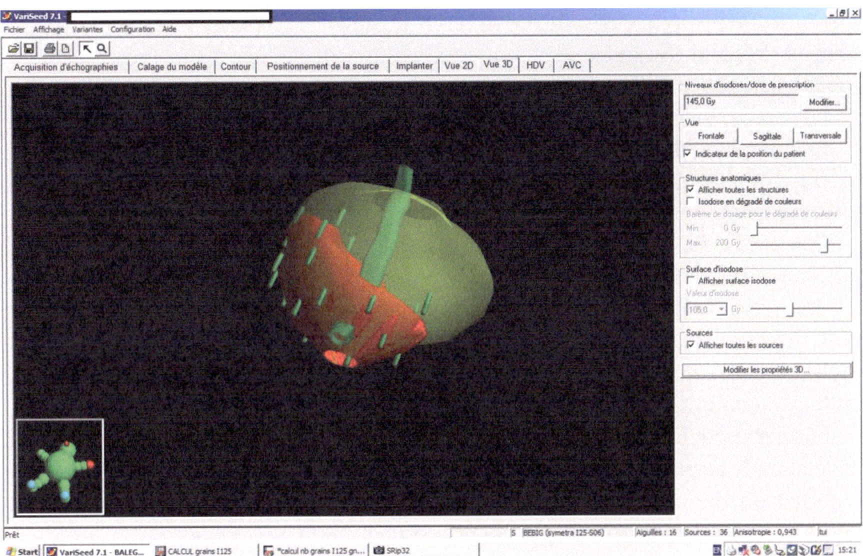

Fig. 13.1 Focal brachytherapy of the right apex; Choice of the volume and preplanning

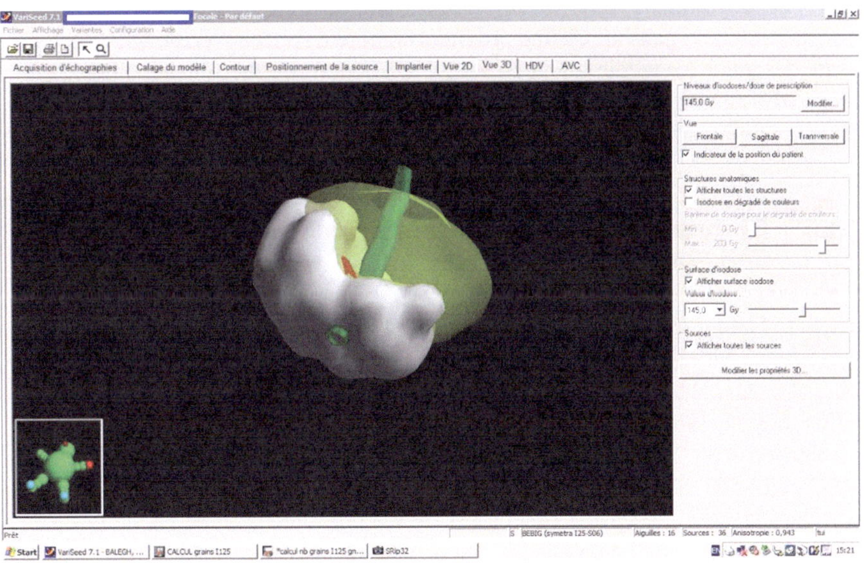

Fig. 13.2 Focal brachytherapy of the right apex; Isodose 145 Gy

Either a set of equally-spaced needles is implanted within the chosen volume, or a first set of needles is implanted at the periphery of the focal volume (focal "peripheral" needles), with a second set subsequently implanted according to a preplanning. Once the preplanning for the focal volume is performed, loose seeds can be implanted in a single step, with continuous dosimetric feedback as each iodine-125 seed is dropped. Stranded seeds, a combination of stranded and loose seeds, or seeds intercalated with "spacers" can also been proposed, mostly for "focal" (hemi-gland) brachytherapy.

In contrast with conventional whole-prostate brachytherapy, where the seeds are usually implanted at the periphery of the prostate, for those ultrafocal or hemifocal [14] implantations, the seeds are evenly distributed within the focal volume.

The dose to be delivered to the focal volume is usually the dose recommended by ABS and GEC-ESTRO for the whole prostate (145 Gy) [4, 5]. The dose constraints for the rectum and the urethra remained the same as those advised by ABS and GEC-ESTRO. The already-mentioned consensus paper [14] insists on the fact that high consideration should be given to the organs at risk: urethra, rectum, penile bulb, and contralateral neurovascular bundle at the apex.

Further modeling may be required for prescription dose recommendations. We have already seen details of the types of focal brachytherapy (Sect. 13.4). A group reported on the validation of a radiobiological model for low-dose-rate prostate boost focal therapy treatment planning [28].

Finally, post-implant dosimetry remains mandatory in all cases; it should be conducted at least at 4–8 weeks, with or without an early control at 24 h.

Focal high-dose rate (HDR) is an alternative; in the model proposed by Kamrava et al. [29], hemi-gland (HG) plans yielded a statistically significant decreased radiation dose to the organs at risk and provided complete target coverage with a catheter array designed for whole-gland coverage. The good dosimetry results obtained in this study support the feasibility of hemi-gland brachytherapy by using a subset of the whole-gland catheter array.

13.6 Review of Literature: Oncological and Functional Outcomes

13.6.1 First-Line Focal Brachytherapy

Very few series have been reported so far on focal brachytherapy being proposed as a first monotherapy.

Nguyen et al. [30] updated the results of a cohort of 318 patients treated between 1997 and 2007. The selection criteria were clinical T1c, prostate-specific antigen less than 15 ng/ml, Gleason 3+4 or less. All patients received magnetic resonance imaging-guided brachytherapy in which only the peripheral zone was targeted. Median follow-up was 5.1 years (maximum 12.1 years). For intermediate-risk cases, survival was 73.0 % (55.0–84.8) at 5 years and 66.4 % (44.8–81.1) at 8 years. The author concludes that further follow-up will determine whether magnetic resonance imaging-guided brachytherapy targeting the peripheral zone produces comparable cancer control to whole-gland treatment in men with low-risk disease. However, they believe that at this time the technique does not appear adequate for men with even favorable intermediate-risk disease. Of note, this type of "partial" (peripheral only) implantation is rather different from the various current proposals of "focal" brachytherapy [14].

The Paris group [19] published a preliminary series of 21 patients who underwent focal brachytherapy between February 2010 and March 2012. This highly selected series represented only 3.7 % of the cases treated by the group during that period; patient selection was based on (at least) two series of prostate biopsies and on a high-resolution magnetic resonance imaging (MRI). Only patients with very limited and localized tumors, according to strict criteria (see Sect. 13.3), were selected for the procedure. The technique used a real-time procedure with the implantation of free iodine-125 seeds, and dynamic dose calculation. The prescribed dose for the focal volume was 145 Gray (Gy).

In terms of dosimetry, the treated volume corresponded to a mean value of 34 % of the total prostatic volume (range 20–48 %). For the focal volume, mean D90 was 183.2 Gy (range 176–188 Gy), and the mean V100 was 99.3 % (range 98.8–100 %).

In terms of biological evolution, the mean initial PSA was 6.9 ng/mL (range 3.6–13.9). At 2 months, the mean PSA was 5.5 (range 1.8–14.2) with five patients experiencing a moderate increase from the initial value. At 12 months, the mean value dropped to 2.6 ng/mL. The follow-up of this series is far too short to allow any conclusions, apart from the observation of a PSA decrease in all cases at 1 year.

A systematic histologic follow-up was planned in the study, with post-implant biopsies to be performed 12–24 months after the focal treatment. Six patients underwent control biopsies 14–27 months after the implantation. In five of them, the biopsies were negative; in one patient, on biopsies performed at 2 years, a Gleason 6 (3+3) lesion measuring less than 1 mm was found at the right base. The focal brachytherapy had targeted the left base. Of note for this patient, the PSA dropped from an initial value of 5.44 to 1.25 ng/mL at 2 years post-implant. After discussion, it was decided to offer this patient a strict active surveillance of this microlesion, with regular PSAs and MRIs.

In terms of toxicity, when compared with a previous cohort treated by whole-prostate brachytherapy, at 6 months urinary toxicity (International Prostate Symptom Score) was borderline reduced ($p=0.04$), while the recovery of the International Index of Erectile Function (IIEF5) was better ($p=0.014$). The Incontinence Score (ICS) was nil in almost all cases, as was rectal toxicity.

The question of post-focal therapy morbidity was also addressed by Barret et al. [31] in a series of 106 patients treated by various focal procedures; overall morbidity was acceptable with less than 2 % major complications.

13.6.2 Focal Brachytherapy for Salvage

Salvage *whole-prostate* permanent implant brachytherapy after failure of a previous external irradiation has been proposed by several authors, with results that were sometimes encouraging [32], but sometimes less so [33]. Other groups have used HDR techniques with interesting preliminary results [34, 35]. A clear limit of these procedures involving the whole prostate is their toxicity.

In such a context, Wallace et al. [36] postulated that the use of multiparametric MRI-directed focal salvage permanent interstitial brachytherapy for locally recurrent adenocarcinoma of the prostate is a promising strategy for avoiding more aggressive and expensive treatments that are associated with increased morbidity, potentially improving survival at potentially lower costs.

Reporting on 15 patients who underwent MRI/magnetic resonance spectroscopy (MRS) planning for salvage brachytherapy, Hsu et al. [37] specified that a full dose was prescribed to "areas of recurrence and underdosage, without entire prostate implantation" (thus a "focal" salvage treatment). He concludes that such a technique is feasible with short-term control comparable to conventional salvage, with less toxicity.

Conclusion

In conclusion, focal brachytherapy is still in its infancy; very few results are available to date, and most of them lack sufficient follow-up. Only the preliminary toxicity data appears to be encouraging, with a (logical) trend toward less pronounced urinary and sexual toxicity, which will have to be confirmed. In such a context, focal brachytherapy must be implemented with great care in very select patients.

However, due to its ability to treat a well-defined partial prostatic volume with a precise dose, also due to the possibility of treating a few millimeters outside the prostate adjacent to the lesion, focal brachytherapy could stand as one of the best focal techniques to be proposed to carefully selected patients.

It remains clear in 2013 that more follow-up and more cases are necessary to demonstrate that focal brachytherapy could achieve the same satisfactory results in terms of relapse-free survival as the conventional "whole" prostate brachytherapy in selected patients, with hopefully less toxicity and easier salvage treatment in case of a relapse.

References

1. Crook J. The role of brachytherapy in the definitive management of prostate cancer. Cancer Radiother. 2011;15(3):230–7.
2. Cosset JM, Hannoun-Lévi JM, Peiffert D, Delannes M, Pommier P, et al. Permanent implant prostate cancer brachytherapy: 2013 state-of-the art. Cancer Radiother. 2013;17(2):111–7.
3. Grimm P, Billiet I, Bostwick D, Dicker AP, Frank S, Immerzeel J, et al. Comparative analysis of prostate-specific antigen free survival outcomes for patients with low, intermediate and high risk prostate cancer treatment by radical therapy. Results from the Prostate Cancer Results Study Group. BJU Int. 2012;109 Suppl 1:22–9.
4. Salembier C, Lavagnini P, Nickers P, Mangili P, Rijnders A, Polo A, et al.; For the GEC ESTRO PROBATE Group. Tumour and target volumes in permanent prostate brachytherapy: a supplement to the ESTRO/EAU/EORTC recommendations on prostate brachytherapy. Radiother Oncol. 2007;83(1):3–10.
5. Davis BJ, Horwitz EM, Lee WR, Crook JM, Stock RG, Merrick GS, et al. American Brachytherapy Society consensus guidelines for transrectal ultrasound-guided permanent prostate brachytherapy. Brachytherapy. 2012;11(1):6–19.

6. Hoskin PJ, Rojas AM, Bownes PJ, Lowe GJ, Ostler PJ, Bryant L. Randomised trial of external beam radiotherapy alone or combined with high-dose-rate brachytherapy boost for localised prostate cancer. Radiother Oncol. 2012;103(2):217–22.

7. Ghilezan M, Martinez A, Gustason G, Krauss D, Antonucci JV, Chen P, et al. High-dose-rate brachytherapy as monotherapy delivered in two fractions within one day for favorable/intermediate-risk prostate cancer: preliminary toxicity data. Int J Radiat Oncol Biol Phys. 2012;83(3):927–32.

8. Hoskin P, Rojas A, Lowe G, Bryant L, Ostler P, Hughes R, et al. High-dose-rate brachytherapy alone for localized prostate cancer in patients at moderate or high risk of biochemical recurrence. Int J Radiat Oncol Biol Phys. 2012;82(4):1376–84.

9. Sartor AO, Hricak H, Wheeler TM. Evaluating localized prostate cancer and identifying candidates for focal therapy. Urology. 2008;6(Suppl):S12–24.

10. Jayram G, Eggener SE. Patient selection for focal therapy of localized prostate cancer. Curr Opin Urol. 2009;19:268–73.

11. Polascik TJ, Mouraviev V. Focal therapy for prostate cancer is a reasonable treatment option in properly selected patients. Urology. 2009;74:726–30.

12. Mouraviev V, Mayes JM, Polascik TJ. Pathologic basis of focal therapy for early-stage prostate cancer. Nat Rev Urol. 2009;6:205–15.

13. Tsivian M, Kimura M, Sun L, Mouraviev V, Mayes JM, Polascik TJ. Predicting unilateral prostate cancer on routine diagnostic biopsy: sextant vs extended. BJU Int. 2010;105:1089–92.

14. Langley S, Ahmed HU, Al-Qaisieh B, Bostwick D, Dickinson L, Veiga FG, et al. Report of a consensus meeting on focal low dose rate brachytherapy for prostate cancer. BJU Int. 2012;109 Suppl 1:7–16.

15. Bott SR, Henderson A, Halls JE, Montgomery BS, Laing R, Langley SE. Extensive transperineal template biopsies of prostate: modified technique and results. Urology. 2006;68:1037–41.

16. Taira AV, Merrick GS, Galbreath RW, Andreini H, Taubenslag W, Curtis R, et al. Performance of transperineal template-guided mapping biopsy in detecting prostate cancer in the initial and repeat biopsy setting. Prostate Cancer Prostatic Dis. 2010;13:71–7.

17. Rastinehad AR, Baccala Jr AA, Chung PH, Proano JM, Kruecker J, Xu S, et al. D'Amico risk stratification correlates with degree of suspicion of prostate cancer on multiparametric magnetic resonance imaging. J Urol. 2011;185:815–20.

18. Rosenkrantz AB, Scionti SM, Mendrinos S, Taneja SS. Role of MRI in minimally invasive focal ablative therapy for prostate cancer. Am J Roentgenol. 2011;1:W90–6.

19. Cosset JM, Cathelineau X, Wakil G, Pierrat N, Quenzer O, Prapotnich D, et al. Focal brachytherapy for selected low-risk prostate cancers: a pilot study. Brachytherapy. 2013;12(4):331–7.

20. Marberger M, Carroll PR, Zelefsky MJ, Coleman JA, Hricak H, Scardino PT, et al. New treatments for localized prostate cancer. Urology. 2008;72(6 Suppl):S36–43.

21. Ahmed HU, Moore C, Emberton M. Minimally-invasive technologies in uro-oncology: the role of cryotherapy, HIFU and photodynamic therapy in whole gland and focal therapy of localised prostate cancer. Surg Oncol. 2009;18:219–32.

22. Bozzini G, Colin P, Nevoux P, Villers A, Mordon S, Betrouni N. Focal therapy of prostate cancer: energies and procedures. Urol Oncol. 2013;31(2):155–67.

23. Bahn DK, Silverman PD. Focal cryoablation of prostate: a review. ScientificWorldJournal. 2008;8:486–91.

24. Chaussy CG, Thüroff S. Transrectal high-intensity focused ultrasound for local treatment of prostate cancer: current role. Arch Esp Urol. 2011;64:493–506.

25. El Fegoun AB, Barret E, Prapotnich D, Soon S, Cathelineau X, Rozet F, et al. Focal therapy with high-intensity focused ultrasound for prostate cancer in the elderly. A feasibility study with 10 years follow-up. Int Braz J Urol. 2011;37:213–9.

26. Chauveinc L, Flam T, Solignac S, Thiounn N, Firmin F, Debré B, et al. Prostate cancer brachytherapy: is real-time ultrasound-based dosimetry predictive of subsequent CT-based dose

distribution calculation? A study of 450 patients by the Institut Curie/Hospital Cochin (Paris) Group. Int J Radiat Oncol Biol Phys. 2004;59:691–5.

27. Cosset JM, Flam T, Thiounn N, Gomme S, Rosenwald JC, Asselain B, et al. Selecting patients for exclusive permanent implant prostate brachytherapy: the experience of the Paris Institut Curie/Cochin Hospital/Necker Hospital group on 809 patients. Int J Radiat Oncol Biol Phys. 2008;71:1042–8.

28. Haworth A, Williams S, Reynolds H, Waterhouse D, Duchesne GM, Bucci J, et al. Validation of a radiobiological model for low-dose-rate prostate boost focal therapy treatment planning. Brachytherapy. 2013;12:628–36.

29. Kamrava M, Chung MP, Kayode O, Wang J, Marks L, Kupelian P. Focal high-dose-rate brachytherapy: a dosimetric comparison of hemigland vs. conventional whole-gland treatment. Brachytherapy. 2013;12:434–41.

30. Nguyen PL, Chen MH, Zhang Y, Tempany CM, Cormack RA, Beard CJ, et al. Updated results of magnetic resonance imaging guided partial prostate brachytherapy for favorable risk prostate cancer: implications for focal therapy. J Urol. 2012;188(4):1151–6.

31. Barret E, Ahallal Y, Sanchez-Salas R, Galiano M, Cosset JM, Validire P, et al. Morbidity of focal therapy in the treatment of localized prostate cancer. Eur Urol. 2013;63(4):618–22.

32. Gomez-Veiga F, Mariño A, Alvarez L, Rodriguez I, Fernandez C, Pertega S, et al. Brachytherapy for the treatment of recurrent prostate cancer after radiotherapy or radical prostatectomy. BJU Int. 2012;109 Suppl 1:17–21.

33. Peters M, Moman MR, van der Poel HG, Vergunst H, de Jong IJ, Vijverberg PL, et al. Patterns of outcome and toxicity after salvage prostatectomy, salvage cryosurgery and salvage brachytherapy for prostate cancer recurrences after radiation therapy: a multi-center experience and literature review. World J Urol. 2013;31(2):403–9.

34. Jo Y, Fujii T, Hara R, Yokoyama T, Miyaji Y, Yoden E, et al. Salvage high-dose-rate brachytherapy for local prostate cancer recurrence after radiotherapy – preliminary results. BJU Int. 2012;109(6):835–9.

35. Chen CP, Weinberg V, Shinohara K, Roach 3rd M, Nash M, Gottschalk A. Salvage HDR brachytherapy for recurrent prostate cancer after previous definitive radiation therapy: 5-year outcomes. Int J Radiat Oncol Biol Phys. 2013;86(2):324–9.

36. Wallace T, Avital I, Stojadinovic A, Brücher BL, Cote E, Yu J. Multi-parametric MRI-directed focal salvage permanent interstitial brachytherapy for locally recurrent adenocarcinoma of the prostate: a novel approach. J Cancer. 2013;4(2):146–51.

37. Hsu CC, Hsu H, Pickett B, Crehange G, Hsu IC, Dea R, et al. Feasibility of MR imaging/MR spectroscopy-planned focal partial salvage permanent prostate implant (PPI) for localized recurrence after initial PPI for prostate cancer. Int J Radiat Oncol Biol Phys. 2013;85(2):370–7.

Ashley J. Ridout, Mark Emberton, and Caroline M. Moore

14.1 Principles of Photodynamic Therapy (PDT)

The use of light for the treatment of disease has been well reported in historical literature and can be traced back to ancient times. 'Heliotherapy', or whole body sun exposure, was popular in ancient Greece, and other ancient cultures used similar strategies for the treatment of skin diseases such as psoriasis and vitiligo. Sunlight exposure has also been used for treating other conditions, including scurvy, paralysis, oedema and muscle weakness. The potential contribution of light therapy was recognised with a Nobel Prize in 1903, for the use of carbon arc phototherapy in the treatment of cutaneous tuberculosis [1]. Currently, the therapeutic use of light takes various forms, including UVA light exposure for skin disease, phototherapy for jaundice in neonates and photodynamic therapy.

Photodynamic therapy (PDT) uses light of an appropriate wavelength to activate a photosensitising agent in the presence of oxygen, with cytotoxic effect. PDT was first used for the treatment of superficial lesions such as lupus vulgaris and skin cancers. Whilst early work used lamps for light delivery to the skin, the use of lasers for light delivery has allowed PDT to be delivered to both hollow and solid organs, and as a consequence the use of PDT has since expanded to include urological oncology and for benign and malignant disease at other sites. These include interstitial cancers of the head, neck [2] and pancreas [3] and skin conditions such as acne vulgaris [4] and age-related macular degeneration [5].

A.J. Ridout • M. Emberton • C.M. Moore, MD, FRCS (Urol) (⊠)
Division of Surgical and Interventional Science, University College London, London, UK

Department of Urology, University College London Hospitals NHS Foundation Trust,
3rd Floor, Charles Bell House, 67-73 Riding House Street, London W1W 7EJ, UK
e-mail: caroline.moore@ucl.ac.uk; carolinemoore@doctors.org.uk

© Springer-Verlag France 2015
E. Barret, M. Durand (eds.), *Technical Aspects of Focal Therapy
in Localized Prostate Cancer*, DOI 10.1007/978-2-8178-0484-2_14

The first urological use of PDT was for superficial bladder cancer, where light was applied to the bladder after intravenous administration of haematoporphyrin derivative (HpD) [6]. This procedure was complicated by significant side effects, with the potential for allergic reactions, and uptake of the photosensitiser in the skin required protection from light for several weeks. As a consequence, uptake of PDT for treatment of urological conditions was met with some resistance [7]. Technical improvements, including the transperineal approach to the prostate and advances in photosensitising agent properties, have translated into significant advances in the use of PDT in prostate cancer, for both whole gland and focal treatment of primary and recurrent disease. Use of light activation in a more localised area of the prostate offers the potential to provide a focal treatment for prostate cancer.

14.1.1 Mechanism of Action

Photodynamic therapy requires activation of a photosensitising (PS) agent, using light of a particular wavelength, in the presence of oxygen. After intravenous, oral or topical administration of the photosensitiser, the light promotes the photosensitiser (administered in its ground state and pharmacologically inactive until exposed to the appropriate wavelength) to a higher energy (singlet) state through absorption of a luminescent photon. Energy may be released from the activated photosensitiser in three ways – emission of heat, light, or conversion to an intermediate energy state (triplet state), before returning to its stable (ground) state. When in the intermediate state, the photosensitiser can produce hydroxyl and superoxide radicals (type 1 reaction) or convert tissue molecular oxygen to singlet oxygen (type 2 reaction). Singlet oxygen reacts with proteins, lipids and cellular nucleic acids, causing cell death through functional and structural damage (induction of necrosis and/or apoptosis), as well as hydroxyl and superoxide radicals. Singlet oxygen has an extremely short half-life and results in localised tissue damage and subsequent cell death. It is thought that type 2 reactions are more important for many photosensitisers [8]. The photosensitiser is subsequently destroyed by the singlet oxygen and the intermediate oxygen radicals – known as 'photobleaching', where the induced fluorescence decreases over time [9]. An acute inflammatory response is also implicated in tissue destruction, inducing leucocytes such as dendritic cells and neutrophils [10].

14.1.2 Photosensitisers

The ideal photosensitiser agent would be pharmacologically stable, non-toxic and accumulate preferentially in cancer cells. Activation by different wavelengths of light would increase potential therapeutic uses, with longer wavelengths producing deeper tissue penetration and allowing interstitial treatments. After treatment, the agent would quickly be washed out of the body, reducing the potential for side effects associated with residual photosensitivity.

Photosensitiser agents are either activated in the tissue or in the vasculature. Tissue-activated agents are associated with a delay of hours to days between drug administration and treatment (the 'drug-light interval'), whilst the agent reaches optimal tissue concentration. During this time, the agent can also accumulate in other tissues (such as the skin and eyes), causing photosensitivity. These areas must then be protected from light exposure, and this may be required for up to 6 weeks after drug administration. Vascular-activated agents achieve optimal concentration within the vessels within minutes, at which point the activating light can be administered. Resultant toxic radical oxygen species are limited to the vasculature, causing oxidative stress through endothelial effects, vasoconstriction and vessel occlusion [9, 11]. These agents are rapidly washed out from the vasculature, liver and skin. As a result, administration of the photosensitising agent and PDT treatment do not need to be separated in time, and a much shorter period of light protection is required. The first photosensitiser for vascular-targeted PDT (VTP) to be used in large-scale clinical trials in the prostate was WST-09, a palladium bacteriopheophorbide molecule, made from the bacteriochlorophyll a molecule [12]. Subsequently, a water-soluble derivate of palladium bacteriopheophorbide, WST-11, was produced by the same group [13]. Both agents are activated at light wavelengths near the infrared aspect wavelength (763 nm and 753–757 nm, respectively) and so can penetrate more deeply into tissue – this is advantageous for both interstitial treatment and treatment of larger volumes of tissue [11].

14.1.3 Photosensitiser Selectivity

The oncological uses of PDT rely upon the ability to treat tumour tissue whilst sparing normal tissue, and this is particularly relevant to the focal treatment of prostate cancer. This selectivity can be achieved either by use of selective uptake of the photosensitising agent to tumour cells, as happens with ALA for photodynamic diagnosis in the bladder or by the delivery of light selectively to the area to be treated. It has been observed that some photosensitisers preferentially accumulate in malignant cells [14]. Hydrophobic photosensitisers are transported with lipoproteins, and it may be that, due to low-density lipoprotein overexpression in tumours cells, photosensitisers are preferentially accumulated. In addition to this, at physiological pH, most photosensitiser agents are in an ionic state – at the lower pH associated with tumour cells, agents become increasingly lipophilic, and therefore absorption may be further increased [15].

If the photosensitiser agent can be targeted towards tumour cells specifically, there is likely to be a reduction in collateral damage and subsequent side effects. This may be possible through linkage to serum proteins (such as albumin) and subsequent uptake into cells via receptor-mediated endocytosis [16]. One such technique uses monoclonal antibody linkage – the use of prostate-specific membrane antigen (PSMA) has generated interest for both imaging and therapeutic purposes. In vitro studies have shown that photosensitiser-conjugated PSMA inhibitors have potential for the focal targeted treatment of prostate cancer [17]. Once thought of as the 'magic bullet' for targeted cancer therapy, disadvantages to the antibody-targeted approach have emerged. Monoclonal antibody use may be limited by the reduced photosensitivity of the combination as compared to the free photosensitiser agent, and, furthermore, the heterogeneity of antibody expression in prostate cancers may result in incomplete targeting to the tumour tissue. Consequently, interest has necessarily been directed towards other methods of targeting, including delivery of the photosensitiser agent into the cell rather than just to the cell surface. Suggested techniques have included linkage of the agent to serum proteins, annexins, bisphosphonates, steroids, toxins and lectins, epidermal growth factor, insulin and nuclear localisation signals and adenovirus and adenoviral proteins [18].

Other work attempted to increase specificity with development of a group of polymeric protease-specific photosensitiser prodrugs [19]. These incorporate enhanced permeability and retention due to a polymeric carrier; activation via cleavage of peptide linkers by urokinase-type plasminogen activator (uPA), which is overexpressed in prostate cancer tissues; and displaying increased sensitivity and production of toxic radicals when exposed to local irradiation. In vitro and animal studies have shown potential, but further work is required to establish the potential of this strategy for clinical PDT use. The main method of targeting in focal prostate PDT at present is, however, to deliver light only to those areas of the prostate which are to be treated.

14.2 Specific Indications and Limitations

The first clinical use of PDT in prostate cancer was reported in 1990, in two patients who underwent transurethral prostate resection 6 weeks prior to treatment. Each individual was treated transurethrally with a different tissue-based photosensitiser (haematoporphyrin derivative and porfimer sodium) [20]. Both patients showed decreasing PSA levels and were biopsied 3 months after treatment, with no histological evidence of residual disease (although one patient died 6 months after treatment for reasons not related to prostate cancer or his treatment). After this initial work, PDT was used in other solid-organ cancers, and interest in the use of PDT for prostate cancer treatment grew. Now, the use of PDT in prostate cancer has been evaluated for primary and salvage treatment, both on a whole gland and focal basis. It is an area of growing interest, but still remains controversial, and more evidence is required before it is integrated into mainstream practice. It is currently only available in centres participating in clinical trials.

14.2.1 Indications

Since its efficacy was proven in preclinical studies, use of PDT has been studied and reported for both primary prostate cancer treatment and treatment of disease that has recurred after radiotherapy. It has only been used in those with organ-confined disease, although there has been interest in the use of PDT for the treatment of

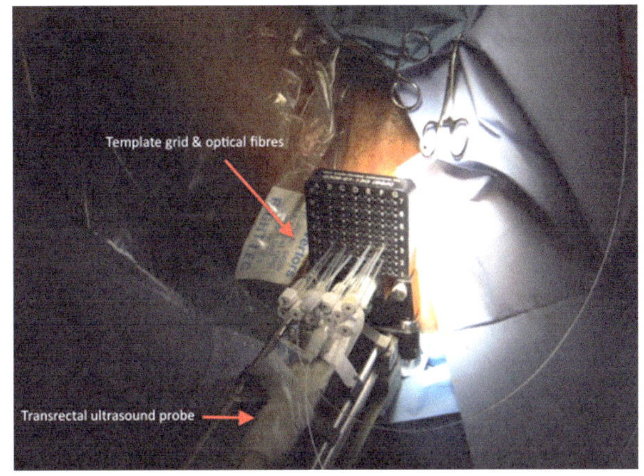

Fig. 14.1 Patient positioned in lithotomy position, with transperineal brachytherapy grid placed over the perineum and optical fibres inserted under transrectal ultrasound guidance

solitary bone metastases and for prostate bed recurrence after radical surgery. The potential advantage of PDT is the ability for selective destruction of tissue, respecting anatomical boundaries and preserving function. Animal model studies have suggested a differential effect between prostate tissue and the supportive stroma, and it was thought that this may preserve important functional structures, such as the urethra and urinary sphincter [21]. Whilst this has been shown in animal studies, it should be noted that in clinical use, care must be taken to ensure that an appropriate drug and light dose combination is used, with the light activating fibres correctly placed in order to avoid unwanted extraprostatic effects.

Advantages

The technical aspects of the procedure involve laser fibre placement (within hollow plastic brachytherapy needles) into the prostate (see Fig. 14.1). Anyone capable of accurate needle placement within the prostate, either from brachytherapy, cryotherapy or transperineal template-guided prostate biopsy experience would quickly be able to learn the technical aspects of delivery of photodynamic therapy. The transperineal placement of light delivery fibres also allows treatment of the anterior zones of larger prostates that may be out of reach of other transrectally delivered modalities, such as high-intensity focused ultrasound (HIFU), although needle placement in these individuals may be anatomically limited by the pubic arch. This can often be overcome by patient positioning, with legs in an extreme hip flexion modified lithotomy position, and occasionally by use of a sandbag or 1 litre bag of normal saline, to raise the pelvis.

As photosensitiser agents with short drug-light intervals are developed, PDT treatments can be carried out in a single session, without the need for multiple visits, making it an attractive option for patients who choose focal treatment in a day case setting [16]. Furthermore, it has been shown in a small study that PDT treatment can be repeated in the same region of the prostate, even in those who have been previously exposed to radiotherapy treatment, as it does not show the cumulative toxicity of ionising radiation [22].

Limitations

Clinical experience with this technique is limited to a small number of centres which have taken part in clinical trials. When using a new photosensitiser, it is necessary to do careful dose-escalation studies of both drug and light dose, in order to establish the most effective combination for a given drug. The dose response for this needs to be evaluated soon after the treatment, for example, with dynamic contrast-enhanced MR imaging at 1 week. This means that a dose-escalation programme in itself can be an expensive clinical research programme, even before true efficacy studies can be started.

14.3 Preclinical and Clinical Evidence for the Use of PDT in Prostate Cancer

14.3.1 Preclinical Studies

The canine prostate provides the closest anatomical animal model to the human prostate and so has been used as a disease model in both its benign condition and with spontaneously occurring prostate cancer. Feasibility for interstitial treatment of the prostate, using laser fibres placed within the gland, was demonstrated, and haemorrhagic necrosis and subsequent fibrosis and prostate volume reduction caused by the PDT procedure were shown [23]. Although never extending their results to clinical studies, this group modelled photosensitiser distribution, light penetration and PDT effect. Serial studies showed haemorrhage and necrosis around the light fibres with an average radius of 6 mm. They were able to closely predict necrosis in the canine model to within 2 mm [24]. This group suggested the importance of real-time monitoring, with analysis of the attenuation coefficient during treatment, and demonstrated the minimum energy required to produce tissue necrosis in their study, necessary to predict the area of ablation, and therefore to prevent damage to surrounding structures [25].

A variety of photosensitiser agents have been used in preclinical feasibility studies, including tin ethyl etiopurpurin dichloride [26], motexafin lutetium [27], porfimer sodium [28], disulphonated aluminium phthalocyanine and 5-aminolevulinic acid-induced protoporphyrin IX [21] and meso-tetra-(m-hydroxyphenyl) chlorin [29]. The vascular-activated agent, Tookad/WST-09, was first assessed in the canine prostate after radiation therapy [30]. This work was valuable in that it concluded that there was no difference in side effects between PDT used as a primary treatment and PDT used for salvage treatment in the canine prostate and showed that PDT could be used to ablate prostate tissue previously treated with ionising radiation. This highlighted the potential for the use of this form of PDT in the salvage treatment of radio-recurrent prostate cancer in humans. In this study, four dogs were pretreated with 20 fractions of ionising radiation to the prostate. Twenty to twenty-three weeks afterwards, they were treated with WST-09 PDT at 2 mg/kg, with escalating light doses of 50, 100 and 200 J/cm. There were no episodes of urinary retention, and histopathological analysis showed that lesion size correlated with light dose and the acute PDT effect could be clearly distinguished from the effects of previous radiation.

This group also showed gadolinium contrast-enhanced MRI most accurately corresponded to volume of PDT effect on whole-mount histopathology specimens, when compared with diffusion-weighted and T2-weighted imaging at 1 week after treatment [31]. They identified a central core of haemorrhagic necrosis, surrounded by atrophic glandular tissue, fibromuscular hyperplasia, neovascularisation, oedema and dilated glandular structures. The same group also reported an apparent resistance of peripheral nerves to PDT, compared to prostate, at corresponding drug and light dose levels [32]. It was hypothesised that this could eventually correspond to a 'nerve-sparing' approach in the clinical scenario, contextually similar to that employed during the radical prostatectomy, offering the chance to preserve erectile function.

Several of these animal model studies used the transperineal technique of laser fibre insertion (in contrast to the open technique of fibre insertion) [21, 23, 26, 27], which is much more clinically relevant to the treatment of humans. The transurethral delivery of light was also evaluated (although these studies revealed increased side effects due to urethral necrosis, including urinary retention and stricture formation, so the transurethral technique has not been further evaluated [24].

14.3.2 Clinical Studies

Although mostly carried out in the benign canine prostate, animal models helped to improve understanding of photosensitiser agent use, appropriate light doses and drug-light intervals, and this was subsequently translated into clinical studies. After the initial report of two patients treated with PDT [20], a clinical study into the use of PDT in patients with radio-recurrent disease was undertaken, and work was later extended to include those with previously untreated prostate cancer.

14.3.3 Radio-Recurrent Disease Treatment

The first formal study of patients with radio-recurrent disease was reported by Nathan et al. [22] – 14 patients with rising PSA and biopsy-proven local recurrence of prostate cancer after radiotherapy were treated with the tissue-activated photosensitiser agent meso-tetra-hydroxylphenyl-chlorin; mTHPC (temoporfin/'Foscan') at dose 0.15 mg/kg. This was activated 2–5 days after administration by laser light with wavelength 652 nm, transmitted through both bare fibres and cylindrical diffusing transperineal fibres inserted freehand in an open MRI scanner. Initially, lower light doses were used (based on canine studies), but the light dose was escalated, and 9/13 patients who received this higher light dose showed a PSA reduction (by up to 96 %) in the first 3–6 months after treatment, with negative biopsies in four of these men. Eventually all men showed a PSA rise, with ten requiring androgen therapy. Reported morbidities included five patients who reported skin sensitivity reactions after treatment and all patients reporting irritative symptoms during the first month after treatment. Four out of seven men with previously acceptable erectile function reported loss of sexual function. One individual developed a rectourethral fistula, following a posttreatment rectal biopsy of a red patch seen at proctoscopy. MR and CT imaging was used at an interval after the procedure (from several days to 2 months), and up to 91 % prostatic necrosis was seen on posttreatment imaging.

Other groups have used the photosensitiser motexafin lutetium (mLu/LuTex) in treatment of radio-recurrent disease. Studies were carried out to evaluate the feasibility [33] and maximally tolerated dose of this agent [34] and the time course of PSA response to treatment with this agent [35], although no posttreatment imaging was carried out in these studies. Various drug doses, fluences and drug-light intervals were assessed. Reports from 17 treated patients showed that, although there is initially a large increase in PSA, higher-dose PDT resulted in a longer period before biochemical relapse. It was concluded that oncological outcome was better in the group treated with a high-dose protocol –2 mg/kg photosensitiser dose, fluence 150 J/cm^2 and drug-light interval of 3 h, who showed the greatest delay to biochemical progression.

The vascular-activated agent WST-09 (Tookad) has been used in treatment of both recurrent and primary disease. Initial work reporting 24 patients treated with WST-09 first demonstrated drug safety, with a dose-escalation protocol of 0.1, 0.25, 0.5 and 2 mg/kg, respectively, with a fixed light dose of 100 J/cm, and then evaluated light dose-escalation protocols with treatment at 2 mg/kg drug dose with light escalation from 230 to 360 J/cm [36]. Eligibility criteria included histological evidence of radio-recurrent prostate cancer (Gleason >6). Additional criteria included life expectancy greater than 5 years, exclusion of metastatic disease with CT and bone scan, PSA <20 ng/ml and prostate volume <50 cm^3. The procedure was carried out under general anaesthesia with the patient in the lithotomy position. Optical fibres were placed transperineally, using a standard brachytherapy template. Hydrodissection (infiltration of saline between the rectum and prostate) was used to reduce light exposure to the rectum, with optical monitoring fibres in the prostate, rectum and urinary catheter. Intra-operative assessment of light dose was monitored, with removal or repositioning of the optical fibres if the rectal light dose exceeded that of the prostate by more than 10 %. No significant drug-related adverse effects were reported at the highest dose of 2 mg/kg, although there were several episodes of transient hypotension after drug infusion was commenced. Urinary, bowel and rectal functions were not significantly different between baseline and 6-month assessment [11], although most did report urinary symptoms in the initial weeks after treatment.

The same group went on to report their study of the efficacy of 2 mg/kg WST-09 for treatment of the whole prostate in 28 patients with radio-recurrent prostate cancer [37]. Doses and treatment plans were individually calculated with computer assistance prior to treatment, and up to six fibres were inserted per prostate lobe. Contrast-enhanced MRI was done at 7 days after the procedure, and patients were also followed up with PSA and prostate biopsy at 6 months after the procedure. As the study progressed, the light dose was increased, which tended to result in larger avascular areas demonstrated with MRI. They concluded that whole gland treatment was possible, with increased tissue response achieved with increased light dose. For complete response at 6-month biopsy, they suggest that light doses of at least 23 J/cm^2 were required in at least 90 % of the prostate volume.

14.3.4 Primary Disease Treatment

Zaak et al. reported their experience with six patients with localised prostate cancer, treated with 5-aminolevulinic acid (5-ALA) PDT at the dose of 20 mg/kg [38]. 5-ALA is a precursor of the haem synthesis pathway and is metabolised to the endogenous photoactive agent protoporphyrin IX (PPIX). Their first treatment was carried out during a radical prostatectomy, with drug delivery 4 h before the procedure, and light delivery (633 nm) with fluence of 140 J/cm^3. Subsequent treatments were done transurethrally, after TURP, and then transperineally with ultrasound guidance. They report variable PSA reduction at 6 weeks post-procedure; average PSA reduction was 55 % for those treated transurethrally and 30 % for those treated transperineally. There were no reported urinary side effects, skin photosensitivity or other side effects.

Moore et al. reported treatment of six men with previously untreated, histologically confirmed, Gleason $3 + 3$, organ-confined prostate cancer (defined with MRI and bone scan staging investigations), using temoporfin (mTHPC), at dose 0.15 mg/kg^2 [39]. Drug-light intervals were between 2 and 5 days, with quadrantic biopsies taken just prior to light delivery and assessed for fluorescence, compared in normal prostate and prostate cancer tissues. Patients underwent unilateral treatment, depending on the side of biopsy-detected prostate cancer. All patients had cancer identified on biopsy at 2 months post-procedure, with areas of established fibrosis and increased vascularity. Four out of six patients subsequently underwent a second PDT treatment, resulting in a total of ten reported treatments in this study. This group also reported their use of MRI for post-procedure imaging – by 2–3 months after treatment, there was an overall prostate volume reduction from 21 to 35 %. Excluding the two treatments for one individual with exposure to hormone therapy prior to PDT, there was an overall average PSA reduction of 48.3 % for the remaining eight treatments. Reported side effects were reasonably low, with irritative urinary symptoms persisting for 2 weeks after treatment, urinary retention requiring catheterisation in two treatments and one episode of sepsis.

Several Phase II trials have been carried out to evaluate the optimal photosensitiser dose using vascular targeted photodynamic therapy – these trials used padeliporfin (WST-11), due to episodes of intra-operative hypotension associated with padoporfin (WST-09). PCM201 followed a dose-escalation protocol, and PCM203 was a fixed-dose study using 4 mg/kg activated by light dose 200 J/cm with computer-aided light dose planning. A cohort of 40 men showed good correlation between energy delivered and volume of prostatic necrosis, with 200 J applied with a photosensitiser dose of 4 mg/kg produced approximately 1 cm^3 necrosis [40].

They did not report any urinary incontinence, rectal fistulae, hypotension or cardio-vascular/hepatic toxicity. Further reports of a cohort of 85 patients in the PCM203 study reported mean percentage of ablated tissue as 77 % for all patients and 87 % for those who underwent unilateral treatment at the 4 mg/kg dose [41]. Oncological outcomes for this cohort are awaited. A European Phase III randomised trial is currently under way (PCM301), comparing VTP and active surveillance in men with low-risk prostate cancer diagnosed on TRUS biopsy, with 400 men having been included in May 2013.

Further studies will provide more mature data and evidence for oncological control and functional outcomes. These studies will help to further define the role of PDT in the management of prostate cancer.

14.4 Technique

14.4.1 Treatment Planning

A number of factors must be considered when planning PDT treatment. These include total drug dose, drug delivery rate, light dose and dose per unit length of treatment fibre and rate of energy delivery. Planning can either be done prior to treatment, using a 'rule-based' approach based on pretreatment magnetic resonance (MR) and ultrasound imaging or using real-time feedback based upon drug, light and oxygen measurements, where light dosages are modified during treatment [24]. The largest trials of vascular-targeted photodynamic therapy in prostate cancer have used pretreatment MRI to plan the placement of light delivery fibres. These plans have been developed by a small number of radiology and urology experts (a treatment planning committee) with a local study site receiving an MR-based treatment plan. Whilst this is of use in large multi-centre trials where local investigators may otherwise have differed in their treatment approach, it is not necessary for the technique to be widely adopted.

VTP treatment is carried out under ultrasound guidance, in the operating theatre, and therefore the potential for inaccuracy in orientation exists when relating an MR-based treatment plan to a live ultrasound image. During treatment, prostate swelling and the influence of the transrectal ultrasound probe will result in changes in prostate shape during the course of the procedure and treatment. Several methods have been proposed in order to overcome this, including direct ultrasound planning, image modality comparing software or undertaking the procedure within an open core MRI magnet with compatible equipment [16]. There is potential for real-time monitoring of optical and physiological parameters, such that inaccuracies can be detected and amended during the procedure, without relying on pretreatment planning alone. As PDT effect is not evaluable by ultrasound in real time, it has been necessary to identify and monitor presumed surrogate markers of treatment, such as light and oxygen levels, and intraprostatic drug concentration.

The first reported clinical use of patient-specific pretreatment planning for PDT was from the Tookad study of radio-recurrent prostate cancer [42]. Individualised pretreatment planning accounts for the anatomical variation between prostates and increases treatment specificity, with calculation of light characteristics and number and position of treatment fibres. Factors such as light dosimetry, concentration of photosensitiser agent and oxygen availability are also important to consider [43], as well as the optical properties of light scattering and absorption [44]. The optical characteristics of the prostate are variable, impacting both wavelengths of light which are absorbed by haemoglobin and those longer wavelengths which are not [45]. Some groups have used steady-state light fluence measurements, combined with diffusion modelling, to assess a real-time model suitable for treatment modification, but this is affected by needle passages and bleeding. Svensson et al. describe a method, using time-resolved spectroscopy, to assess treatment effect in the human prostate, which they conclude provides a complete optical characterisation of human prostate tissue [46]. Another group has developed a real-time method of treatment feedback, based on a light dose threshold model [47], and concluded that their system could allow delivery of a particular light dose to a target tissue, taking into account variability in optical properties at the therapeutic wavelength. If effectively incorporated into clinical use, these systems may allow the operator to vary the light dose during the procedure, with the potential for increased treatment accuracy, and reduce the chance of treatment-associated morbidities, through sparing of surrounding structures. However, this approach currently lacks adequate evidence that this causes effective ablation volumes [47].

The method used for pretreatment planning of fibre number and placement in the Tookad studies involved assessment of the prostate shape on MRI prior to treatment, with the treatment planned according to a predetermined treatment effect for each optical fibre. A retrospective review of patients treated in Phase I and II studies with WST-11 was used to produce a software-based model for pretreatment PDT planning, and correlation between the pretreatment plan and posttreatment MRI imaging was shown [48]. Real-time feedback treatment planning involves modification of light dose according to feedback during the procedure. Canine studies have been used to demonstrate feasibility of this technique – Jankun et al. used a computer-assisted method for real-time optical fibre placement [49]. The first reported clinical use of real-time dosimetry was reported by Swartling et al. who used a software programme to calculate and adapt the light doses during treatment based on 3D tissue models from ultrasound imaging in four patients [50]. Although residual cancer was detected in 3/4 patients from this study, the authors believe they describe a feasible treatment planning option, but consider that the light dose used was insufficient.

14.4.2 Light Delivery

The photosensitiser agent is usually administered intravenously, with insertion of fibres using a transperineal (brachytherapy) template, guided by transrectal ultrasound (see Fig. 14.1). The patient is placed in the lithotomy position, under general anaesthetic, in a darkened room with the skin and eyes protected from light. A urinary catheter is inserted during the procedure and usually removed on the same day. Appropriate protection from light is important after the procedure, and the patient must be made aware of this during the consent process. Although in studies of PDT for skin conditions white light was used for activation of the photosensitiser agent, it is more efficient to use a single wavelength of light for maximum effect for a given photosensitiser, and this is administered using light produced from a laser guided along optical fibres. These fibres may be either bare ended (where light is emitted directly from the end of the fibre) or cylindrical fibres with a 1–5 cm diffusing end, like the light emitted from a strip light. For bare-ended fibres, the light dose is commonly expressed as J/cm^2 – these fibres can be used for treatment of superficial lesions or lesions within a hollow organ. Cylindrical diffusing fibres are more commonly used in solid organs, such as the prostate – light dose is expressed as J/cm, with the length of fibre corresponding to the required length of treatment. Previously, the 'pull back' technique could be used if the prostate was long and could not be included in a single fibre position. This is now limited by photosensitiser drugs with shorter drug-light intervals, and cylindrical diffusing fibres are more commonly used [51].

14.4.3 Treatment Effect

One of the determinants of the PDT effect (along with the available drug and oxygen) is 'fluence' – defined as the light available to activate the photosensitiser agent in a given volume of tissue. This is a property of both the energy applied to the tissue and the translucency of the tissue. Light penetration depth is defined as the distance from the source at which 67 % of light fluence is lost – this varies with both different tissues and different light wavelengths. A study assessing penetration depth of 763 nm light from a diode laser through the prostate [52], in men undergoing hollow needle insertion for brachytherapy, showed considerable variability between light penetration. This suggests that overlapping treatment zones should be used for PDT, in order to fully cover the desired treatment area. Furthermore, given the considerable variation, it may be that even real-time treatment planning would provide a challenge, given the rapidly changing optical properties over small areas of the prostate. However, this needs to be further assessed in the clinical scenario, taking into account the PDT effect.

14.4.4 Future Developments

Work continues to investigate methods to improve the specificity of photosensitiser agents for prostate cancer cells. The potential for attachment to monoclonal antibodies or other agents, or techniques to increase permeability and retention of agents within cells which are yet to be studied in vivo, provides hope for future treatment, but this technique is yet to be integrated into routine clinical use. With increased specificity, the potential for focal treatment is enhanced, aiming to provide oncological control, whilst reducing the potential side effects of whole gland treatment.

Table 14.1 Summary of PDT studies and reported morbidities

Study	Disease	Number of patients	Reported morbidities
Windahl et al. [20]	Primary	2	None reported
Nathan et al. [22]	Recurrent	14	3 – acute urinary retention; 2 – stress urinary incontinence; 1 – rectourethral fistula (after rectal biopsy); 5 – photosensitivity reactions; all – irritative urinary symptoms
Moore et al. [39]	Primary	6 (10 treatments)	1 – sepsis; 2 – recatheterisations; 1 – temporary erectile dysfunction; all – irritative urinary symptoms
Zaak et al. [38]	Primary	6	None reported
Verigos et al. [34]/ Patel et al. [35]	Recurrent	17	1 – urinary urgency, irritative urinary symptoms
Weersink et al. [51]/ Trachtenberg et al. [36, 37]	Recurrent	24 – 2 optical fibres, 28 – multiple fibres (up to 6)	2 – rectourethral fistulae; intra-operative hypotension; irritative urinary symptoms

14.5 Complications

As with all interventional treatments for prostate cancer, consideration must be given to the potential side effects. This is increasingly important as evidence arises to challenge the role of radical interventions, such as radical prostatectomy, in improving survival for low-risk prostate cancer [53], and as patients become increasingly aware of the wide range of treatment options available to them. Focal treatment aims to offer a minimally invasive method of treatment for localised prostate cancer, with good cancer control and low morbidity. Side effects of PDT are reported on a per-study basis and numbers are still relatively low – longer-term functional data are required, and ongoing studies will help to provide this. Table 14.1 provides a summary of reported morbidities in the studies reported to date – although irritative voiding symptoms do occur, these seem to settle over time in most men. More concerning is the incidence of rectourethral fistulae in several studies, although one of these was attributed to an inappropriate rectal biopsy after treatment. The results of a large European multi-centre trial of PDT versus active surveillance for localised prostate cancer are awaited – in order for PDT to keep pace with other minimally invasive therapies for prostate cancer, and methods of reporting morbidities and oncological outcomes should be formalised.

References

1. Ackroyd R, Kelty C, Brown N, Reed M. The history of photodetection and photodynamic therapy. Photochem Photobiol. 2001;74(5):656–69.
2. Lou PJ, Jäger HR, Jones L, Theodossy T, Bown SG, Hopper C. Interstitial photodynamic therapy as salvage treatment for recurrent head and neck cancer. Br J Cancer. 2004;91(3):441–6.

3. Bown SG, Rogowska AZ, Whitelaw DE, Lees WR, Lovat LB, Ripley P, et al. Photodynamic therapy for cancer of the pancreas. Gut. 2002;50(4):549–57.

4. Gold MH. Acne vulgaris: lasers, light sources and photodynamic therapy–an update 2007. Expert Rev Anti-Infect Ther. 2007;5(6):1059–69.

5. Wormald R, Evans J, Smeeth L, Henshaw K. Photodynamic therapy for neovascular age-related macular degeneration. Cochrane Database Syst Rev. 2007;(3):CD002030.

6. Kelly JF, Snell ME. Hematoporphyrin derivative: a possible aid in the diagnosis and therapy of carcinoma of the bladder. J Urol. 1976;115(2):150–1.

7. Pinthus JH, Bogaards A, Weersink R, Wilson BC, Trachtenberg J. Photodynamic therapy for urological malignancies: past to current approaches. J Urol. 2006;175(4):1201–7.

8. Dougherty TJ. Photodynamic therapy. Photochem Photobiol. 1993;58(6):895–900.

9. Bozzini G, Colin P, Betrouni N, Nevoux P, Ouzzane A, Puech P, et al. Photodynamic therapy in urology: what can we do now and where are we heading? Photodiagnosis Photodyn Ther. 2012;9(3):261–73.

10. Castano AP, Mroz P, Hamblin MR. Photodynamic therapy and anti-tumour immunity. Nat Rev Cancer. 2006;6(7):535–45.

11. Lepor H. Vascular targeted photodynamic therapy for localized prostate cancer. Rev Urol. 2008;10(4):254–61.

12. Schreiber S, Gross S, Brandis A, Harmelin A, Rosenbach-Belkin V, Scherz A, Salomon Y. Local photodynamic therapy (PDT) of rat C6 glioma xenografts with pd-bacteriopheophorbide leads to decreased metastases and increase of animal cure compared with surgery. Int J Cancer. 2002;99(2):279–85.

13. Mazor O, Brandis A, Plaks V, Neumark E, Rosenbach-Belkin V, Salomon Y, Scherz A. WST11, a novel water-soluble bacteriochlorophyll derivative; cellular uptake, pharmacokinetics, biodistribution and vascular-targeted photodynamic activity using melanoma tumors as a model. Photochem Photobiol. 2005;81(2):342–51.

14. Figge FH, Weiland GS, Manganiello LO. Studies on cancer detection and therapy; the affinity of neoplastic, embryonic, and traumatized tissue for porphyrins, metalloporphyrins, and radioactive zinc hematoporphyrin. Anat Rec. 1948;101(4):657.

15. Pottier R, Kennedy JC. The possible role of ionic species in selective biodistribution of photochemotherapeutic agents toward neoplastic tissue. J Photochem Photobiol B. 1990;8(1):1–16.

16. Arumainayagam N, Moore CM, Ahmed HU, Emberton M. Photodynamic therapy for focal ablation of the prostate. World J Urol. 2010;28(5):571–6.

17. Liu T, Wu LY, Berkman CE. Prostate-specific membrane antigen-targeted photodynamic therapy induces rapid cytoskeletal disruption. Cancer Lett. 2010;296(1):106–12.

18. Sharman WM, van Lier JE, Allen CM. Targeted photodynamic therapy via receptor mediated delivery systems. Adv Drug Deliv Rev. 2004;56(1):53–76.

19. Zuluaga MF, Sekkat N, Gabriel D, van den Bergh H, Lange N. Selective photodetection and photodynamic therapy for prostate cancer through targeting of proteolytic activity. Mol Cancer Ther. 2013;12(3):306–13.

20. Windahl T, Andersson SO, Lofgren L. Photodynamic therapy of localised prostatic cancer. Lancet. 1990;336(8723):1139.

21. Chang SC, Buonaccorsi GA, MacRobert AJ, Bown SG. Interstitial photodynamic therapy in the canine prostate with disulfonated aluminum phthalocyanine and 5-aminolevulinic acid-induced protoporphyrin IX. Prostate. 1997;32(2):89–98.

22. Nathan TR, Whitelaw DE, Chang SC, Lees WR, Ripley PM, Payne H, et al. Photodynamic therapy for prostate cancer recurrence after radiotherapy: a phase I study. J Urol. 2002;168(4 Pt 1):1427–32.

23. Selman SH, Keck RW, Hampton JA. Transperineal photodynamic ablation of the canine prostate. J Urol. 1996;156(1):258–60.

24. Moore CM, Emberton M, Bown SG. Photodynamic therapy for prostate cancer–an emerging approach for organ-confined disease. Lasers Surg Med. 2011;43(7):768–75.

25. Jankun J, Lilge L, Douplik A, Keck RW, Pestka M, Szkudlarek M, et al. Optical characteristics of the canine prostate at 665 nm sensitized with tin etiopurpurin dichloride: need for real-time monitoring of photodynamic therapy. J Urol. 2004;172(2):739–43.
26. Selman SH, Albrecht D, Keck RW, Brennan P, Kondo S. Studies of tin ethyl etiopurpurin photodynamic therapy of the canine prostate. J Urol. 2001;165(5):1795–801.
27. Hsi RA, Kapatkin A, Strandberg J, Zhu T, Vulcan T, Solonenko M, et al. Photodynamic therapy in the canine prostate using motexafin lutetium. Clin Cancer Res. 2001;7(3):651–60.
28. Lee LK, Whitehurst C, Chen Q, Pantelides ML, Hetzel FW, Moore JV. Interstitial photodynamic therapy in the canine prostate. Br J Urol. 1997;80(6):898–902.
29. Chang SC, Buonaccorsi G, MacRobert A, Bown SG. Interstitial and transurethral photodynamic therapy of the canine prostate using meso-tetra-(m-hydroxyphenyl) chlorin. Int J Cancer. 1996;67(4):555–62.
30. Huang Z, Chen Q, Trncic N, LaRue SM, Brun PH, Wilson BC, et al. Effects of pd-bacteriopheophorbide (TOOKAD)-mediated photodynamic therapy on canine prostate pretreated with ionizing radiation. Radiat Res. 2004;161(6):723–31.
31. Huang Z, Haider MA, Kraft S, Chen Q, Blanc D, Wilson BC, Hetzel FW. Magnetic resonance imaging correlated with the histopathological effect of pd-bacteriopheophorbide (tookad) photodynamic therapy on the normal canine prostate gland. Lasers Surg Med. 2006;38(7):672–81.
32. Huang Z, Chen Q, Dole KC, Barqawi AB, Chen YK, Blanc D, et al. The effect of tookad-mediated photodynamic ablation of the prostate gland on adjacent tissues–in vivo study in a canine model. Photochem Photobiol Sci. 2007;6(12):1318–24.
33. Du KL, Mick R, Busch TM, Zhu TC, Finlay JC, Yu G, et al. Preliminary results of interstitial motexafin lutetium-mediated PDT for prostate cancer. Lasers Surg Med. 2006;38(5):427–34.
34. Verigos K, Stripp DC, Mick R, Zhu TC, Whittington R, Smith D, et al. Updated results of a phase I trial of motexafin lutetium-mediated interstitial photodynamic therapy in patients with locally recurrent prostate cancer. J Environ Pathol Toxicol Oncol. 2006;25(1–2):373–87.
35. Patel H, Mick R, Finlay J, Zhu TC, Rickter E, Cengel KA, et al. Motexafin lutetium-photodynamic therapy of prostate cancer: short- and long-term effects on prostate-specific antigen. Clin Cancer Res. 2008;14(15):4869–76.
36. Trachtenberg J, Bogaards A, Weersink RA, Haider MA, Evans A, McCluskey SA, et al. Vascular targeted photodynamic therapy with palladium-bacteriopheophorbide photosensitizer for recurrent prostate cancer following definitive radiation therapy: assessment of safety and treatment response. J Urol. 2007;178(5):1974–9; discussion 1979.
37. Trachtenberg J, Weersink RA, Davidson SR, Haider MA, Bogaards A, Gertner MR, et al. Vascular-targeted photodynamic therapy (padoporfin, WS109) for recurrent prostate cancer after failure of external beam radiotherapy: a study of escalating light doses. BJU Int. 2008;102(5):556–62.
38. Zaak D, Stroka R, Hoppner M. Photodynamic therapy by means of 5 ALA induced protoporphyrin IX in human prostate cancer e preliminary results. Med Laser Appl. 2003;18:91–5.
39. Moore CM, Nathan TR, Lees WR, Mosse CA, Freeman A, Emberton M, Bown SG. Photodynamic therapy using meso tetra hydroxy phenyl chlorin (mthpc) in early prostate cancer. Lasers Surg Med. 2006;38(5):356–63.
40. Arumainayagam N. Tookad soluble second generation vascular targeted photodynamic therapy (VTP) for prostate cancer: safety and feasibility. EAU Meeting, Barcelona, 2010.
41. Azzouzi. Results of tookad soluble vascular targeted photodynamic therapy (VTP) for low risk localised prostate cancer (PCM203). AUA Meeting, Washington, DC, 2011.
42. Davidson SR, Weersink RA, Haider MA, Gertner MR, Bogaards A, Giewercer D, et al. Treatment planning and dose analysis for interstitial photodynamic therapy of prostate cancer. Phys Med Biol. 2009;54(8):2293–313.
43. Wilson BC, Patterson MS, Lilge L. Implicit and explicit dosimetry in photodynamic therapy: a new paradigm. Lasers Med Sci. 1997;12(3):182–99.

44. Svensson T, Alerstam E, Einarsdóttír M, Svanberg K, Andersson-Engels S. Towards accurate in vivo spectroscopy of the human prostate. J Biophotonics. 2008;1(3):200–3.
45. Moore CM, Hoh IM, Bown SG, Emberton M. Does photodynamic therapy have the necessary attributes to become a future treatment for organ-confined prostate cancer? BJU Int. 2005;96(6):754–8.
46. Svensson T, Andersson-Engels S, Einarsdóttír M, Svanberg K. In vivo optical characterization of human prostate tissue using near-infrared time-resolved spectroscopy. J Biomed Opt. 2007;12(1):014022.
47. Johansson A, Axelsson J, Andersson-Engels S, Swartling J. Realtime light dosimetry software tools for interstitial photodynamic therapy of the human prostate. Med Phys. 2007;34(11):4309–21.
48. Betrouni N, Lopes R, Puech P, Colin P, Mordon S. A model to estimate the outcome of prostate cancer photodynamic therapy with TOOKAD soluble WST11. Phys Med Biol. 2011;56(15):4771–83.
49. Jankun J, Keck RW, Skrzypczak-Jankun E, Lilge L, Selman SH. Diverse optical characteristic of the prostate and light delivery system: implications for computer modelling of prostatic photodynamic therapy. BJU Int. 2005;95(9):1237–44.
50. Swartling J, Axelsson J, Ahlgren G, Kälkner KM, Nilsson S, Svanberg S, et al. System for interstitial photodynamic therapy with online dosimetry: first clinical experiences of prostate cancer. J Biomed Opt. 2010;15(5):058003.
51. Weersink RA, Bogaards A, Gertner M, Davidson SR, Zhang K, Netchev G, et al. Techniques for delivery and monitoring of TOOKAD (WST09)-mediated photodynamic therapy of the prostate: clinical experience and practicalities. J Photochem Photobiol B. 2005;79(3):211–22.
52. Moore CM, Mosse CA, Allen C, Payne H, Emberton M, Bown SG. Light penetration in the human prostate: a whole prostate clinical study at 763 nm. J Biomed Opt. 2011;16(1):015003.
53. Wilt TJ, Brawer MK, Jones KM, Barry MJ, Aronson WJ, Fox S, et al. Radical prostatectomy versus observation for localized prostate cancer. N Engl J Med. 2012;367(3):203–13.

Focal Laser Interstitial Thermotherapy

15

Nacim Betrouni and Pierre Colin

15.1 Introduction

Currently, different energies are experienced for prostate cancer focal treatment, and thermotherapy includes all the methods aiming to induce coagulative necrosis. Laser is one the energies able to perform this kind of treatment. This technique, known also as focal laser ablation (FLA), has many benefits, such as its ease of use, low cost, and less cumbersome workstation. The following sections discuss the mechanisms, history, and components of FLA, with an account of current clinical experience for prostate cancer.

15.1.1 Mechanisms

Principles

LITT action is based on a photothermal effect. The thermal action results from the absorption of radiant energy by tissue receptive chromophores, inducing heat energy in a very short time (a few seconds) [1]. This increased temperature may cause irreversible damage and remote in vivo destruction (Fig. 15.1). The thermal effect

N. Betrouni, PhD
Inserm (French National Institute of Health and Medical Research), U703,
152 rue du Docteur Yersin, Lille 59120, France

Université Lille Nord de France, Lille F-59000, France

P. Colin, MD, PhD (✉)
Inserm (French National Institute of Health and Medical Research), U703,
152 rue du Docteur Yersin, Lille 59120, France

Department of Urology, La Louvière Private Hospital, Générale de Santé,
Lille F-59000, France
e-mail: docpierrecolin@gamil.com

© Springer-Verlag France 2015
E. Barret, M. Durand (eds.), *Technical Aspects of Focal Therapy in Localized Prostate Cancer*, DOI 10.1007/978-2-8178-0484-2_15

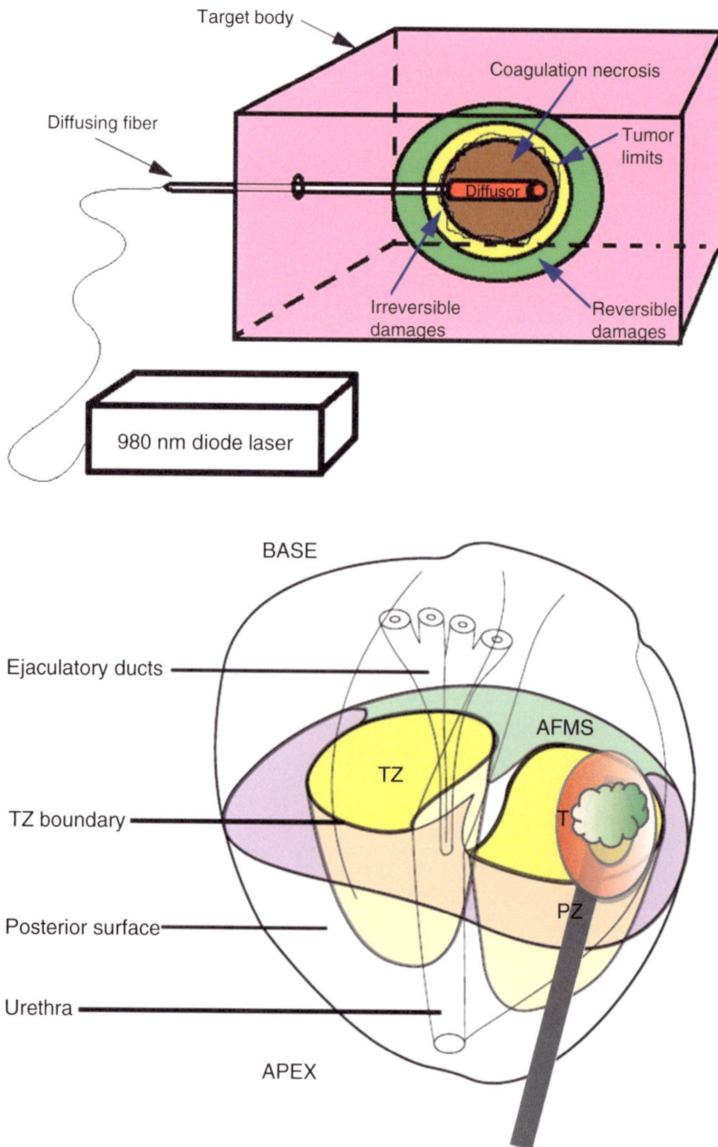

Fig. 15.1 Laser interstitial thermotherapy principles and its applications for focal ablation of prostate cancer

depends not only on the amount of heat energy delivered but also on the depth of light distribution. Consequently, the deep tissue damage is dependent on the wavelength of the laser in action. Due to weak absorption by water or hemoglobin, wavelengths between 590 and 1,064 nm are classically used to obtain deeper tissue penetration.

The extension of thermal tissue damage depends on both temperature and heating duration. Cell viability is related to the thermostability of several critical proteins, and irreversible protein denaturation may occur at around 60 °C [2]. When over 60 °C, coagulation is quasi-instantaneous, between 42 and 60 °C, thermal damage is obtained with longer heating periods. The area submitted to supraphysiological hyperthermia at less than 60 °C will develop coagulative necrosis 24–72 h after treatment [3, 4]. The macroscopic appearance of coagulation areas of FLA correspond to well-demarcated foci of necrosis surrounded by a small rim of hemorrhage with no viable glandular tissue (benign or malignant) after vital staining, based on immunoreactivity with cytokeratin [5, 6].

Thermal Damage

Thermal damage in cells and tissue can be described mathematically by a first-order thermochemical rate equation, in which temperature history determines damage. Damage is considered to be a unimolecular process whereby native molecules are transformed into a denatured/coagulated state through an activated state leading to cell death. Damage is quantified using a single parameter Ω, which ranges on the entire positive real axis, and it is calculated according to the Arrhenius law [7].

$$\Omega(r,\tau) = \ln\left(\frac{C(r,0)}{C(r,\tau)}\right) = A_f \int_0^\tau \exp\left(\frac{-E_a}{RT(r,t)}\right)dt$$

(15.1)

where

- $C(r, 0)$, $C(r, \tau)$ are the concentrations of the undamaged molecules at the beginning and at time τ, respectively.
- A_f (s^{-1}) is the frequency factor,
- E_a (J·mole^{-1}) is the activation energy,
- R (J·mole^{-1}·°K^{-1}) is the universal gas constant, and
- T (°K) is the temperature.

The parameters A_f, E_a, called the kinetic parameters, are temperature dependent and can be determined empirically.

Previous theoretical models of prostate treatment have generally assumed threshold damage temperatures of 50 °C. These values are based on studies involving exposure durations of seconds or greater. For instance, histological evaluation performed by Peters et al. showed that the thermal-injury boundary can be predicted from a threshold-maximum temperature of approximately 51 °C or an equivalent Arrhenius t (43) period of 200 min [4, 8, 9].

Components

Dosimetric Planning

Dosimetric planning of FLA requires three steps to predict the extent of the coagulated necrosis [1]: light distribution, rise in temperature, and the extent of thermal damage. Light distribution could be obtained using Monte Carlo simulation to estimate photon distribution in irradiated tissue. This process is based on tissue optical properties at the laser wavelength used.

The absorption of light in tissue causes a local elevation in temperature. Tissue heat transfer that is due to the energy of light deposited is described by the bioheat transfer equation (Pennes equation):

$$C_p \cdot \frac{\partial T_{(r,t)}}{\partial t} - \nabla \cdot \left(\mathcal{K} \cdot \nabla T_{(r,t)} \right) = W_b \cdot C_p \cdot \left[T_b - T_{(r,t)} \right] + Q_{abs}\left(r,t\right) + Q_{met} \tag{15.2}$$

where

- T is temperature (°K)
- $C_p = C * \rho$ is heat capacity (J·mm^{-3}·°K^{-1}),
- ρ is tissue density (g·mm^{-3}),
- C is specific heat of tissue (J·g^{-1}·°K^{-1}),
- $\mathcal{K}$ is thermal conductivity of tissue (W·mm^{-1}·°K^{-1}),
- w_b is blood flow rate (ml·g^{-1}·min^{-1}),
- T_b is the blood temperature,
- t is time (s),
- Q_{abs} is the heat source (W·mm^{-3}), and
- Q_{met} is the metabolic heat source (W·mm^{-3}).

The third step thermal damage is deduced from the temperature distribution map and estimated using the Arrhenius law (Eq. 15.1).

Sources

As indicated above, most often wavelengths in the red and intra-red spectra (590–1,064 nm) are used to allow deep penetration in tissue. At the beginning of interstitial laser coagulation development, Nd:YAG laser (1,064 nm) was used. This laser source allowed deep penetration into the tissue (10 mm); however, this kind of material is cumbersome due to the need for cooling systems.

In 1998, with the development of lasers for benign prostate hypertrophy (BPH) treatment, small diode lasers appeared allowing interstitial laser coagulation at 830 nm with transurethral application of diffusing fibers [10, 11]. Thereafter these diode lasers were used for hepatic and brain tumor treatment in near-infrared wavelenghts (800–980 nm) [12]. With these wavelengths, while tissue penetration is weaker (5 mm) in comparison with Nd:YAG lasers, the diodes present an excellent energy efficiency permitting the minimization of their cooling system. Improvements in the design of high-power diode laser sources have made medical laser systems smaller, more portable, more powerful, and less expensive than previous generations. Since 2011, diode lasers emitting at 1,064 nm ± 10 nm have been proposed and could replace the Nd:YAG laser.

Diffusers

Light is delivered via flexible quartz fibers from 300 to 600 μm in diameter. Conventional bare-tip fibers provide a spherical lesion of about 15 mm in diameter at their ends, but have been largely replaced by interstitial fibers consisting of cylindrical diffusing tips of 10–40 mm in length. These needles provide a larger ablative area of up to 50 mm [13, 14].

Temperature Monitoring

Temperature can be monitored by three different techniques:

1. Thermocouples placed at the laser probe and used to control the laser power in the adaptive monitoring mode. Usually, the initial laser power is set to 15 W for each fiber and the control temperature is set to 100 °C. As the temperature measured by the laser fiber probe quickly increases to 100 °C, the power delivered by the laser quickly decreases and stabilizes at about 2 W [15].
2. Fluoroptic temperature probes used to control the temperature of specific structures. Due to their technology, theses probes (Model 3100, Luxtron Corp., Santa Clara, California) are insensitive to the magnetic fields. The probes can be used to validate the measurements performed by MR thermometry. They are usually placed at the expected ablation boundary to ensure that therapeutic temperatures (55 °C or greater) are reached at the target borders, and to guarantee that near-critical structures remain unaffected by heat (by maintaining temperatures lower than 42 °C) [16].
3. Real-time MRI control. This technique allows fiber guidance and control of coagulative necrosis after FLA [9, 17]. During the procedure, real-time 3-D temperature maps can be obtained by using the proton resonance frequency (PRF) shift. For MRI thermometry, a gradient-recalled echo pulse sequence is rapidly repeated during FLA procedure. With dedicated specifically developed software, the acquired MR images are analyzed in real time to estimate the thermal images, and also, to compute the ablation zone maps using the Arrhenius model of thermal tissue ablation.

15.2 Clinical Trials

Table 15.1 summarizes the various clinical studies about FLA that have been published.

Several clinical studies in North America have been reported [5, 15, 16, 18]. An initial phase I study (NCT00448695) was published by the team of Professors Trachtenberg and Haider in Toronto; they used a laser diode of 830 nm that had already been used for the treatment of prostatic hyperplasia (Indigo Laser®) [15]. After preplanning using MR images, the laser fibers were placed transperineally; the real-time monitoring was achieved by Contrast-Enhanced UltraSonography (CEUS). Necrotic lesions were visible on this examination (hypovascular zone) and the volumes obtained were consistent with those obtained on the control MRI.

Postoperative morbidity was negligible. The adverse events most frequently reported were of perineal discomfort (25 %) and mild hematuria (16 %). Seventy-five percent of patients treated were able to leave hospital the day after the procedure. At 6 months, there was no significant decrease in erectile dysfunction scores

Table 15.1 Clinical studies concerning Laser Interstitial Thermotherapy for Focal Ablation of Prostate Cancer

Reference	Number of patients	Wavelength Type of laser source	Number of fibers	Energy (Joules) Power (Watt) Time (seconds)	Real-time imaging monitoring	Adverse events	Carcinologic results/remarks
Amin et al. [33]	1 patient	805 nm (Diomed diode laser)	3	3,000 J 2 W 500 s	US and CT scan	Mild dysuria	Feasibility of FLA Biopsies at 10 days: necrotic tissue in targeted area, cancer cells in other area
Atri et al. [15], Lindner et al. [16]	12 patients	830 nm (Indigo diode laser)	1 or 2	2,880 J	CEUS and fluoroptic temperature probes	Perineal discomfort (3patients) mild hematuria (2 patients) hematospermia (2 patients) fatigue (1 patient)	Biopsies at 6 months
				2–15 W (temperature control at 100 °C) 720 s	7 day follow-up 1.5T MRI		67 % of patient free of tumor in the targeted area 50 % of patients free of disease
Raz et al. [18]	2 patients	980 nm (Visualase diode laser)	≥2	Unknown	3D 1.5T MRI control (thermometry, cellular damage planning) and CEUS just after procedure 15 day follow-up 1.5 T MRI	No adverse event	Feasibility to immediately repeat the procedure

Lindner et al. [5]	4 patients	980 nm (Visualase diode laser)	2 or 3	3,260–5,900 J	CEUS and fluoroptic temperature probes	Not describe	Strong correlation between MRI findings and vital stain histopathology images (Pearson correlation index = 0.89)
					7 day 1.5 T MRI control follows by radical prostatectomy		
Lindner et al. [19]	2 patients	980 nm (Visualase diode laser)	Unknown	Unknown	3D Robotic 1.5 T MRI control (thermometry, cellular damage planning)	Improvement of IPSS score (1 patient)	Safe and precise robotic guidance of laser fiber
						No change of IIEF-5 score	Possible oblique insertion angles to provide adequate dose
Woodrum et al. [20]	1 patient with locally recurrence prostate cancer after prostatectomy	980 nm (Visualase diode laser)	2	Unknown	3T MRI control (thermometry, cellular damage planning)	No change of potency or continence	Feasibility of FLA for locally recurrence of prostate cancer
Oto et al. [21]	9 patients	980 nm (Visualase diode laser)	1 diffusing fiber of 1 cm length	Unknown	1.5T MRI control (thermometry, cellular damage planning)	No major complication or adverse event	Biopsies at 6 months: 77 % of patient free of tumor in the targeted area
						No change of IPSS score	
						No change of SHIM score	

(IIEF-5) or worsening of urinary symptoms as assessed by the International Prostate Symptom Score (IPSS).

On 6-month biopsies, the short-term oncological results seemed promising, with 67 % of patients without tumor recurrence in the treated area [16].

Three other studies demonstrate the feasibility of focal treatment of cancer by the MRI-guided LITT system at 980 nm with the Visualase® system (NCT00805883, NCT01094665, and NCT01192438) [15, 18]. In a phase I trial (NCT00805883) that included four patients, the laser fibers' guidance was performed as previously reported [5]. A radical prostatectomy was performed 1 week after the LITT procedure. Analysis of the surgical specimens showed a good correlation between the volumes of thermal damage visible on MRI and those actually recorded on the vital stain histopathological parts set (Pearson coefficient $R=0.89$). In the thermal ablation zone, the lack of viable tumor cells seen after immunostaining for cytokeratin 8 validates the scientific relevance of this minimally invasive treatment modality [5, 6].

In a phase I trial (NCT01094665), Raz et al. described fiber guidance under 3-D MRI reconstruction by the transperineal approach in two patients. MRI thermometry and thermal damage planning were calculated using the Visualase® system. Transrectal CEUS was achieved immediately after the FLA procedure and in case of residual vascularized target tissue, another procedure with new fiber positioning was performed. The patients were discharged home within 3 h and no adverse events or complications were noted at ≤ 1 month following treatment [18].

The same research team described the feasibility of robotic MRI-guided FLA in one case [19].

In another phase I trial (NCT01192438), Oto et al. described the feasibility and safety of FLA (with the Visualase system) under MRI guidance in nine patients [21]. The procedure was performed under conscious light sedation in all patients with a Gleason score of 7 or less in 3 or fewer biopsy cores. The mean laser ablation duration was 4.3 min for a procedure time of 2.5–4 h. No major complications or serious adverse effects were observed. Urinary function (IPSS) and sexual score (SHIM) were not significantly different between preoperative and control examinations at 1, 3, and 6 months after the procedure. A hypovascular defect was immediately noticed on posttreatment contrast-enhanced MR imaging in 88.9 % of patients. MR imaging-guided biopsy of the ablation area was performed at 6 months and showed persistent Gleason 6 adenocarcinoma in two patients (22 %). For the authors, these two failures could be explained by problems in targeting, suboptimal temperature mapping, or an insufficient ablation zone leading to positive margins.

Woodrum et al. reported the case of one patient with locally recurrent prostate cancer after radical prostatectomy treated by FLA under 3T MRI guidance [20]. The authors reported no change in continence or potency after the MRI-guided FLA procedure.

Today, three phase 1 trials are recruiting in Canada (NCT01094665) and the USA (NCT01377753); many American centers are already equipped with the Visualase® system and have begun publishing about the LITT technique for focal treatment.

15.3 Discussion

FLA could be one of the partial prostate cancer treatment modalities [5]. FLA is a minimally invasive technique that is under development for in situ destruction of solid-organ tumors. Based on the use of low-power lasers, which deliver luminous energy using an adapted optical system, FLA produces a controlled coagulative necrosis zone, reducing the risk to the healthy adjacent structures (nerves, blood vessels, sphincters) [3, 5, 15, 16, 18].

Before the generalization of this concept, many issues have to be addressed. The first concerns the ability to place the laser-diffusing fiber precisely within the target area. According to the results of the first clinical trials, one part of treatment failure can be explained by the problem of correct targeting of the visible lesion on MRI. This limitation exists for the FLA but also for the all other interstitial techniques (e.g., photodynamic therapy, cryoablation, radiofrequency, or definitive electroporation).

Using a brachytherapy stabilizing apparatus with modified template grid and VariSeed® system, Atri et al. were able to target in transrectal ultrasonography a suspicious area visible in MRI after rigid body registration [15]. Also, to compensate prostate deformation using transrectal sonography, the authors planned a target volume four times greater than the MRI suspicious area. In a phase I (NCT00448695) trial, Lindner et al. described the same transperineal technique using 3-D US and deformable registration for MR image fusion [16]. The authors concluded that improved deformable registration techniques might be able to minimize registration errors and improve targeting. The development of such commercial devices with laser-intagrated platform has now been achieved (e.g., Echolaser® by Esaote®). However, to the best of our knowledge, no data are available regarding FLA of prostate application.

Thereafter, to enhance accuracy and facilitate real-time assessment of lesion sizes, the same team performed fiber placement manually under MRI procedure [18, 21]. They used an MRI-compatible template grid and multiplanar images to obtain virtual 3-D representation of the template with insertion paths and fiber placement within the prostate. The accuracy of MRI template-based manual with the targeted area was tested in a preclinical study concluding to a fiber placement error of about 1.1 ± 0.7 mm [22].

Recently, the robotic guidance emerged as a possibility to achieved the procedure under MRI. In the last few years, robotic MR-guided biopsy of the prostate has been reported to be technically safe and there has been a high degree of accuracy in biopsy needle placement [23, 24]. Linder et al. described the first case of robotic MRI-guided FLA [19]. Moreover, with the accurate placing of the diffusing part of the laser fiber within the prostate cancer, the authors demonstrated that the robot can be used to produce oblique insertion angles to provide adequate dose coverage of low-volume tumors or tumors in a difficult location (anterior). This placement technology could be used for FLA under 3-D-CEUS too, but as far as we know it was not previously described with this energy source [25].

The second issue is the treatment planning required to optimize therapy parameters to ensure the optimal coverage of the area while sparing surrounding tissue.

This issue is challenging and still needs the development of dedicated dosimetric tools, as was the case for radiotherapy and brachytherapy. Recent key advances in MRIs allowed the opening of some technological locks in FLA monitoring and guidance. With computer modeling development for thermal damage and multiplanar MR temperature imaging, it is now possible to accurately determine the expected thermal necrosis in regions of interest and to control in real time the photothermal effect on homogeneous tissue [21, 22, 26, 27]. The commercialization of integrated systems (laser source and fiber, computerized planning and monitoring solution) has made MRI-guided FLA clinically relevant [16, 18, 21]. However, some limitations are still present. Principal variability observed between predicted and obtained ablation areas is due to tissue heterogeneity; this is in relation firstly to the relaxation properties of the tissue (dependent on zonal anatomy, presence of tumor, vascularization, etc.) and secondly with the change of the tissular thermal conductivity during increases in temperature. New nonlinear calibrated computational models of the bioheat transfer may provide a reasonable approximation of the laser-tissue interaction, which could be useful for treatment planning in heterogeneous areas such as prostate cancer [26, 28]. Another limitation for thermal necrosis prediction is related with cooled applicators. To avoid charring or photovaporization, most teams use cooled applicators to maintain a temperature between 60 and 100 °C during the heating phase. The use of these kinds of applicators needs computer modeling of the temperature rise of the in situ fluid to reduce systematic errors [28, 29].

To reduce morbidity for healthy adjacent structures and reinforce specificity of FLA for cancer cells, recent preclinical developments using nanoparticles have been described [30–32]. The goal of this technique is to produce photothermal coagulation in prostate tissue containing nanoparticles by Near InfraRed (NIR) activation. As cancer cells accumulate more nanoparticles than healthy tissue (passive diffusion in tumor neovasculature by enhanced permeability and retention effect), the NIR illumination activates a specific coagulation of the cancer cells. Indeed, photoactivation of nanoparticles is made at power levels that do not generate significant damage in normal tissue.

In conclusion, FLA is a potential tool for focal therapy of low-risk prostate cancer. Precision, real-time monitoring, MRI compatibility and the low cost of the integrated system are principal factors in this minimally invasive therapy. The feasibility and safety of this technique have been reported in phase I assays. Further trials are required to show the technique's long-term oncologic effectiveness.

References

1. Mordon SR, Wassmer B, Reynaud JP, Zemmouri J. Mathematical modeling of laser lipolysis. Biomed Eng Online. 2008;7:10.
2. Ritchie KP, Keller BM, Syed KM, Lepock JR. Hyperthermia (heat shock)-induced protein denaturation in liver, muscle and lens tissue as determined by differential scanning calorimetry. Int J Hyperthermia. 1994;10(5):605–18.
3. Colin P, Nevoux P, Marqa M, Auger F, Leroy X, Villers A, et al. Focal laser interstitial

thermotherapy (LITT) at 980 nm for prostate cancer: treatment feasibility in Dunning R3327-AT2 rat prostate tumour. BJU Int. 2012;109:452–8.

4. van Nimwegen SA, L'Eplattenier HF, Rem AI, van der Lugt JJ, Kirpensteijn J. Nd:YAG surgical laser effects in canine prostate tissue: temperature and damage distribution. Phys Med Biol. 2009;54(1):29–44.

5. Lindner U, Lawrentschuk N, Weersink RA, Davidson SR, Raz O, Hlasny E, et al. Focal laser ablation for prostate cancer followed by radical prostatectomy: validation of focal therapy and imaging accuracy. Eur Urol. 2010;57(6):1111–4.

6. Evans AJ, Ryan P, Van derKwast T. Treatment effects in the prostate including those associated with traditional and emerging therapies. Adv Anat Pathol. 2011;18(4):281–93.

7. Jankun J, Keck RW, Skrzypczak-Jankun E, Lilge L, Selman SH. Diverse optical characteristic of the prostate and light delivery system: implications for computer modelling of prostatic photodynamic therapy. BJU Int. 2005;95(9):1237–44.

8. Bhowmick S, Swanlund DJ, Coad JE, Lulloff L, Hoey MF, Bischof JC. Evaluation of thermal therapy in a prostate cancer model using a wet electrode radiofrequency probe. J Endourol Endourol Soc. 2001;15(6):629–40.

9. Peters RD, Chan E, Trachtenberg J, Jothy S, Kapusta L, Kucharczyk W, et al. Magnetic resonance thermometry for predicting thermal damage: an application of interstitial laser coagulation in an in vivo canine prostate model. Magn Reson Med. 2000;44(6):873–83.

10. Issa MM, Townsend M, Jiminez VK, Miller LE, Anastasia K. A new technique of intraprostatic fiber placement to minimize thermal injury to prostatic urothelium during indigo interstitial laser thermal therapy. Urology. 1998;51(1):105–10.

11. Issa MM. The evolution of laser therapy in the treatment of benign prostatic hyperplasia. Rev Urol. 2005;7 Suppl 9:S15–22.

12. Carpentier A, McNichols RJ, Stafford RJ, Itzcovitz J, Guichard JP, Reizine D, et al. Real-time magnetic resonance-guided laser thermal therapy for focal metastatic brain tumors. Neurosurgery. 2008;63(1 Suppl 1):ONS21–8; discussion ONS8–9.

13. Huang GT, Wang TH, Sheu JC, Daikuzono N, Sung JL, Wu MZ, et al. Low-power laserthermia for the treatment of small hepatocellular carcinoma. Eur J Cancer. 1991;27(12):1622–7.

14. Muralidharan V, Malcontenti-Wilson C, Christophi C. Interstitial laser hyperthermia for colorectal liver metastases: the effect of thermal sensitization and the use of a cylindrical diffuser tip on tumor necrosis. J Clin Laser Med Surg. 2002;20(4):189–96.

15. Atri M, Gertner MR, Haider MA, Weersink RA, Trachtenberg J. Contrast-enhanced ultrasonography for real-time monitoring of interstitial laser thermal therapy in the focal treatment of prostate cancer. Can Urol Assoc J. 2009;3(2):125–30.

16. Lindner U, Weersink RA, Haider MA, Gertner MR, Davidson SR, Atri M, et al. Image guided photothermal focal therapy for localized prostate cancer: phase I trial. J Urol. 2009;182:1371.

17. Woodrum DA, Gorny KR, Mynderse LA, Amrami KK, Felmlee JP, Bjarnason H, et al. Feasibility of 3.0T magnetic resonance imaging-guided laser ablation of a cadaveric prostate. Urology. 2010;75(6):1514 e1–6.

18. Raz O, Haider MA, Davidson SR, Lindner U, Hlasny E, Weersink R, et al. Real-time magnetic resonance imaging-guided focal laser therapy in patients with low-risk prostate cance. Eur Urol. 2010;58(1):173–7.

19. Lindner U, Louis AS, Colquhoun AJ, Boström PJ, Davidson SR, Raz O, et al. First robotic magnetic resonance-guided laser focal therapy for prostate cancer: a case report and review of the literature. Interv Oncol Soc J. 2011;1(1):69–77 [Review Article].

20. Woodrum DA, Mynderse LA, Gorny KR, Amrami KK, McNichols RJ, Callstrom MR. 3.0T MR-guided laser ablation of a prostate cancer recurrence in the postsurgical prostate bed. J Vasc Interv Radiol. 2011;22(7):929–34.

21. Oto A, Sethi I, Karczmar G, McNichols R, Ivancevic MK, Stadler WM, et al. MR imaging-guided focal laser ablation for prostate cancer: phase I trial. Radiology. 2013;267(3):932–40.

22. Stafford RJ, Shetty A, Elliott AM, Klumpp SA, McNichols RJ, Gowda A, et al. Magnetic resonance guided, focal laser induced interstitial thermal therapy in a canine prostate model. J Urol. 2010;184(4):1514–20.

23. Song SE, Cho NB, Fischer G, Hata N, Tempany C, Fichtinger G, et al. Development of a pneumatic robot for MRI-guided transperineal prostate biopsy and brachytherapy: new approaches. IEEE Int Conf Robot Autom. 2010;2010:2580–5.
24. Zangos S, Melzer A, Eichler K, Sadighi C, Thalhammer A, Bodelle B, et al. MR-compatible assistance system for biopsy in a high-field-strength system: initial results in patients with suspicious prostate lesions. Radiology. 2011;259(3):903–10.
25. Ho H, Yuen JS, Mohan P, Lim EW, Cheng CW. Robotic transperineal prostate biopsy: pilot clinical study. Urology. 2011;78(5):1203–8.
26. Marqa MF, Colin P, Nevoux P, Mordon SR, Betrouni N. Focal laser ablation of prostate cancer: numerical simulation of temperature and damage distribution. Biomed Eng Online. 2011;10:45.
27. McNichols RJ, Gowda A, Kangasniemi M, Bankson JA, Price RE, Hazle JD. MR thermometry-based feedback control of laser interstitial thermal therapy at 980 nm. Lasers Surg Med. 2004;34(1):48–55.
28. Fuentes D, Oden JT, Diller KR, Hazle JD, Elliott A, Shetty A, et al. Computational modeling and real-time control of patient-specific laser treatment of cancer. Ann Biomed Eng. 2009;37(4):763–82.
29. Fuentes D, Walker C, Elliott A, Shetty A, Hazle JD, Stafford RJ. Magnetic resonance temperature imaging validation of a bioheat transfer model for laser-induced thermal therapy. Int J Hyperthermia. 2011;27(5):453–64.
30. Feng Y, Fuentes D, Hawkins A, Bass J, Rylander MN, Elliott A, Shetty A, Stafford RJ, Oden JT. Nanoshell-mediated laser surgery simulation for prostate cancer treatment. Eng Comput. 2008;25:3–13.
31. Stern JM, Stanfield J, Kabbani W, Hsieh JT, Cadeddu JA. Selective prostate cancer thermal ablation with laser activated gold nanoshells. J Urol. 2008;179(2):748–53.
32. Schwartz JA, Price RE, Gill-Sharp KL, Sang KL, Khorchani J, Goodwin BS, et al. Selective nanoparticle-directed ablation of the canine prostate. Lasers Surg Med. 2011;43(3):213–20.
33. Amin, Z., W.R. Lees, and S.G. Bown, Technical note: interstitial laser photocoagulation for the treatment of prostatic cancer. Br J Radiol, 1993.

Emerging Energies for Focal Ablation of Prostate Cancer

16

Y. Ahallal and Eric Barret

16.1 Introduction

Prostate cancer (PCa) is currently being diagnosed at an earlier clinical stage, lower risk grade, and smaller tumor volume compared with 20 years ago [1]. Meanwhile, there is increased evidence that a significant amount of overtreatment in patients who undergo radical treatment does not lead to survival benefits [2]. Furthermore, it has been clearly established that radical treatments carry the risk of treatment-related toxicity, which can also lead to negative effects on the patient's quality of life [3, 4]. Bearing in mind the potential morbidity of radical prostatectomy (RP) and radiation, and to avoid the overtreatment of low-risk localized PCa, an increasing number of patients are thus considering focal therapy (FT) as an alternative primary approach to radical treatments. FT is an emerging alternative treatment option that offers great hope for the management and control of PCa because of the decreased morbidity of treated patients. The key challenge for current FT modalities is to treat only localized tumors, sparing any surrounding tissues, especially near the neurovascular bundles and the urethral sphincter, to minimize the potential morbidity.

There are four energy modalities that are available for use in focal therapy. Cryotherapy is the elective destruction of tissue by low temperature and thawing. High-intensity focused ultrasound is also suitable for FT; with this, the targeted ultrasound waves generate high temperature in a localized area, causing tissue damage. Vascular-targeted photodynamic therapy is an ablative technology that uses photosensitizers caught by tissues producing radical oxygen species when exposed to light of a specific wavelength, resulting in tissue destruction. FT can also be

Y. Ahallal • E. Barret, MD (✉)
Department of Urology, Institut Montsouris,
Paris-Descartes University, 42 bd Jourdan, Paris 75014, France
e-mail: eric.barret@imm.fr

© Springer-Verlag France 2015
E. Barret, M. Durand (eds.), *Technical Aspects of Focal Therapy
in Localized Prostate Cancer*, DOI 10.1007/978-2-8178-0484-2_16

performed using brachytherapy in which "free" iodine-125 seeds are placed in the hypothetical cancer location (defined by the site of positive biopsies and MRI images), under the guidance of ultrasound.

In this section, we review the emerging FT energies that are suitable for use in the treatment of localized PCa.

16.2 Irreversible Electroporation for the Ablation of Prostate Cancer

Applications of current radical and ablative techniques for the treatment of PCa induce relatively high risks of erectile dysfunction and incontinence in patients. The aforementioned toxicity is due to procedure-related damage of the blood vessels, the urethra and/or the neurovascular bundle. The relatively high incidence of erectile dysfunction is due to the damage of the neurovascular nerve bundle and/or blood flow to the penis, whereas incontinence is primarily due to the damage of the distal urethral smooth-muscle sphincter and the striated muscle. Finding new procedures that can limit damage to these structures will lead to the potential to improve patients' treatment outcomes. It was demonstrated that ablation with a nonthermal energy called "irreversible electroporation" (IRE) is effective in destroying the cancer cells and has the advantage of sparing surrounding tissue such as blood vessels and neurons – which surgical and other ablation techniques are unable to achieve. We can therefore hypothesize that using ablation with IRE as opposed to traditional surgical techniques might help to reduce treatment-related toxicity.

16.2.1 IRE Principles

In 1965 Coster first observed the phenomenon of a "punch-through" of the cell membrane by an electric current, following which the term "electroporation" was defined as the formation of pores in the cell membrane due to an electric field [5]. Electroporation, or electropermeabilization, is the phenomenon by which cell membrane permeability to ions and macromolecules is increased by exposing the cell to short electric current pulses. The permeabilization can be temporary (reversible electroporation) or permanent (irreversible electroporation), depending on the electric field magnitude and duration, period, and number of pulses [6].

Reversible electroporation has been used to transfer macromolecules into target cells in vitro, using an electric field to induce reversible membrane permeability. The pulsed electric fields increase the permeability of the cell membrane by a phenomenon known as electroporation, a process that can be reversible or irreversible, depending on the combination of the following variables: the pulse duration, the electric field intensity, and the number of pulses [7]. Reversible electroporation, which makes the cell membrane more permeable, has been used in electrochemotherapy to facilitate the uptake of chemotherapeutic agents into cells [8]. Reversible electroporation was also used in the gene therapy [9].

Recently, the electric field has been modulated to produce permanent membrane permeability and cell death. IRE was initially developed as a technique for ablation in the liver, pancreas, kidney, and prostate in animal test subjects [10–12], and was found to be successful in inducing hepatocellular, breast, and sarcoma tumor deaths in those test subjects [13, 14].

In vitro, IRE has been used to sterilize water, because the IRE leads to bacteria and yeast death. In vivo, the destroyed cells are left in situ and are removed by the immune system [9].

In animal experiments, IRE has been shown to effectively ablate tumor cells in vitro [15]. IRE experiments in both animals and humans have shown that the surrounding connective tissue structure is preserved and there is no damage to the associated blood vessels or neural tissue [15]. It is therefore assumed that the preservation of the surrounding tissue will reduce treatment-related toxicity inherent in current prostate cancer therapies.

16.2.2 IRE Device and Procedure

IRE is performed using the Angiodynamics Nanoknife System (Angiodynamics, Latham, NY). This system is the first available technological platform based on the IRE principles, and it is manufactured and distributed by Angiodynamics Inc. under the trade name of Nanoknife™. Nanoknife has been approved by the regulatory authorities in Europe (CE certificate), as well as the U.S. Food and Drug Administration, for marketing under those jurisdictions.

The Nanoknife system consists of a computer-controlled pulse generator that delivers 3,000 V pulses to the IRE probes. Typically, 90 pulses (which last from 20 to 100 µs each) are delivered. Shorter durations may be utilized in cases where high electrical resistance is encountered. The pulse voltages and duration are based on preclinical studies [12, 16]. Treatment planning is based on preoperative imaging with preplanning ultrasound and MRI. From the preoperative imaging, the tumor dimensions are inputted into the pulse generator, which will calculate the number and spacing of probes needed to create the ablation zone, based on a computer algorithm. Patients will have an ultrasound of the prostate whereby the imaging data will be entered into the planning software system, which will determine the volume and shape of the prostate; following this, one specified area will be chosen for ablation. IRE electrodes consist of insulated 19-gauge or larger needles with an exposed active portion of 1–4 cm. For most applications, multiple electrodes are required; these are spaced 1–3 cm apart to provide sufficient electric field strengths for irreversible cell damage.

The needle electrodes are percutaneously placed in the tumor under ultrasound (US) image guidance and the tumor cells are destroyed by disrupting the cell membrane with short-duration, high-voltage direct current. Either a single bipolar or multiple monopolar probe may be used, with greater numbers of probes needed for larger ablation zones. Probe spacing typically varies from 0.5 to 2 cm apart, with the specific distance determined by computer algorithm. The probes are radiopaque to aid in intraprocedural identification of the probe tip. The proper distance between probes is measured at the tip, and the probes must be placed within 10° of parallel for irreversible electroporation to occur. Small deviations in probe placement can lead to areas of reversible electroporation which are likely to result in PCa recurrence.

Delivery of the pulses is synchronized to the patient's ECG, which is an incorporated feature of the Nanoknife pulse generator.

The pulses are timed to be delivered during the absolute myocardial refractory period 50 μs after the R-wave, in order to prevent the generation of arrhythmias. Due to this synchronization, the patient must have a pulse rate of under 115. Higher pulse rates will cause the pulse generator to suppose that an arrhythmia is occurring, therefore ceasing to deliver further pulses. During the procedure, the progress of the ablation is followed by tracking the actual current delivered, which should increase throughout the procedure, as ablated tissue has lower resistance.

16.2.3 Advantages of IRE Compared to Current FT Energies

In a canine test subject, Onik et al. reported IRE to be feasible and efficient for the treatment of localized PCa [13]. Their literature demonstrated in addition that IRE is safe in humans. IRE actually spares blood vessels, renal structures, gastrointestinal structures and neurons. Fifty-four percent of the patients treated experienced no pain postoperatively, while 39 % experienced minimal pain [15, 17].

Recently, Schoellnast et al. reported the results of an animal study that demonstrated that neurons were spared post- IRE. The study performed IRE on the sciatic nerves of six pigs that were euthanized 2 months later, and enabled histological analysis of the targeted nerves. The experiment showed that the endoneurial architecture of all nerves had been preserved, and various small-caliber axons demonstrated axonal regeneration. Schoellnast et al. found that the endoneurium and perineurium remained intact, even when signs of injury (axonal swelling and inflammatory infiltrates) were present at all time points. Moreover, the pigs were able to stand without assistance after 3 days [18]. In a similar report, Li et al. have reported on the effects of IRE on rats after applying IRE to their sciatic nerves; the authors reported a full recovery of the rats' functioning and activities after less than 7 weeks post-ablation [19].

The selective tissue ablation has important clinical implications, such as decreasing the incidence of urethral or neurovascular bundles damage in focal IRE of localized prostate cancer and therefore potentially preserving erectile function. There has been no direct study addressing these concerns in humans.

In another preclinical canine study using 12 dogs, Tsivian et al. evaluated histological changes, erectile function, and side effects of bilateral focal ablation. The postoperative course was uneventful in all of the test subjects. All the dogs were fully potent, even as early as 5 days after ablation, while histological examinations showed inflammatory changes in the targeted area at 7 days, and replacement by fibrosis occurred at 30 days. Overall histological damage to the capsule, urethra, rectal wall, or nerves was not identified [20].

Moreover, IRE has numerous advantages over thermal ablation techniques, including smaller needle probes; availability of radiology guidance; no thermal damage to adjacent structures; rapid disappearance of targeted cells; no residual cavity; and little postoperative pain.

IRE was shown to provide short treatment times, and it is expected that the use of IRE for the treatment of PCa will significantly improve outcomes and quality of life for patients undergoing PCa treatment. These reported advantages over conventional thermal ablative techniques make IRE ablation an attractive technique for targeted focal destruction of prostate cancer.

The results of preclinical studies can be used as a foundation for future research and translation of the potential benefits of this technology to focal PCa treatment. Along with the ability to spare the adjacent tissues, coupled with the excellent preservation of erectile function after bilateral focal ablation, recent data indicate that IRE is a promising technology for targeted ablation of the prostate.

One of the main disadvantages of this procedure is the risk of reflex movements induced by the electrical impulse that could lead to needle displacement, which could potentially cause damage to healthy structures [13].

16.3 Interstitial Microwave Thermal Therapy (IMT)

IMT is experimental for the treatment of prostate cancer with the aim of curing the disease while causing less morbidity than other conventional therapies (i.e., surgery, radiation).

16.3.1 Principles of IMT

Microwave antennas launch electromagnetic waves in the frequency range of 300–2,450 MHz into the targeted tissue. Microwave heating is produced as a result of dielectric hysteresis. When electromagnetic energy is applied to tissue, some of the energy is used to force molecules with an intrinsic dipole moment to continuously realign with the applied field. This rotation of molecules represents an increase in kinetic energy, and hence an elevation in local tissue temperatures. The waves cause small electric currents to propagate through tissue, inducing an increase of temperature [21].

The goal of developing IMT is to heat the area potentially harboring prostatic cancer cells to a cytotoxic temperature of 55–70 °C, while protecting critical adjacent tissues, such as the rectum, bladder, and urethra. Microwave needles, each housed within a water-cooling jacket, are inserted in the prostate through the perineum under transrectal ultrasound guidance; the urethra can be cooled using saline serum irrigation. The heating pattern of the needle is peanut-shaped with a maximum diameter of 50 % power deposition contour of 0.75 cm. Microwave energy is delivered at a frequency of 915 MHz. The generator is a model 500 Precision Hyperthermia System (BSD Medical Corp., Salt Lake City, Utah), and the power delivered to each antenna is adjustable up to a maximum of 25 W.

16.3.2 Potential Therapeutic Applications of IMT

To date, IMT has mainly been performed for recurrent cancers after external beam radiation, and no attempt of focal therapy is yet available.

Sherar et al. reported the safety and feasibility of IMT for recurrent PCa after radiation therapy. This trial showed that at 6 months posttreatment, 52 % of patients had PSA levels lower than 0.5 ng/mL and 64 % of patients had negative biopsies. In a longer follow-up period of 2 years, 42 % of patients were found to be biochemically recurrence-free after the ablation [22].

Lancaster et al. reported one patient with localized PCa who had a whole-gland microwave thermal therapy. After 18 months, there was no biochemical recurrence [23].

On a preclinical dog test subject, Cheng et al. successfully monitored an IMT procedure using MRI and contrast-enhanced ultrasound [24].

The realization of focal microwave thermal therapy will be made possible by the development of medical imaging and biopsy techniques.

16.4 Radiofrequency Interstitial Tumor Ablation (RITA)

Radiofrequency energy has been used to focally destroy tissues in animals as well as in humans. The safety and efficacy of this method were first demonstrated in the treatment of liver cancers and osteoid osteomas [25, 26]. The targeted tissue was irreversibly destroyed by coagulative necrosis.

Radiofrequency energy is used extensively to treat benign prostatic hyperplasia using the transurethral needle ablation (TUNA) device. Through a transurethral approach, coagulative necrosis is produced around the needles inserted into the prostate adenoma [27].

RITA energy is launched by a radiofrequency generator that can reach 50 W with a frequency of 460 kHz. Through 15-gauge needles, which are introduced into the prostate using the transperineal approach under TRUS guidance, this energy is administered with monopolar triple-hook electrodes separated by a 120° angle, describing a 2 cm volume sphere.

The urethra is protected by a Foley catheter irrigated with cold saline. Rectal temperature is monitored using thermocouples. RITA induces an irreversible destruction of tissue by increasing temperatures to around 100 °C, which induces a coagulative necrosis in the tumoral area without any evidence of venous thrombosis or significant hemorrhages at the tumoral borders [28].

Many teams have demonstrated RITA to be feasible, safe, and reproducible for the treatment of localized PCa [28–30].

In a phase 1 trial, Djavan et al. showed RITA to be safe, feasible, and efficient in accurately destroying tissue. A total of ten patients had RITA of localized PCa prior to MRI and radical prostatectomy. After ablation, MRI accurately visualized the foci of coagulative necrosis as documented in histology [28].

Shariat et al. reported focal RITA outcomes in 11 patients with localized PCa. Ninety percent of the patients showed a more than 50 % decrease in postoperative PSA, and PSA doubling time after RITA was longer than that before RITA. At 1-year follow-up biopsies, 55 % of patients were free of cancer. Minor complications occurred with hematuria in two patients, bladder spasms in one patient and burning sensation during micturition in another patient. Shariat et al. did not report whether there were changes in the patient's continence and erectile function as a result of this treatment. Two procedures had to be aborted because of the increase of temperature showed by the rectal probe [30].

Due to the incompleteness of evidence towards its benefits and risks, further studies are needed to evaluate the real potential of focal RITA.

Conclusion

Abundant debates exist with regard to the appropriate patient selection for focal therapy; however, there is almost no discussion on the ideal focal therapy energy. The latter must meet several criteria: (1) to be able to target and treat a specific area of the prostate; (2) to accurately shape the targeted area with no significant effect on the surrounding tissue; (3) to be minimally invasive with a low morbidity; and (4) to be reproducible.

References

1. Stattin P, Holmberg E, Johansson JE, Holmberg L, Adolfsson J, Hugosson J. Outcomes in localized prostate cancer: National Prostate Cancer Register of Sweden follow-up study. J Natl Cancer Inst. 2010;102(13):950–8. Epub 2010/06/22.
2. Loeb S, Vonesh EF, Metter EJ, Carter HB, Gann PH, Catalona WJ. What is the true number needed to screen and treat to save a life with prostate-specific antigen testing? J Clin Oncol. 2011;29(4):464–7. Epub 2010/12/30.
3. Wallace M. Uncertainty and quality of life of older men who undergo watchful waiting for prostate cancer. Oncol Nurs Forum. 2003;30(2):303–9. Epub 2003/04/15
4. Cooperberg MR, Lubeck DP, Meng MV, Mehta SS, Carroll PR. The changing face of low-risk prostate cancer: trends in clinical presentation and primary management. J Clin Oncol Off J Am Soc Clin Oncol. 2004;22(11):2141–9. Epub 2004/06/01.
5. Coster HG. A quantitative analysis of the voltage-current relationships of fixed charge membranes and the associated property of "punch-through". Biophys J. 1965;5(5):669–86. Epub 1965/09/01.
6. Neumann E, Schaefer-Ridder M, Wang Y, Hofschneider PH. Gene transfer into mouse lyoma cells by electroporation in high electric fields. EMBO J. 1982;1(7):841–5. Epub 1982/01/01.
7. Al-Sakere B, Andre F, Bernat C, Connault E, Opolon P, Davalos RV, et al. Tumor ablation with irreversible electroporation. PLoS One. 2007;2(11):e1135. Epub 2007/11/09.
8. Thomson KR, Cheung W, Ellis SJ, Federman D, Kavnoudias H, Loader-Oliver D, et al. Investigation of the safety of irreversible electroporation in humans. J Vasc Interv Radiol JVIR. 2011;22(5):611–21. Epub 2011/03/29.
9. Davalos RV, Mir IL, Rubinsky B. Tissue ablation with irreversible electroporation. Ann Biomed Eng. 2005;33(2):223–31. Epub 2005/03/18.
10. Lee EW, Loh CT, Kee ST. Imaging guided percutaneous irreversible electroporation: ultrasound and immunohistological correlation. Technol Cancer Res Treat. 2007;6(4):287–94. Epub 2007/08/03.

11. Edd JF, Horowitz L, Davalos RV, Mir LM, Rubinsky B. In vivo results of a new focal tissue ablation technique: irreversible electroporation. IEEE Trans Biomed Eng. 2006;53(7):1409–15. Epub 2006/07/13.

12. Charpentier KP, Wolf F, Noble L, Winn B, Resnick M, Dupuy DE. Irreversible electroporation of the liver and liver hilum in swine. HPB. 2011;13(3):168–73. Epub 2011/02/12.

13. Onik G, Mikus P, Rubinsky B. Irreversible electroporation: implications for prostate ablation. Technol Cancer Res Treat. 2007;6(4):295–300. Epub 2007/08/03.

14. Al-Sakere B, Bernat C, Andre F, Connault E, Opolon P, Davalos RV, et al. A study of the immunological response to tumor ablation with irreversible electroporation. Technol Cancer Res Treat. 2007;6(4):301–6. Epub 2007/08/03.

15. Ball C, Thomson KR, Kavnoudias H. Irreversible electroporation: a new challenge in "out of operating theater" anesthesia. Anesth Analg. 2010;110(5):1305–9. Epub 2010/02/10.

16. Bower M, Sherwood L, Li Y, Martin R. Irreversible electroporation of the pancreas: definitive local therapy without systemic effects. J Surg Oncol. 2011;104(1):22–8. Epub 2011/03/02.

17. Stock RG, Kao J, Stone NN. Penile erectile function after permanent radioactive seed implantation for treatment of prostate cancer. J Urol. 2001;165(2):436–9. Epub 2001/02/15.

18. Schoellnast H, Monette S, Ezell PC, Maybody M, Erinjeri JP, Stubblefield MD, et al. The delayed effects of irreversible electroporation ablation on nerves. Eur Radiol. 2013;23(2):375–80. Epub 2012/09/27.

19. Li W, Fan Q, Ji Z, Qiu X, Li Z. The effects of irreversible electroporation (IRE) on nerves. PLoS One. 2011;6(4):e18831. Epub 2011/05/03.

20. Tsivian M, Polascik TJ. Bilateral focal ablation of prostate tissue using low-energy direct current (LEDC): a preclinical canine study. BJU Int. 2013;112(4):526–30. Epub 2013/07/25.

21. Bozzini G, Colin P, Nevoux P, Villers A, Mordon S, Betrouni N. Focal therapy of prostate cancer: energies and procedures. Urol Oncol. 2013;31(2):155–67. Epub 2012/07/17.

22. Sherar MD, Gertner MR, Yue CK, O'Malley ME, Toi A, Gladman AS, et al. Interstitial microwave thermal therapy for prostate cancer: method of treatment and results of a phase I/II trial. J Urol. 2001;166(5):1707–14. Epub 2001/10/05.

23. Lancaster C, Toi A, Trachtenberg J. Interstitial microwave thermoablation for localized prostate cancer. Urology. 1999;53(4):828–31. Epub 1999/04/10.

24. Cheng HL, Haider MA, Dill-Macky MJ, Sweet JM, Trachtenberg J, Gertner MR. MRI and contrast-enhanced ultrasound monitoring of prostate microwave focal thermal therapy: an in vivo canine study. J Magn Reson Imaging. 2008;28(1):136–43. Epub 2008/06/27.

25. Rossi S, Di Stasi M, Buscarini E, Cavanna L, Quaretti P, Squassante E, et al. Percutaneous radiofrequency interstitial thermal ablation in the treatment of small hepatocellular carcinoma. Cancer J Sci Am. 1995;1(1):73–81. Epub 1995/05/01.

26. de Berg JC, Pattynama PM, Obermann WR, Bode PJ, Vielvoye GJ, Taminiau AH. Percutaneous computed-tomography-guided thermocoagulation for osteoid osteomas. Lancet. 1995;346(8971):350–1. Epub 1995/08/05.

27. Xylinas E, Le Gal S, Descazeaud A. Transurethral needle ablation Prostiva for treating symptomatic benign prostatic hyperplasia: a review. Progres en urologie. 2010;20(8):566–71. Epub 2010/09/14. Traitement de l'hyperplasie benigne de la prostate par radiofrequence monopolaire type Prostiva.

28. Djavan B, Zlotta AR, Susani M, Heinz G, Shariat S, Silverman DE, et al. Transperineal radiofrequency interstitial tumor ablation of the prostate: correlation of magnetic resonance imaging with histopathologic examination. Urology. 1997;50(6):986–92; discussion 92–3; Epub 1998/01/14.

29. Zlotta AR, Djavan B, Matos C, Noel JC, Peny MO, Silverman DE, et al. Percutaneous transperineal radiofrequency ablation of prostate tumour: safety, feasibility and pathological effects on human prostate cancer. Br J Urol. 1998;81(2):265–75. Epub 1998/03/06.

30. Shariat SF, Raptidis G, Masatoschi M, Bergamaschi F, Slawin KM. Pilot study of radiofrequency interstitial tumor ablation (RITA) for the treatment of radio-recurrent prostate cancer. Prostate. 2005;65(3):260–7. Epub 2005/07/15.

Lukman Hakim[$], Lorenzo Tosco, Wahjoe Djatisoesanto,
Thomas Van den Broeck, Willemien van den Bos,
Maarten Albersen, Hein Van Poppel, and Steven Joniau[$]

17.1 Purpose of Focal Treatment Follow-Up

Focal therapy as a treatment for localized prostate cancer (PCa) aims to completely destroy all malignant cells within the tumor area (oncological goal) while preserving surrounding nonmalignant tissue and physiological function (functional goal) such as urinary and erectile function [1]. The ideal imaging technology to support focal therapy would permit reliable contouring of the tumor area (target tissue) in order to target the treatment and evaluate tissue changes. Furthermore, it would permit to identify tumor growth following treatment [2]. Referring to these goals, the follow-up strategies after focal therapy generally aim at identifying the effectiveness of cancer control (oncological outcome), the functional outcomes, and adverse events. Additionally, follow-up strategy needs to cover the monitoring of disease progression and the option for salvage treatment when failure occurs.

[$]Author contributed equally with all other contributors.

L. Hakim, MD
Department of Urology, University Hospitals Leuven, Herestraat 49, Leuven 3000, Belgium

Department of Urology, Airlangga University/Dr. Soetomo General Hospital,
Mayjen Moestopo 6 – 8, Surabaya 60286, Indonesia

L. Tosco, MD • T. Van den Broeck, MD • M. Albersen, MD, PhD • H. Van Poppel, MD, PhD
S. Joniau, MD, PhD (✉)
Department of Urology, University Hospitals Leuven, Herestraat 49, Leuven 3000, Belgium
e-mail: steven.joniau@uzleuven.be

W. Djatisoesanto, MD, PhD
Department of Urology, Airlangga University/Dr. Soetomo General Hospital,
Mayjen Moestopo 6 – 8, Surabaya 60286, Indonesia

W. van den Bos, MD
Department of Urology, Academic Medical Center Amsterdam,
Meibergdreef 9, Amsterdam 1105 AZ, The Netherlands

© Springer-Verlag France 2015
E. Barret, M. Durand (eds.), *Technical Aspects of Focal Therapy
in Localized Prostate Cancer*, DOI 10.1007/978-2-8178-0484-2_17

Until recently, no universal follow-up protocol was agreed upon. Previous studies led to differences in outcomes as a result of the lack of uniform patient selection criteria, pre- and posttreatment evaluation, and the diversity of end point definition.

17.2 How to Follow Up Patients After Focal Therapy

The follow-up after focal therapy for PCa entails various aspects: the definition of therapy failure and disease recurrence, the follow-up intervals, the methods and technologies to use for accurate outcome measurement, etc. Various follow-up plans have been proposed in published series of focal therapy for localized PCa, starting at 1 month following focal therapy, with 3 monthly intervals in the first year, 6 monthly in the second year, and annually thereafter [3, 4]. In some studies, the proposed follow-up intervals differed, but with a similar consideration that intervals become longer as the follow-up time lengthens.

Prostate-specific antigen (PSA), transrectal ultrasound (TRUS), and ultrasound (US)-guided biopsy, multiparametric magnetic resonance imaging (mpMRI), and validated questionnaires were commonly used methods to identify and monitor oncological and functional outcomes as well as disease progression. The basic concept of the follow-up is to design a standardized protocol that may be individualized, based on patient and disease characteristics.

A recent consensus of experts from around the world that involved a multidisciplinary panel of 48 experts in the field of focal therapy agreed that PSA measurement should be part of the follow-up schedule. They proposed measurements at 3 monthly intervals in the first year, biannually in the second, annually in the third, and based on the investigators' discretion thereafter. TRUS-guided systematic whole-gland biopsies are recommended between 6 and 12 months following treatment. Furthermore, the panel proposed performing an mpMRI (T2 weighted images combined with at least two functional MRI techniques) before follow-up biopsies [5]. These aspects of oncological follow-up will be discussed below.

17.2.1 PSA Monitoring

Since its introduction in 1987, PSA has been used increasingly and has led to the detection of less aggressive disease at an earlier (localized) stage, lower grade, and smaller volume. PSA is commonly used for screening, diagnosis, and follow-up after whole-gland treatment to detect treatment failure or disease recurrence. This gland-driven marker has been validated in several surgical and radiotherapy studies with large sample sizes. However, PSA measurement might not be of benefit in indicating incomplete tumor destruction in the follow-up setting of focal therapy, since the remaining benign glandular tissue as well as possible residual tumor cells keep on secreting PSA [2]. Furthermore, the mechanisms of cell death are likely to be different when comparing whole-gland treatments such as surgery or radiotherapy to focal ablation. As a result, PSA kinetics (PSA density, PSA doubling time, and PSA velocity) are also likely to differ [4].

PSA is currently used as one criterion for biochemical failure following whole-gland ablation. Most of the published studies have used either the Phoenix (ASTRO) definition, which defined failure as $\geq$PSA nadir + 2 ng/ml, or the Stuttgart definition, which defined failure as $\geq$PSA nadir + 1.2 ng/ml. The first was developed and validated for radiotherapy but not for other treatment options, while the later was generated from HIFU-based whole-gland ablation. Unfortunately, the latter definition has not been externally validated. In a first attempt to find a reliable definition of biochemical failure following peripheral zone brachytherapy as zonal ablation, Nguyen et al. [6] refined the Phoenix criteria by adding PSA velocity to the definition. In their series on zonal brachytherapy, PSA nadir + 2 + PSA velocity 0.75 ng/ml per year was shown to perform better in predicting clinical failure compared to the Phoenix definition [6].

Despite the recommendation of 48 multidisciplinary-experts regarding PSA, the panel members also acknowledged that the use of PSA in the follow-up of focal therapy lacks evidence and needs further validation. Therefore, the interpretation of PSA as a stand-alone parameter in the follow-up setting should be avoided [5].

17.2.2 Imaging

TRUS and Derivates

Imaging technology for prostate diseases was initially influenced by the introduction of TRUS in the early 1970s and was later considered to be the gold standard platform for needle biopsy-based PCa diagnosis [7]. Since then, the technology of US has developed rapidly, not only for the detection of cancer foci, but also for therapy planning, guidance, and monitoring during brachytherapy and ablative (whole-gland and focal) therapy and thereafter in follow-up programs. However, a multidisciplinary meeting of experts reached a consensus in 2012 that none of the currently available US-based imaging techniques should be used to decide for or against focal therapy. US-based imaging modalities cannot replace TRUS-guided biopsy as the basis for focal therapy treatment decisions [2, 8]. Conventional TRUS should only be used to identify the prostate, to guide the biopsy procedure, to assess the prostate volume and to identify anatomical variations [8]. Referring to this consensus, the use of US imaging alone in posttreatment follow-up is equally meaningless without a biopsy, given the fact that anatomy and vascularity of the prostate and possible remaining cancer are more difficult to image and interpret following ablation due to posttreatment effects.

Besides the fact that TRUS largely underperforms in localizing PCa foci and cannot be used as a sole technique in focal treatment follow-up, TRUS-guided biopsy is also flawed by inherent random and systematic sampling errors when used after focal therapy and may not be reliable in determining the absence of residual disease [4]. A systematic review conducted by Valerio et al. involving a total of 2,350 cases of localized PCa observed that 14 of the 29 (48 %) previous studies in focal therapy reported their usage of US imaging following focal therapy to evaluate the effectiveness of ablation; of them, 13 (93 %) used TRUS as a guidance for biopsy and 1 (7 %) used transperineal template-mapping biopsy (TTMB) [4].

New techniques have emerged to address these limitations. Current available technologies to improve the diagnosis of PCa are either contrast-enhanced ultrasound (CEUS) [9], real-time US elastography [10], computer-aided US that extracts and analyzes data to identify cancer tissue using pre-developed software [11], or MRI-based technology that uses various modalities to increase cancer detection rates [12–16].

CEUS was previously used within the context of PCa detection and localization. Although CEUS technology is advantageous to MRI as it may provide real-time assessment of cancer destruction during or immediately after treatment, its use for evaluating the effectiveness of focal therapy without biopsy lacks evidence. Rouvière et al. studied the use of CEUS to distinguish between ablated (devascularized) and viable (enhanced) tissue post-HIFU treatment, and observed a significant correlation between the CEUS predetermined parameters and the biopsy results. CEUS clearly depicted devascularized areas within minutes of ablation, up until 45 days thereafter [17]. 3-D-US, in combination with systematic biopsy, may increase the accuracy of evaluating destruction zones after focal ablation. To increase diagnostic accuracy, some authors used a 3-D-constructed map that enables displaying the most frequent locations of PCa based on the 3-D reconstruction of prostatectomy specimens [18, 19]. Although these novel imaging technologies are promising, the lack of evidence in prospective trials and absence of external validation are their major limitations at this moment.

mpMRI

MRI-based technology has become the imaging option of choice for the evaluation of the effectiveness of focal therapy, given the uncertainty of post-ablation PSA and the risk of sampling errors when using TRUS-guided biopsy. mpMRI is considered the gold-standard imaging technique following HIFU treatment, and it integrates T2-weighted imaging combined with at least two functional MRI techniques (diffusion-weighted MRI (DW-MRI), dynamic contrast-enhanced MRI (DCE-MRI), or MRI spectroscopy) [20]. mpMRI aims to increase the detection rate of remaining or recurrent cancers within the destroyed zone following focal therapy. In two studies of HIFU-treated patients, Ahmed et al. observed no significant cancer in the treatment area when mpMRI showed no signs of a remaining cancer. The sensitivity of MRI for the detection of residual disease ranged from 73 to 87 %, and the specificity from 73 to 82 %, with good agreement between readers [22]. Taken together, mpMRI appears to be the optimal imaging modality in the follow-up of patients' post-focal therapy, as it reliably detects high-grade tumors (GS ≥ 7) and anterior tumors, and also shows significant correlation with the results of post-ablation biopsy results. On the other hand, mpMRI overlooks some low-grade tumors, and it is sometimes difficult to interpret post-ablation tissue changes. Therefore, the use of mpMRI in post-ablation treatment follow-up still needs confirmed standardized criteria [22].

There was a multidisciplinary consensus in 2013 regarding the role of mpMRI in the follow-up of focal therapy for localized PCa. mpMRI should be performed 6 months after treatment and followed by a yearly mpMRI. It was also agreed that adverse mpMRI findings should be further confirmed by biopsy before re-treatment, and that mpMRI should be interpreted by experienced radiologists or uro-oncologic radiologists [5, 23]. What should be kept in mind is that mpMRI cannot be a substitute for prostate biopsy in the follow-up setting, but needs to be seen as a tool to support the prostate biopsy findings.

17.2.3 Prostate Biopsy

Since the transrectal sextant prostate biopsy was introduced by Hodge in 1989, this procedure has become a robust method for the diagnosis of PCa, but the rate of missed cancers observed in that study was found to be quite high (14 of 57 biopsies or >25 %) [24]. Many later studies focused on how to increase the detection rate by increasing the number of biopsy cores, adapting the number of cores to the prostate size and using different systematic templates. Tsivian et al. [25] showed an increase of sensitivity, specificity, and accuracy to detect unilateral PCa from 84.1 to 88 %; 37.1 to 53.9 %, and 49 to 59 %, respectively, when comparing sextant and extended core biopsies [25]. Other studies have shown that by using a 10–14 core biopsy protocol, only 20–35 % of unilateral PCa on biopsies (proposed as the best candidates for focal therapy) have true unilateral disease at radical prostatectomy [2]. The correlation of the Gleason biopsy score and Gleason surgery score were also shown to be low [26, 27]. These facts show that conventional and even more extended templates of prostate biopsy (up to 14 cores) are not sensitive enough to detect unilateral PCa and do not correlate well with radical prostatectomy specimens, which may lead to undertreatment of the disease. Saturation biopsy schemes, which refer to a systematic biopsy procedure with ≥20 cores, may offer a better option, increasing the detection rate of PCa with 30–40 % in men who had a prior negative biopsy, but with twofold higher morbidity rates (urinary retention 10 % vs. 1 %, hematuria requiring treatment 4 % vs. 0 %; $p < 0.001$) compared to 12–18 core biopsies [27–29]. These facts suggest that a higher number of biopsies might result in a higher detection rate, which is important for patient selection in focal therapy schemes. Nevertheless, saturation biopsy was also shown to miss significant cancers, with as much as 83 % of overlooked contralateral cancers and 8 % of missed stage pT3 cancers. Finally, transperineal template-mapping biopsy under 3-D ultrasound guidance (3-D-TTMB) might further increase the detection rate by at least 40 % following previous negative transrectal biopsy [30–32].

In terms of follow-up after focal therapy, prostate biopsy is an option for evaluating or detecting remaining cancers within the ablated tissue and identifying missed or new cancers in the untreated gland. Since PSA and imaging have not been proven reliable in ruling out remaining or recurrent cancers, a systematic prostate biopsy will still be necessary to identify incomplete tumor destruction or tumor recurrence following focal ablation. Here, a systematic 3-D-TTMB might be helpful, whereas a conventional random core biopsy might miss remaining cancers at a higher percentage [30–33]. Up until now, this technique appears to be one of the most accurate tools for confirming the effectiveness of focal therapy, with only a <5 % risk of missing significant PCa [4]. The need for general anesthesia for performing 3D-TTMB is still an issue given the nature of the noninvasiveness of focal therapy.

17.3 Definitions of Treatment Failure

The definitions of treatment failure in the focal therapy setting have not yet been standardized. Previous researchers used varying outcome parameters, such as survival outcomes (biochemical recurrence-free survival, overall survival, or PCa-specific survival) or positive biopsies at the treatment area or in the ipsilateral or contralateral lobe. Other researchers used the need for further treatment (salvage therapy) as the definition of failure [34].

As mentioned in the PSA section above, several criteria have been developed to define failure following focal therapy, and most researchers used either the Phoenix, Stuttgart, or Nguyen criteria. The lack of evidence and validation remain the main problems regarding these criteria, so that prospective studies with adequate sample sizes and similar end points need to be establish in order to validate PSA-based outcome definitions. The use of hard survival end points that would allow comparison with active surveillance or accepted radical treatments would require large-scale RCTs with a minimum of 5 years to recruit a sufficient number of patients and another 10–15 years of follow-up [4].

In order to overcome some of the difficulties related to outcome definitions, an international multidisciplinary consensus on trial design suggested the following for future focal therapy trials [5]:

- In-field failure: either (1) cancer of a higher Gleason grade; (2) persistent cancer of similar or lower grade after repeat focal therapy to the same area; or (3) the need for additional PCa treatment other than focal therapy because of objective findings elsewhere in the gland (e.g., high-grade cancer).
- Low-grade, low-volume tumor foci <3 mm, Gleason $3+3$ found out-of-field is not considered a failure.
- Selection failure: any cancer characteristic that matches the inclusion criteria for focal therapy as recommended by the panel and located out-of-field.
- The panel also agreed that biochemical failure currently should not be used as an outcome definition in upcoming trials, because of insufficient data.

Since histopathological criteria are currently used to determine treatment failure, the technique of biopsy is also of importance. Based on recent evidence, a 3-D/4-D-TTMB as mentioned in the imaging section above may provide the highest accuracy for this purpose. Nevertheless, the consensus panel agreed that TRUS-guided systematic whole-prostate biopsy and additionally targeted biopsy to the area of the focal ablation, taken between 6 and 12 months following focal therapy, would be the optimal strategy [5].

In summary, the failure criteria for focal therapy at this moment seem to rely on consensus and are based on histopathology, until PSA or other biochemical markers show strong evidence as reliable and validated outcome parameters. This situation may remain for the next 5–7 years, until some ongoing phase 2 and 3 comparative trials in focal therapy will be published [5].

17.4 Definition of Recurrence

The terminology of recurrence and failure are interchangeably used in cancer treatment. However, failure represents incomplete ablation, while recurrence represents a relapse of cancer following a successful ablation. As mentioned in the section above, various failure criteria were used following focal therapy.

Villers et al. studied 117 prostate specimens from 234 prostatectomy-treated patients and observed that 80 % of additional incidental cancers were <0.5 ml while fewer than 20 % of index tumors were <0.5 ml. It was concluded that additional incidental tumors are common in PCa patients, but their volume was rarely similar to the volume of the index lesions [35].

On the other hand, Stamey et al. studied prostate specimens following cysto-prostatectomy and concluded that 0.5 ml could be used as a volume cut-off for a clinically significant PCa. The authors proposed that cancer progression is proportional to cancer volume, and observed that 80 % of PCas smaller than 0.5 ml are not likely to ever reach a clinically significant size in view of the long PSA doubling time [36].

Previous studies in focal therapy have used 0.5 ml as an end point to evaluate treatment, and a dominant tumor of >0.5 ml is also recommended by an international expert consensus of focal therapy as a primary end point for future trials [5]. Referring to this evidence, one should consider that a tumor size with a cut-off of 0.5 ml should be considered as a criterion for recurrence following treatment, but on the contrary this was not recommended by the international experts, based on the current consensus of focal therapy trial design.

Bahn et al. studied the outcomes of 73 unilateral localized PCas following cryotherapy and observed that among the biopsy-proven recurrences, the range of PSA was between 0 and 1.5 ng/ml, suggesting that biopsy revealed cancer recurrence before it was detected by PSA [34]. Histopathology results following focal therapy are currently considered to be highly accurate in identifying both failure and local recurrence.

Conclusion

Considering the lack of evidence supporting the concept of focal therapy in localized PCa, well-designed, prospective trials using standardized in- and exclusion criteria and outcome definitions are necessary. PSA and various imaging technologies are nowadays commonly used in the follow-up after focal therapy, but none of these are externally validated yet. Ideally, focal therapy outcomes should be compared with the outcomes of radical whole-gland treatment, such as radical prostatectomy and radiotherapy, and with those of active surveillance. However, results from such trials are expected to become available only in the future.

In the meantime, applying in- and exclusion criteria and follow-up plan as recommended by a recent consensus paper by multidisciplinary experts in the field of focal therapy provides the means to achieve outcomes from future trials that may allow comparison between studies and standardization of outcome parameters.

We propose a follow-up plan based on the recommendations of the recently published multidisciplinary consensus paper (Fig. 17.1) [5].

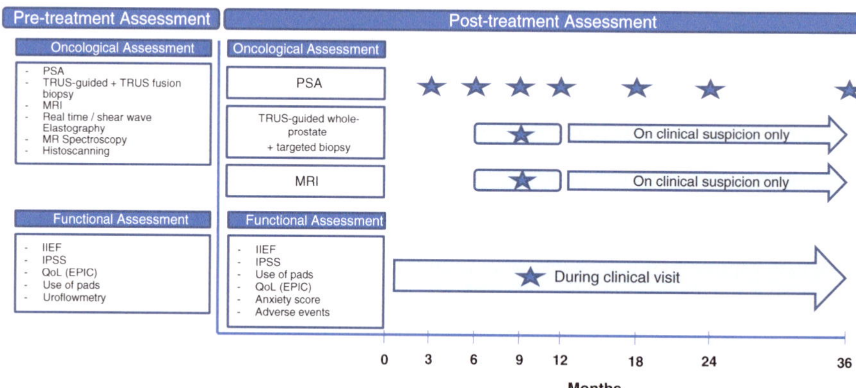

Fig. 17.1 A schematic pre and posttreatment assessment based on the International Multidisciplinary Consensus on Trial Design in Focal Therapy of Prostate Cancer. *Left side*: Pre-assessment should at least consist of oncological assessment: PSA TRUS-guided systematic biopsy + targeted biopsy of the whole prostate and MRI (the best characteristic possible, prefera-bly mpMRI) which can be performed prior to biopsy or 4–8 weeks thereafter. MP spectroscopy, elastography, and histoscanning may be performed to provide more information on location, aggressiveness and extent of tumor; Functional assessment should be performed using currently validated questionnaires: The International Index of Erectile Function (*IIEF*) and International Prostate Symptoms Score (*IPSS*). Quality of life (*QoL*) assessment should also be performed using the Expanded PCa Index Composite (*EPIC*) questionnaire. Incase incontinence occurs, the use of pads should be measured. Uroflowmetry is not essential, but may provide additional data on outlet obstruction and postvoiding residual. *Right side*: The posttreatment assessment should consist of oncological and functional assessments, adverse events, and optionally anxiety scores. The PSA measurement should be performed at 3-month interval during the first year of follow-up, biannu-ally in the second year and yearly in the third year. After 3 years, PSA evaluation can be performed based on clinician's discretion. TRUS-guided systematic whole-prostate biopsy + targeted biopsy to the suspicious areas should be performed between 6 and 8-month following focal therapy, while mpMRI should be performed prior to biopsy or 6–8 weeks thereafter by a uro-oncologic radiolo-gists. After this period, biopsy should only be performed based on based on clinical suspicion only. mpMRI should be performed in addition to biopsy. Functional assessment includes all the ques-tionnaires of the pretreatment, while adverse events should be observed in addition. Anxiety scores is an option to assess during the follow-up. Since there is no consensus on the time of functional assessment should be performed in the follow-up setting, it can be assess based on patients com-plaints or clinicians discretion during the clinical visit

References

1. Mouraviev V, Mayes JM, Polascik TJ. Pathologic basis of focal therapy for early-stage prostate cancer. Nat Rev Urol. 2009;6:205–15.
2. Rouvière O, Gelet A, Crouzet S, Chapelon J-Y. Prostate focused ultrasound focal therapy-imaging for the future. Nat Rev Clin Oncol. 2012;9:721–7.
3. Ahmed HU, et al. Focal therapy for localised unifocal and multifocal prostate cancer: a prospective development study. Lancet Oncol. 2012;13:622–32.
4. Valerio M, et al. The role of focal therapy in the management of localised prostate cancer: a systematic review. Eur Urol. 2013;44:1–20.
5. Van den Bos W, et al. Focal therapy in prostate cancer: international multidisciplinary consensus on trial design. Eur Urol. 2014;65:1078–83. doi:10.1016/j.eururo.2014.01.001.
6. Nguyen PL, et al. Updated results of magnetic resonance imaging guided partial prostate brachytherapy for favorable risk prostate cancer: implications for focal therapy. J Urol. 2012;188:1151–6.
7. Heidenreich A, et al. EAU guidelines on prostate cancer. Part 1: screening, diagnosis, and treatment of clinically localised disease. Eur Urol. 2011;59:61–71.
8. Smeenge M, et al. Role of transrectal ultrasonography (TRUS) in focal therapy of prostate cancer: report from a Consensus Panel. BJU Int. 2012;110:942–8.
9. Smeenge M, Mischi M, Laguna Pes MP, de la Rosette JJMCH, Wijkstra H. Novel contrast-enhanced ultrasound imaging in prostate cancer. World J Urol. 2011;29:581–7.
10. Walz J, et al. Identification of the prostate cancer index lesion by real-time elastography: considerations for focal therapy of prostate cancer. World J Urol. 2011;29:589–94.
11. Simmons LA, et al. Detection, localisation and characterisation of prostate cancer by prostate HistoScanning(™). BJU Int. 2012;110:28–35.
12. Girouin N, et al. Prostate dynamic contrast-enhanced MRI with simple visual diagnostic criteria: is it reasonable? Eur Radiol. 2007;17:1498–509.
13. Fütterer F, et al. Prostate cancer localization with dynamic contrast- enhanced MR imaging and purpose: methods: results: conclusion. Radiology. 2006;241:449–58.
14. Katahira K, et al. Ultra-high-b-value diffusion-weighted MR imaging for the detection of prostate cancer: evaluation in 201 cases with histopathological correlation. Eur Radiol. 2011;21:188–96.
15. Reinsberg SA, et al. Combined use of diffusion-weighted MRI and 1H MR spectroscopy to increase accuracy in prostate cancer detection. AJR Am J Roentgenol. 2007;188:91–8.
16. Tan CH, Wang J, Kundra V. Diffusion weighted imaging in prostate cancer. Eur Radiol. 2011;21:593–603.
17. Rouviere O, et al. Prostate cancer ablation with focused ultrasound: assessment of tissue destruction with purpose : methods: results: conclusion. Radiology. 2011;259:583–91.
18. Narayanan R, et al. Adaptation of a 3D prostate cancer atlas for transrectal ultrasound guided target-specific biopsy. Phys Med Biol. 2008;53:N397–406.
19. Zhan Y, et al. Targeted prostate biopsy using statistical image analysis. IEEE Trans Med Imaging. 2007;26:779–88.
20. Cordeiro ER, et al. High-intensity focused ultrasound (HIFU) for definitive treatment of prostate cancer. BJU Int. 2012;110:1228–42.
21. Ahmed HU, et al. Focal therapy for localized prostate cancer: a phase I/II trial. J Urol. 2011;185:1246–54.
22. Punwani S, et al. Prostatic cancer surveillance following whole-gland high-intensity focused ultrasound: comparison of MRI and prostate-specific antigen for detection of residual or recurrent disease. Br J Radiol. 2012;85:720–8.
23. Muller B, et al. The role of multiparametric magnetic resonance imaging in focal therapy for prostate cancer: a delphi consensus project. BJU Int. 2014;114:698–707. doi:10.1111/bju.12548.

24. Lehana Yeo, Dharmesh Patel, Christian Bach, Athanasios Papatsoris, Noor Buchholz, Islam Junaid, Junaid Masood. The Development of the Modern Prostate Biopsy, Prostate Biopsy, Dr. Nabil K. Bissada (Ed.), ISBN: 978-953-307-702-4, InTech, Available from: http://www.intechopen.com/books/prostate-biopsy/the- development-of-the-modern-prostate-biopsy.
25. Tsivian M, et al. Predicting unilateral prostate cancer on routine diagnostic biopsy: sextant vs extended. BJU Int. 2010;105:1089–92.
26. Taneja SS, Mason M. Candidate selection for prostate cancer focal therapy. J Endourol. 2010;24:835–41.
27. Walz J, et al. High incidence of prostate cancer detected by saturation biopsy after previous negative biopsy series. Eur Urol. 2006;50:498–505.
28. Shariat SF, Roehrborn CG. Using biopsy to detect prostate cancer. Rev Urol. 2008;10:262–80.
29. Ashley RA, et al. Reassessing the diagnostic yield of saturation biopsy of the prostate. Eur Urol. 2008;53:976–81.
30. Igel TC, et al. Systematic transperineal ultrasound guided template biopsy of the prostate in patients at high risk. J Urol. 2001;165:1575–9.
31. Sartor AO, et al. Evaluating localized prostate cancer and identifying candidates for focal therapy. Urology. 2008;72:S12–24.
32. Merrick GS, et al. Prostate cancer distribution in patients diagnosed by transperineal template-guided saturation biopsy. Eur Urol. 2007;52:715–23.
33. Taira AV, et al. Performance of transperineal template-guided mapping biopsy in detecting prostate cancer in the initial and repeat biopsy setting. Prostate Cancer Prostatic Dis. 2010;13:71–7.
34. Bahn D, et al. Focal cryotherapy for clinically unilateral, low-intermediate risk prostate cancer in 73 men with a median follow-up of 3.7 years. Eur Urol. 2012;62:55–63.
35. Villers A, McNeal JE, Freiha FS, Stamey TA. Multiple cancers in the prostate morphologic features of clinically recognized versus incidental tumors. Cancer. 1992;70(9):2313–8.
36. Stamey TA, Yang N, Hay AR, McNeal JE, Freiha FS, Redwine E. Prostate-specific antigen as a serum marker for adenocarcinoma of the prostate. N Engl J Med. 1987;317(15):909–16.

18

Adil Ouzzane, Pierre Colin, Nacim Betrouni,
and Arnauld Villers

18.1 Introduction

Focal therapy (FT) is a novel therapeutic approach for investigating localized prostate cancer and consists of the ablation of all known clinically significant cancer foci within the prostate gland while sparing the rest of the gland to avoid urinary and sexual side effects [1]. Compared to whole-gland treatment approaches such as radical prostatectomy or external radiation beam therapy, FT is not a definitive local therapy, and re-treatment seems feasible in cases of treatment failure or local recurrence. However, the definition of treatment failure and local recurrence is not yet clearly documented because FT strategies range from true focal ablation of the index tumor or hemiablation to subtotal ablation of three-quarters of the gland [2]. Prostate-specific antigen (PSA) monitoring is not accurate for outcome assessment

A. Ouzzane • P. Colin
Department of Urology, CHU Lille, Université de Lille, Lille F-59000, France

Inserm (French National Institute of Health and Medical Research),
U1189-ONCO-THAI, Lille, France

Department of Urology, Université de Lille, Lille, France

N. Betrouni
Inserm (French National Institute of Health and Medical Research),
U1189-ONCO-THAI, Lille, France

Université de Lille, Lille, France

A. Villers, MD, PhD (✉)
Department of Urology, CHU Lille, Université de Lille, Lille F-59000, France

Inserm (French National Institute of Health and Medical Research),
U1189-ONCO-THAI, Lille, France

Université de Lille, Lille, France

Department of Urology, Hôpital Claude Huriez, Rue Michel Polonovski, Lille 59000, France
e-mail: arnauld.villers@wanadoo.fr

© Springer-Verlag France 2015
E. Barret, M. Durand (eds.), *Technical Aspects of Focal Therapy
in Localized Prostate Cancer*, DOI 10.1007/978-2-8178-0484-2_18

because a proportion of prostate tissue is left untreated after FT. Moreover, PSA kinetics for success and failure are not well defined, and magnetic resonance imaging (MRI) evaluation in combination with biopsy results are the most relevant tools available for the diagnosis of failure. The goal of this chapter is to summarize the limited data available on failure or recurrence after focal ablation of prostate cancer and to issue recommendations for the second therapy strategy.

18.2 Treatment of Histological Recurrence

Over the last few years, the interest on focal therapy for prostate cancer has dramatically increased. In a recent systematic review, nine series using variable sources of energy with post-focal therapy biopsies were reported [3]. Positive biopsies ranged from 4 to 50 %, with clinically significant cancer ranging from 0 to 17 %. Only two series evaluated the presence of residual tumors in the treated area, and this amounted from 3 to 14 %, with the need for secondary focal treatments ranging from 0 to 33 % in them. However, except for these early feasibility studies, which verified the effect of tissue ablation or reporting biochemical non-validated outcomes, only a few series with clinically relevant sample size and follow-up biopsy data were published (Table 18.1). Failure or recurrence can be detected by MRI and proven by positive biopsies in the treated lobe, while positive biopsies or a

Table 18.1 Key studies reporting histologic control and recurrence management after focal therapy for localized prostate cancer

Series	Modality and selection criteria	Follow-up	Failure and recurrence	Failure and recurrence management
Ahmed et al. [4] (*n*=42)	HIFU, cancer on MRI and TMB, Gleason 4+3 or less, T2 stage or less, PSA 15 ng/ml or less	TMB, MRI and targeted biopsies at 6 months, MRI and targeted biopsies at 12 months	9/39 (3 significant)	AS: 5
			MRI+:7/9 positive biopsies	Re-HIFU: 4
			MRI−: 2/30 positive biopsies	
Bahn et al. [5] (*n*=73)	Cryotherapy, unilateral T1-T2b cancer, Gleason ≤7, PSA ≤20 ng/ml	TRUS biopsies at 6, 12 months and yearly	12/48 biopsied had cancer (1 treated lobe, 11 untreated lobe)	ADT: 1
				AS: 8
				Re-treatment: 3 (2 cryotherapy and 1 RT)
Unpublished ongoing study by the AFU (*n*=87)	HIFU, unilateral cancer at MRI and 12 biopsies, Gleason score ≤3+4, PSA <10 ng/ml	MRI and SB at 6 or 12 months	6/25 biopsied had cancer (2 treated lobe, 4 untreated lobe)	AS: 2
				Re-treatment: 2
				RP: 1
				EBRT: 1

PSA prostate-specific antigen, *TMB* transperineal mapping biopsies, *SB* systematic biopsies, *AS* active surveillance, *ADT* androgen deprivation therapy, *EBRT* external radiation beam therapy, *RP* radical prostatectomy, *AFU* French association of urology suspicious MRI in the contralateral lobe can be explained by a secondary tumor (preexisting or de novo occurrence). Indeed, decision-making criteria include the number and location of positive biopsy cores, tumor grade, and MRI findings, and may lead to active surveillance, re-treatment with focal approach or salvage radical treatment. Reported secondary treatment modalities in key studies are summarized in Table 18.1. Beyond their feasibility, outcomes of secondary treatment after histological recurrence are not documented since they concern only a few cases.

18.3 Treatment of De Novo Lesion Occurrence: Possibilities and Results

Prostate cancer is a multifocal disease, as demonstrated by radical prostatectomy and autopsy series. However (and despite this multifocality), the prognosis is mainly due to the index tumor that represents the largest tumor within the gland harboring the highest grade and is eventually responsible for adverse pathological features (extraprostatic extension, nodal and metastatic spread, etc.) [6]. The goal of focal therapy is to target and destroy the index lesion in the prostate, sparing the rest of the gland, including small secondary tumor foci, that can be followed for progression. In a series of 215 cancer foci detected in an unselected population of 96 cysto-prostatectomy specimens, prostate cancer was multifocal in 58 % of the cases, including 79 % of bilateral cases [7]. Consequently, a second cancer can potentially be detected in 58 % of cases after focal therapy of prostate cancer, including 79 % in the contralateral lobe and 21 % in the same lobe. However, 33 % of cancers are anteriorly located beyond the area sampled by systematic biopsies while the remaining 67 % are posterior and can be incidentally detected at systematic biopsies. These second tumors are insignificant in volume (less than 0.5 cc) in 86 % [8] of cases and are undetectable with current imaging techniques in the majority of cases. In clinical practice, failure or recurrence is defined by positive biopsies in the treated lobe while positive biopsies in the untreated lobe are related to secondary preexisting or de novo tumors. Moreover, differentiating de novo occurrence and a preexisting secondary tumor is not possible with today's available diagnostic tools. If secondary treatment is needed, the prostate may be treated in similar fashion with serial treatments or repeat treatment. The treatment of de novo lesion occurrence should follow the same rules as the primary tumor. Hence, FT can be part of the therapeutic arsenal as well as active surveillance and whole-gland treatment (Table 18.2). However, potential bilateral damage of the neurovascular bundle after second contralateral FT would make FT less attractive due to the lack of functional benefits and the risk of recurrence or undertreatment. This situation may lead to considering whole-gland therapy to be an alternative to FT for a secondary approach.

18.4 Management of PSA-Relapse After FC

Unlike for whole-gland therapies, there is no consensus in the literature for biochemical-recurrence definition after FT. This is mainly explained by the variable proportion of preserved prostate tissue after FT which is related to prostate size at

Table 18.2 Patient selection criteria for FT

Criteria	Best selection criteria for FT	Comments
Age	No limits	Life expectancy >5 years might be added
Urinary function	No limits	IPSS DM to inform about the risk of AUR
Prostate size	Depends upon modality	In small glands <20 cc (or previous TURP) FT may damage periprostatic: striated sphincter
MRI and MR-targeted biopsies	Yes (some not MRI seen cancers could be eligible for FT)	MRI best modality to see index tumor and check rest of gland is free of tumor
		MR-targeted biopsies necessary to diagnose 20 % of tumors missed by posterior systematic biopsies
Index tumor >0.5 cc or 7 mm diameter	Yes	Represents the limit of detection by MRI. Could be 2 index tumors need to be treated
Tumor grade	Grades 3 or 4	If well circumscribed and located of grade 4 <50 % is not a contraindication (4 + 3 or 4 + 4 reserved in phase III FT vs RP)
Tumor volume	0.5–2 cc [1]	Should be less than 2/3 of a lobe in height, and less than half of a lobe in thickness. Otherwise, it should be subtotal therapy
DRE, T stage	Could be T1c or T2 or T3a	DRE could be suspicious or not. Best criteria is location and size at imaging and biopsies
PSA	3–10 ng/ml or 10–20 ng/ml in concordance with tumor grade and volume	PSA value should be concordant with tumor size and grade and gland size. If PSA close to 20 ng/ml, with a kinetics >1 ng/ml/year in case of a 0.5 cc grade 3 + 3 tumor, there is discordance
Location	Not at the apex	Ablation of lesion plus margin located the apex without sphincter damage has not been validated (based on subsequent radical prostatectomy). Lesion contour at MRI should be >5 mm from apex. Anterior location or close to urethra or bladder neck is not a contraindication
Multifocality	Yes	Not a contraindication if clinically insignificant tumor foci[a]

[a]Clinically insignificant tumor foci defined as a cT1c, DRE negative, one or two positive biopsies <3 mm grade 3 + 3, (Harnden Criteria) not seen at MRI

baseline and the volume of the ablated zone. Despite the lack of a PSA threshold for recurrence after FT, the PSA kinetic should be part from the follow-up setting. The value of ancillary PSA data, such as PSA velocity and slope, free vs. total PSA, PSA doubling time, and PSA density, has not yet been established. Lindner et al. failed to find any correlation between new or residual cancers on post-ablation biopsy and nadir PSA, time to nadir PSA, or PSA velocity following interstitial photothermal FT [9]. From a practical point of view, PSA measurement can be used as a predictor of local cancer recurrence. PSA relapse should be considered as a histological progression of cancer or BPH following FT, and patients should be assessed with combined MRI and biopsies, which remain the gold standard tests. The accuracy of PSA kinetics or threshold will be assessed prospectively in ongoing trials.

18.5   Treatment of Progression of Primary Lesion: Possibilities and Results

There is a notable lack of a standardized approach to decision-making in managing the progression of primary lesions after FT, and the techniques vary widely from AS or re-FT to whole-gland treatment (Table 18.1). Two parameters should be taken into consideration: tumor characteristics, and functional evaluation of the patient. If FT selection criteria can be respected (Table 18.2), salvage FT should be considered. If criteria for FT selection cannot be fulfilled, whole-gland therapy should be carried out. Regarding the functional results, if no expected benefit of second FT is likely to occur (functional sequel already present or very likely to occur), this situation may lead to considering whole-gland therapy.

Conclusion

Compared to whole-gland treatment approaches such as radical prostatectomy or external radiation beam therapy, FT is not a definitive local therapy and re-treatment seems feasible in cases of treatment failure or local recurrence. Failure or recurrence after focal therapy can be detected by MRI and proven by positive biopsies in the treated lobe, while positive biopsies or suspicious MRIs in the contralateral lobe can be explained by secondary tumors (pre-existing or de novo occurrence). Decision-making criteria for failure or recurrence management include functional evaluation of the patient, number and location of positive biopsy cores, tumor grade, and MRI findings, and may lead to active surveillance, re-treatment with focal approach, or salvage radical treatment.

References

1. Crawford ED, Barqawi A. Targeted focal therapy: a minimally invasive ablation technique for early prostate cancer. Oncology (Williston Park). 2007;21(1):27–32; discussion 3–4, 9.
2. Polascik TJ, Mouraviev V. Focal therapy for prostate cancer is a reasonable treatment option in properly selected patients. Urology. 2009;74(4):726–30.
3. Valerio M, Ahmed HU, Emberton M, Lawrentschuk N, Lazzeri M, Montironi R, et al. The role of focal therapy in the management of localised prostate cancer: a systematic review. Eur Urol. 2014;66(4):732–51. pii: S0302-2838(13)00557-5. 2014;66(4):732–51.
4. Ahmed HU, Hindley RG, Dickinson L, Freeman A, Kirkham AP, Sahu M, et al. Focal therapy for localised unifocal and multifocal prostate cancer: a prospective development study. Lancet Oncol. 2012;13(6):622–32.
5. Bahn D, de Castro Abreu AL, Gill IS, Hung AJ, Silverman P, Gross ME, et al. Focal cryotherapy for clinically unilateral, low-intermediate risk prostate cancer in 73 men with a median follow-up of 3.7 years. Eur Urol. 2012;62(1):55–63.

6. Ahmed HU. The index lesion and the origin of prostate cancer. N Engl J Med. 2009;361(17): 1704–6.
7. Nevoux P, Ouzzane A, Ahmed HU, Emberton M, Montironi R, Presti Jr JC, et al. Quantitative tissue analyses of prostate cancer foci in an unselected cystoprostatectomy series. BJU Int. 2012;110(4):517–23.
8. Mouraviev V, Villers A, Bostwick DG, Wheeler TM, Montironi R, Polascik TJ. Understanding the pathological features of focality, grade and tumor volume of early-stage prostate cancer as a foundation for parenchyma-sparing prostate cancer therapies: active surveillance and focal targeted therapy. BJU Int. 2011;108(7):1074–85.
9. Lindner U, Weersink RA, Haider MA, Gertner MR, Davidson SR, Atri M, et al. Image guided photothermal focal therapy for localized prostate cancer: phase I trial. J Urol. 2009;182: 1371–7.

Salvage Focal Therapy for Prostate Cancer

Rajan Ramanathan and J. Stephen Jones

19.1 Introduction

Radiation therapy (RT) is one of the treatment options for prostate cancer and around a third of patients opt to have RT (either external beam RT (EBRT) or brachytherapy); of these, approximately 30–40 % patients develop biochemical failure (BF) [1].

BF after RT may be related to the dose of radiation used [2, 3], stage at presentation, disease burden (cancer volume), and grade of the disease.

Salvage treatment options for patients who relapse after RT can be excisional (salvage radical prostatectomy (RP)) or can ablative (non-excisional, e.g., salvage cryoablation, salvage RT, or salvage high-intensity focused ultrasound (HIFU) ablation). A reasonable volume of experience has been accrued in the areas of salvage cryoablation and salvage brachytherapy; however, experience with salvage HIFU is still evolving.

The most appropriate therapy for a given patient will depend on the nature of the relapse, age of the patient, rise in PSA, PSA doubling time and the Gleason score on repeat biopsies, and to a major extent personal treatment preference of the physician. In this chapter, we will review the role of focal salvage therapy.

19.2 Pathophysiology and Principles of Focal Salvage Therapy

Modalities used for focal salvage therapy, like cryoablation, that aim to minimize complications by using urethral warming or sphincter-sparing approaches may end up undertreating these areas in the prostate. Studies have shown that recurrences

R. Ramanathan, MD • J.S. Jones, MD, FACS, MBA (✉)
Department of Urology, Glickman Urological and Kidney Institute,
Cleveland Clinic, 9500 Euclid Avenue, Cleveland, OH 44195, USA
e-mail: JONESS7@ccf.org

© Springer-Verlag France 2015
E. Barret, M. Durand (eds.), *Technical Aspects of Focal Therapy
in Localized Prostate Cancer*, DOI 10.1007/978-2-8178-0484-2_19

after RT are multifocal and often occur exactly in the areas that get undertreated by some of these salvage modalities. There are also challenges with following up patients after salvage treatments since the criteria used for identifying recurrence after failed salvage treatments have not been standardized. This is partly because of differences in the disease characteristics, and a PSA of 10 ng/ml in the setting of salvage therapy is not equivalent in terms of disease or pathology to a patient with a PSA of 10 ng/ml before RT [4]. It is therefore essential to understand the pathophysiology of the disease in this group of patients, in order to appreciate the challenges faced during salvage focal therapy.

19.2.1 Patterns of Failure: Lessons Learned from Salvage RP and Whole-Mount Prostate Examinations

Early studies based on whole-mount examination of the prostate after RP described patterns in the distribution of cancer [5]. The authors evaluated 112 sagittally sectioned whole-mount RP specimens for prostate cancer volume, multifocality, and location of the cancer foci, with the primary aim of proposing modifications to the technique of prostate cryoablation. Multifocal cancers were seen in 79.5 % of the specimens, and the authors felt that modifications designed to reduce urethral injury could affect cancer eradication since 66 % of cases were found to have cancer less than 5 mm from the urethra [5]. In another series comprising of 350 RP specimens, again using whole-mount examinations, the cancers were found to be 0–18 mm away from the urethra (mean distance of 3 mm) and 17 % of the tumors were in contact with the urethra. Apical cancers were very common, seen in 290/350 (74 %) cases, and these were more likely to be closer to the urethra (median distance 2 mm versus 3 mm; $P < 5$ 0.004) [6]. Patterns of recurrence after RT were also found to be similar [7]. Whole-mount specimen examinations of salvage prostatectomies showed multifocal cancers in 28 %, and 93 % of specimens contained cancer in the apical regions. Approximately two thirds (65 %) of cancers were found to be 0–5 mm from the urethra, with 7 % of cancers found to be involving the urethra [7]. Seminal vesicle involvement (SVI) was seen in 28 % [7] and this is an important consideration when selecting candidates for salvage cryoablation. In a review of literature, Touma et al. looked at a salvage prostatectomy series and reported an SVI rate of 28.9–62.5 %, and only 25–40 % patients had organ confined disease [8].

Huang et al. also showed that radiation failures often have more aggressive pathological characteristics. In their series they noted signs of locally advanced disease such as extraprostatic extension (ECE) in 43 % or SVI in 28 %, and 11 % of patients had lymph node-positive disease (LNI). One fourth of patients (25 %) had a Gleason grade ≥ 8, and a third (33 %) were upgraded on the final pathology after prostatectomy, and this was even noted in 3/4 cases who started out with a biopsy Gleason grade of 6 [7].

Many cryoablation failures occur in the prostate apex and the SV, and given the similarity in the distribution of radio-recurrent cancers, risks of undertreatment are high. The proportion of unaltered prostate epithelium in the post ablation biopsy may indicate the degree of undertreatment and can be seen in over 50 % patients [9]. In another study, 67/113 (59 %) patients had viable epithelial tissue or residual cancer after cryoablation [10]. The residual cancer rate was found to be proportional to the extent of unaltered prostatic glandular tissue per core of biopsy. At an average of 10 % unaltered tissue per core, 8.4 % showed residual tumor on the biopsy, but when the percent normal epithelium per core increased, the residual cancer rate increased to 43.6 % [9]. However, some feel that although atypical or normal prostatic glandular tissue is seen on biopsies, after salvage cryoablation, this finding is not a very accurate predictor of BF [10].

It is therefore crucial to understand the patterns of recurrence and select patients carefully for salvage therapy since all forms of salvage therapy have a higher incidence of complications.

19.2.2 Challenges with Identifying Failures that Are Localized to the Prostate Alone

Patients with failures that are localized to the prostate alone are the most optimal candidates for salvage focal therapy. However, identifying these patients can be a challenge. Extraprostatic extension, SVI, and occult nodal metastatic disease can be extremely difficult to identify. In almost all forms of focal therapy, these areas can end up being undertreated. It is essential to use more extensive biopsies of the prostate in order to identify multifocality. Template perineal biopsies may be better at detecting apical cancers than standard transrectal biopsies. Seminal vesicle biopsies should be done routinely and one should consider doing a lymph node dissection or pelvic imaging in order to identify microscopic or gross lymph node-positive disease. The presence of lymph node disease, distant disease, or a positive bone scan rules out organ confined disease and should be considered a contraindication for salvage focal therapy.

19.2.3 Challenges with Identifying Recurrence After Salvage Focal Therapy

PSA cutoff points are different for different modalities.

Currently, it is challenging enough to accurately detect biochemical failure (BF) after primary RT. The ASTRO definition was described in a consensus conference in 1996 and published in 1997 [11]. The sensitivity and specificity of the ASTRO definition are estimated to be around 60 % and 72 %, respectively [12]. In their study, Horwitz et al. described the following three definitions that had better sensitivity and specificity than the ASTRO: PSA greater than current nadir plus 3 ng/ml (sensitivity 66 % and specificity 77 %), dated at call; PSA greater than absolute nadir plus 2 ng/ml (sensitivity 64 % and specificity 74 %), dated at call; or two consecutive increases of at least 0.5 ng/ml, backdated (sensitivity 67 % and specificity 78 %) [12]. The Phoenix definition was then described during a consensus conference in 2005 and published in 2006 [13], and both ASTRO and Phoenix criteria may not be the most ideal way to identify radiation failures [14]. It is, however, even more difficult to accurately identify recurrence after salvage focal therapy, since there are no clear guidelines for the definition of biochemical failure after salvage focal therapy. If these failures cannot be accurately identified, then it is difficult to assess the true efficacy of these salvage treatment options.

It is rational to assume that criteria used for defining BF after RP could be extended to the scenario involving salvage excisional forms of treatment like salvage RP: if the recurrence of the disease is entirely limited to the prostate gland and the whole gland is removed, the PSA patterns should be identical in both circumstances.

However, the situation is more complex when dealing with non-excisional salvage treatment. Again, the ASTRO and Phoenix definition for RT failure can be applied by extrapolation, in the follow-up of patients post salvage brachytherapy. However, for other modalities, it is extremely difficult to adjust for the effect of PSA producing residual benign tissue, and many authors continue to extend the currently available definitions of BF after RT, or modifications thereof, to studies analyzing or reporting on results of salvage focal therapy.

For cryoablation after RT failure, authors have reported results using ASTRO and Phoenix definitions for biochemical failures. Chin et al. showed in their study that with the PSA cutoff set to >4, >2, or >0.5 ng/ml, 68 %, 55 %, or 34 % of patients, respectively, were considered to be BF-free [15]. Based on a 7-year retrospective study, the BF-free rates for the groups with pretreatment PSAs of <4 ng/ ml, 4–10 ng/ml, and >10 ng/ml and for the whole group were 61, 62, 50, and 59 %, at a PSA cutoff of >0.5 ng/ml. When the PSA cutoff was increased to >1 ng/ml, these corresponding figures increased to 78, 74, 46, and 69 %, respectively [16]. A PSA cutoff of <0.6 ng/ml has been described, and these authors also showed that an initial PSA level of <0.6 ng/ml after salvage cryoablation predicts favorable (67 % at 36 months) BF-free survival [17]. Biopsy failure also correlates with PSA nadirs and was lowest when the nadirs were <0.1 ng/ml (7 %) but was seen in 60 % of patients with nadir values 0.5 ng/ml or greater [18]. In a systematic review, it was noted that the various salvage cryoablation series used PSA cutoffs of 0.3 ng/ ml, 0.4 ng/ml, and 0.5 ng/ml, ASTRO and Phoenix definitions, to report their results [19].

In a series of patients undergoing HIFU, Blana et al. showed improved sensitivity and specificity at PSA cutoffs ranging between 1.2 and 1.4 ng/ml. When "PSA nadir plus X" values were studied, the specificity expectedly increased with higher values of X, and understandably, the sensitivity was highest closer to the nadir ($X = 0$). In their study, "PSA nadir plus 1.2" and PSA velocity >0.2 ng/ml/year were found to have the highest capacity of predicting failure [20]. The authors suggested that this new definition called the Stuttgart definition (PSA nadir plus 1.2 ng/ml) be added to the assessment of HIFU failures since this does not involve complicated backdating [20].

19.2.4 Principles and Technical Considerations of Focal Therapy

Cryoablation

The first-generation devices used a liquid nitrogen system to produce cooling; however, the more modern devices use an argon-helium system. By using ultrathin needles, multiple probe temperature monitoring, real-time tissue imaging, urethral warming catheters, and more than one freeze-thaw cycle, a more controlled ablation and minimized collateral tissue damage are possible. The efficacy of cryoablation depends on the temperature achieved, the rate of cooling, and the number of freeze-thaw cycles used. Temperatures of −40 °C have been associated with adequate cell destruction. In vitro studies done on an (Narayan and Dahiya) ND-1 prostate cancer cell line showed that changes in the chemical cell milieu are responsible for cell death seen at cooling rates under 5 °C/min, but the mechanism at cooling rates higher than 25 °C/min is from rapid intracellular ice formation [21]. These authors also postulated that intracellular ice formation is a key step for adequate apoptosis, and this can be achieved by using a double (or even triple) freeze/thaw cycle that keeps cells frozen at subzero temperatures for a longer time. Use of efficient combinations of cooling rates and end-point temperatures is also required in order to achieve cell death. For lower cooling rates, temperatures need to go as low as −40 °C, but for higher cooling rates of 25 °C/min, temperatures can be as high as −19 °C and still cause adequate cell kill [21]. Others have also recommended the use of double freeze-thaw [22] and the efficacy of double freeze-thaw cycles has been confirmed in clinical studies. Patients undergoing salvage cryoablation with a double freeze-thaw cycle were found to have better outcomes than those undergoing ablation with a single freeze-thaw cycle, and this reflected in biopsies (93 % negative biopsies versus 71 %, $p < 0.02$) as well as PSA studies (lower BF rates of 44 % versus 65 %, $p < 0.03$) [23]. Many authors now routinely recommend the use of two freeze-thaw cycles, and Izawa recommend a minimum of five cryoprobes during salvage cryoablation [10]. The role of temperature monitoring was addressed by Wong et al., and in their study, 83 % of patients who did not have temperature monitoring had failure confirmed by positive biopsies, compared to only a 10 % positive biopsy rate seen in the group of 71 patients who had temperature monitoring [24].

HIFU

High-intensity focused ultrasound, as the name suggests, is used to cause rapid tissue heating to 70–100 °C thus causing tissue destruction. The zone of tissue destroyed can be varied and multiple elementary lesions can be created using movement of the transducer and the use of phased array [25]. Of the available devices, the Ablatherm machine incorporates safety features that reduce risk of rectal injury by stabilizing the rectal wall and maintaining a constant transducer to rectal wall distance and also a patient motion sensor that turns off the transducer as soon as it detects patient movement during the firing sequence [25]. The lesion size is 19–24 mm × 1.7 mm × 1.7 mm, and for the first session of the primary treatment, 5 s treatment pulses and 5 s shot intervals are used, while for salvage HIFU, 4 s treatment pulse and 7 s shot interval are used [25]. The Sonablate system has different treatment probes that create different elementary lesions: 10 mm×2 mm×2 mm (single beam), 2.5 cm/4.5 cm focal-length probes and 10 mm×3 mm×3 mm (split beam), 3 cm/3.5 cm/4 cm focal-length probes [26]. Larger glands require the use of longer focal lengths. The ablation proceeds in the anteroposterior direction and is done in coronal slices which are 10 mm thick [26].

Brachytherapy

Most salvage brachytherapy reported in the literature has been performed with low-dose rate (LDR) permanent seed implants. However, in a recent meta-analysis, 3 of the 13 articles reviewed from the salvage brachytherapy group used HDR brachytherapy and had a higher complication rate [19] (Table 19.2).

19.3 Indications for Salvage Focal Therapy and Patient Selection

19.3.1 Identifying the Patient Who Has Failed RT: Definitions of BF After RT

After RT, the PSA continues to decrease sometimes for up until 2 years after the RT, although "PSA bounce" can be seen and can cause diagnostic confusion. Currently, the commonly used criteria are based on the principles of waiting for the PSA to settle to the lowest point on the curve, the PSA nadir, and then using predetermined criteria to define a rise. The two commonly used criteria are the ASTRO and the Phoenix definitions (Table 19.1).

When making a treatment decision regarding salvage therapy, the Phoenix and ASTRO criteria may both have limitations, since neither is considered an ideal system capable of monitoring disease progression, and many patients may have missed the window of opportunity for salvage therapy using either criterion [14]. Prostate biopsies may be a better way to assess BF if the PSA fails to reach expected nadirs or starts to rise abnormally [14].

Table 19.1 Criteria for biochemical failure after RT

Criterion	Description	Comments	Limitations
Astro 1997 [11]	Three consecutive increases in PSA after nadir has been reached	Date of failure is backdated	Delayed diagnosis of recurrence
		Taken as the midpoint between the PSA nadir and the first rise	Issues with PSA bounce
RTOG-Astro (Phoenix) 2006 [13]	Increase in PSA of 2 ng/ml above nadir (nadir+2)	Possibly a better predictor of distant metastases cause-specific mortality and overall mortality	May delay salvage treatment opportunity while waiting for the PSA to exceed nadir by +2

19.3.2 Case Selection

Given the patterns of recurrence and aggressive pathological features of radio-recurrent cancers, like higher ECE, SVI, LNI, and Gleason grade, complicated by issues with upgrading of tumors on final pathology in a third of patients, case selection plays a key role. Unfortunately, many of these predictors of BF (like Gleason grade 8 or greater, locally advanced disease ($\geq$pT3) or LNI) cannot all be accurately identified by currently available diagnostic techniques [7, 27]. Could these patients be more accurately identified, they can then be excluded from being offered focal salvage treatment, since the outcomes are expected to be poor and the risks of treatment then outweigh possible benefits. In the next section, we discuss some of the available tools that aid the case selection process.

Prostate Biopsies

Currently, it is unlikely that salvage focal treatment will be offered to any patient without definitive confirmation of recurrence, by a prostate biopsy. The biopsy can be used to differentiate between unifocal versus multifocal recurrence and can help in the decision-making process for focal versus whole-gland ablation. It is now well established that RT induces cytostructural changes that can cause interpretational problems. In the request for pathology, the pathologist must be made aware that the patient received prior radiation, and experience on the part of the pathologist interpreting these biopsies is critical to a correct diagnosis. Crook et al. reported on false-negative biopsies arising out of inadequate sampling. They also reported that delayed tumor regression can cause an initially positive biopsy to revert to a negative one later on. A third category of biopsies, in which clumps of residual tumor cells of uncertain significance, exhibiting radiation-induced changes, commonly cause interpretation problems and get classified as indeterminate [28]. Features of radiation injury that have been described include squamous metaplasia with or without atypia, a decreased ratio of the number of tumor glands to stroma, and atrophy [29].

The timing of the biopsies after RT also needs careful consideration. In a prospective study on 498 men, post-RT protocol prostate biopsies were done starting 12–18 months after RT. In the study, the proportion of indeterminate biopsies decreased with time, being 33 % for biopsy 1 (median 13 months) versus 7 % for biopsy 4 (median 44 months). Over a period of time, 30 % of indeterminate biopsies reverted to negatives, while 18 % progressed to local failure and 34 % remained indeterminate [28]. They found biopsy status at 24–36 months ($p=0.0005$) to be an independent predictor of outcome [28].

This is often considered the rationale for doing biopsies typically after 24 months after the RT. If biopsies need to be done earlier, a pathologist with experience in the field should ideally read the slides. It is also strongly recommended that apical sampling and SV biopsies be done, since, as discussed in the previous section, relapse is not uncommonly seen in these areas. It is generally accepted that SV-positive disease cannot be cured by some modalities offering focal salvage therapy and the risks of performing these on the SV are relatively higher.

PSA

Chin et al. reviewed the literature with respect to primary and salvage cryoablation and found that for salvage cryoablation, patient selection is crucial; when the pre-cryoablation PSA was more than 10 ng/ml and post-cryoablation nadir PSA >1 ng/ml, the outcomes were poor [30]. The outcomes are dependent on the disease burden, and data from our institution looked at surrogate markers of the volume of cancer on prostate biopsy like the total number of positive cores, the ratio of the number of positive cores to the total number of cores, and positive cores expressed as a function of prostate volume and found that the lower the disease burden, the better the outcomes [31].

Studies have looked at PSA levels and PSA doubling times (PSADT). Spiess et al. reported that a pre-salvage cryoablation serum PSA level >10 ng/ml ($P=0.002$) and PSA DT ≤ 16 months ($P=0.06$) were found to be good predictors of BF [32].

PSA velocity has also been looked at. Drawing parallels from studies that have shown poorer outcomes after RT/RP when pretreatment PSA velocity was >2.0 ng/ml/year [33, 34], Nguyen et al. suggested that patients with pretreatment PSA velocity >2.0 ng/ml/year should be considered as having micrometastatic disease at the time of BF [35].

Metastatic Evaluation

It is imperative to rule out local or distant metastatic disease before considering potentially aggressive local salvage therapy. Developments in imaging tools afford better staging, but are still far from being perfect.

Imaging

Of the available tools, conventional CT scans cannot detect lymph node involvement unless there is relatively bulky disease. MRI may be more useful for extraprostatic and multifocal disease, but still has a limited role in the detection of micrometastatic lymph node disease.

Magnetic Resonance Imaging (MRI)

MRI is evolving toward becoming a good imaging tool for the prostate, but accurate evaluation and differentiation of benign versus recurrent cancer is particularly difficult after RT. Assessment of true sensitivities and accuracy of MRI and other imaging modalities is complicated by a verification bias. Biopsies used to confirm true positives are not perfect either. In one study, the authors used focal nodularity showing reduced signal intensity on T2-weighted images, as the criterion for recurrent tumor [36]. Although the sample size was only nine patients, all underwent salvage radical prostatectomies for increasing PSA after RT. MRI and MR spectroscopy were found to have sensitivities of 68 and 77 %, respectively; biopsy was able to detect about half (sensitivity 48 %), but the sensitivity of digital rectal examination was too low (16 %) to be even considered useful. MR spectroscopy appeared to have the lowest specificity of 78 % [36]. Dynamic MRI is another useful tool for the assessment of local recurrence, and a retrospective study looked at three functional MRI sequences, using an identical protocol with 3-T MRI. Diffusion-weighted imaging (DWI), dynamic contrast-enhanced (DCE) MRI, and 3D (1) H-MR spectroscopy (MRS) were assessed on 60 patients (group A, RP, 28 patients; group B, EBRT, 32 patients) with suspicion of local recurrence based on PSA and confirmed on transrectal ultrasound-guided biopsies plus a reduction in PSA level after salvage therapy [37]. Sensitivity with T2-weighted MRI and 3D (1) H-MRS sequences was 57 and 53 %, respectively, for group A and 71 and 78 %, respectively, for group B. DCE-MRI alone showed a sensitivity of 100 and 96 %, respectively, for groups A and B. DWI alone had a higher sensitivity for group B (96 %) than for group A (71 %). The combination of T2-weighted imaging plus DWI plus DCE-MRI provided sensitivity as high as 100 % in group B. The authors felt that T2-weighted imaging, in spite of limited accuracy, often provides essential morphologic information and 3D MRS needs to be improved. They also concluded that the performance of functional imaging sequences for detecting recurrence is different after RP and external beam radiotherapy; while DCE-MRI is efficient in detecting recurrences after RP and after EBRT, the combination of DCE-MRI and DWI may provide the most optimal diagnostic efficacy after RT [37]. Another study found that multiparametric MRI has greater accuracy than T2-weighted imaging alone, for the detection of recurrent prostate cancer after RT, and no additional benefit was noted when T2-weighted imaging and DWI were supplemented with dynamic contrast enhancement [38].

Positron Emission Tomography (PET)

The role of PET/CT has been studied. For the assessment of these patients, 18F-fluorodeoxyglucose (18F-FDG)-PET has a very limited, if any, role. Prostate cancer showed a very low 18F-FDG uptake and in the study was unable to accurately differentiate between postoperative fibrotic changes and local recurrence after RP [39]. The role of 18F-FDG based imaging for detection of LNI has turned up mixed results. Chang et al. compared 18F-FDG with pathology. Of the patients with proven nodal metastatic disease, FDG-avid activity in the corresponding areas was found in 12/16 (75.0 %) patients while four had false-negative scans [40]. There were no false-positive scans, and they calculated the sensitivity, specificity, accuracy, positive predictive value (PPV), and negative predictive value (NPV) of FDG-PET for detecting LNI to be 75.0, 100.0, 83.3, 100.0, and 67.7 %, respectively [40]. Seltzer et al. compared helical CT, 18F-FDG-PET scanning, and 111 indium capromab pendetide scans in 45 patients suspected of having a BF (median PSA 3.8 ng./ml.) after RP (33 patients), RT (9 patients), or cryosurgery (3 patients), with a view to identifying lymph node involvement. Results were verified using fine-needle aspirations in 12 patients having lymph nodes ≥1 cm in size on CT. True positive rates were higher for PET than capromab scans (6/9 for PET versus 1/6 for capromab). The authors concluded that CT and PET were able to detect LNI in 50 % of patients when the PSA >4 ng/ml or a PSA velocity >0.2 ng/ml/month, but both techniques fell short in their abilities to detect LNI in patients who had lower PSA or lower PSA velocities. Capromab monoclonal antibody scan had the lowest detection rates [41].

11C-choline scanning is dependent on the phenomenon of increased uptake and integration of the tracer into phospholipids in the cancer cell membranes, and this activity is possibly dependent on the upregulation of choline kinase [42].

Tracer-based PET scanning, using 11C-choline, 11C-acetate, or 18F-fluoromethyl choline, may have some potential to identify recurrences [43].

In one study, 11C-choline PET had a true positivity rate of 38 % after RP and 78 % after EBRT [44]. But more interestingly, in their study, when the scans were negative (ten patients), no recurrence could be identified clinically or by biopsy [44]. Using 11C-acetate in patients with a rising PSA after treatment (RP-30 cases, RT-16 cases), a study found local, nodal, or bone recurrences in 7, 33, and 7 % of patients, respectively, in the RP groups and in 62, 38, and 13 %, respectively, in the RT group [45]. Sandblom et al. showed that pathologic tracer uptake activity with acetate was seen in 15/20 (75 %) patients, with eight having a solitary lesion (7, prostatic fossa; 1, regional lymph nodes) and seven with multiple lesions [46].

Studies have also looked at the ability of 11C-choline PET/CT to detect LNI. De Jong et al. correlated the imaging findings with pathology, prospectively in 67 patients undergoing surgery, and found that sensitivity for detecting LNI was 80 %, specificity was 96 %, and the accuracy was 93 % [47]. A few cases (5/12) of extra-regional nodal metastases were also picked up [47]. In another similar study, 25 patients with BF after RP who underwent bilateral pelvic node dissection with or without retroperitoneal lymph node dissection also had prior PET/CT. The results of the PET/CT were compared with pathology, and the authors found a sensitivity, specificity, PPV, NPV, and accuracy of 64, 90, 86, 72, and 77 %, respectively [48].

Acetate and choline PET scans can detect lymph node metastases but more studies are required to show the exact benefit of running these expensive tests. Overall, the currently available literature points to a relatively poor yield of positive scans at lower PSA values, and no tracer has been shown to be able to detect local recurrence within the clinically useful PSA levels of ≤ 1 ng/ml [49].

Role of PLND

PLND is another way to detect LNI. This is an invasive surgical option with associated complications and proper case selection is essential. PSA levels and other non-invasive studies can be used to identify patients who would be good candidates for this.

Assessment of Distant Metastases with Imaging

Bone scans have a low diagnostic yield in asymptomatic prostate cancer patients with PSA levels below 10 ng/ml. Although the risk of a positive bone scan increases with increasing PSA levels, elevated PSA levels are not very good positive predictors of positive bone scans [50]. The risk of a positive bone scan increased from 8 % for PSA levels 20–50 ng/ml to 40 % for PSA levels over 50 ng/ml. In contrast, lower PSA levels especially below 10 ng/ml were an excellent predictor of a negative bone scan, and in their study no positive scans were found in 290 patients with PSA levels <10 ng/ml [50]. At the PSA levels that are seen after BF, it is unlikely that bone scan would be of tremendous help.

MRI-DWI and 11C-choline PET/CT can also aid in the detection of bone metastases. In one study, DWI appeared to be as effective as short inversion time inversion recovery (STIR), T1-weighted spin echo sequences, and 11C-choline PET/CT for the detection of bone metastatic disease [51]. In another series, 18F-(sodium fluoride) NaF PET studies had an acceptable sensitivity for identifying bone metastatic prostate cancer and in a comparison performed better than whole-body DWI in terms of sensitivity, but DWI had a superior specificity [52]. Although today these are still in early stages of development and experience with these modalities is limited, diffusion-weighted whole-body imaging may someday be used to detect distant disease and monitor progress of bone metastatic disease after systemic treatments.

19.3.3 Summary

Based on a systematic review, Nguyen et al. proposed clinical parameters that could predict bDFS after salvage focal therapy: low-risk disease (like cT1c or cT2a, PSA <10 ng/ml, and Gleason score ≤6) at the time of original diagnosis, PSA velocity before initial RT <2 ng/ml/year, time to post-radiation PSA failure >3 years, post-radiation PSADT >12 months, and negative bone scan and pelvic imaging [35]. Pre-salvage clinical characteristics that portend a poorer prognosis include PSA levels >10 ng/ml, pre-salvage T3/T4 disease, or pre-salvage Gleason scores ≥7 on a re-biopsy, and such patients are unlikely to be cured by salvage local therapy [35].

19.4 Results

Since there are no clear guidelines for the definition for BF after salvage focal therapy, results have not been reported in a standardized fashion. Two excellent systematic reviews have looked at the literature available and attempted to tabulate the results in a more uniform pattern [19, 35]. The results from these articles have been summarized in Table 19.2.

Salvage Brachytherapy: In their systematic review, the authors found that 3/13 publications reported having used HDR [19]. The radioactive dose delivered varies between 108–170 Gy for 125 I and 90–170 Gy for 103 Pd, and this did not seem to affect the outcome [53]. Grado et al. reported an actuarial disease-free survival at 3 years and 5 years of 48 and 34 %, respectively, using the ASTRO definition [54]. Using HDR brachytherapy, a more recent study done on 52 patients reported a 5-year bDFS of 51 % (95 % CI: 34–66 %). Overall biochemical DFS rates reported in literature after salvage brachytherapy have ranged from 70 to 75 % at 4 years and 20 to 87 % at 5 years [53]. See also Table 19.2.

Salvage Cryoablation: There is a wide variation in the reporting of DFS in the cryoablation series, both in terms of the criteria used to define BF and duration of follow-up (Table 19.2). PSA cutoffs used included 0.3 ng/ml, 0.4 ng/ml, and 0.5 ng/ml, ASTRO and Phoenix definitions [19]. Pisters et al. reported a 5-year bDFS of 58.9 %, on a series of 279 patients using the ASTRO definition [55]. The success rates varied between 20 and 70 % (Table 19.2).

Table 19.2 Oncologic outcomes

Author (year) reference	Type of review	# Studies	# Patients range	Therapy type/comments	Median FU range (months)	Failure definition	5-year FFS (%)	Other comments
Salvage brachytherapy								
Parekh (2013) [19]	Systematic review	13	7–49	LDR-10, HDR-3, neoadjuvant ADT in 3	18.7–86	ASTRO-6, Phoenix-2, others-5	34–89	
Nguyen (2007) [35]	Systematic review	10	13–49	NA	19–64	ASTRO-5, Phoenix-1, others-4	20–89	
Boukaram (2010) [49]	General review	11	17–49	NA	19–64	NA	34–89	
Chen (2013) [57]	Retrospective	–	52	HDR	59.6	Phoenix	92	KM estimate
Gomez-Vaiega (2012) [53]	General review	11	17–49	120–200 Gy dosage	19–108	NA	20–89	
Kimura (2010) [58]	General review	8	13–49	NA	19–64	ASTRO-4, Phoenix-1, others-3	34–87	
Peters (2013) [59]	Multicenter, retrospective	–	31	NA	108	Phoenix	85	
Salvage cryoablation								
Parekh (2013) [19]	Systematic review	16	18–279	3rd gen-1, 2nd gen-1, data NA-14	9–113	ASTRO-3, Phoenix-3, others-10	18–83	FFS not always at 5 years but reported in nonuniform manner across series
Nguyen (2007) [35]	Systematic review	9	18–131	3rd gen-1, data NA-8	19–57	Phoenix-1, others-7	18–77	
Boukaram (2010) [49]	General review	6	38–131	NA	19–82	NA	23–74	
Autran-Gomez (2012) [60]	General review	11	19–279	NA	NA	NA	11–74	
Kimura (2010) [58]	General review	8	18–279	3rd gen-5, 2nd gen-2, 1st gen-1	12–82	ASTRO-2, Phoenix-2, others-4	34–74	
Mouraview (2012) [61]	Systematic review	10	29–279	Cryocare-6, seednet-3	17–122	ASTRO-2, Phoenix-2, others-6	34–74	
Finley (2011) [1]	General review	9	15–279	NA	18–82.3	ASTRO-4, Pheonix-1, others-4	34–72.2	

Salvage HIFU

Parekh (2013) [19]	Systematic review	7	31–167	Post RP-2, post EBRT-5	7.4–48	NA	50–84	FFS not at 5 years
Ahmed (2012) [62]	Registry, retrospective	–	39	Hemiablation-16, focal-23	17	Phoenix, Stuttgart, biopsy	69	
Autran-Gomez (2012) [60]	General review	3	50–167	NA	NA	NA	25–54	FFS<3 years
Kimura (2010) [58]	General review	3	32–167	NA	7.4–18.1	NA	46–61	FFS<3 years
Sountoulides (2012) [63]	General review	4	31–167	NA	7.4–19.8	NA	44–92	–

Salvage HIFU: This is a relatively newer modality and follow-ups have been relatively short with most series reporting results at 1, 2, or 3 years. Murat et al. described on 194 HFU sessions on 167 patients and stated a 3-year failure-free survival (FFS) of 53 %. Other series have reported FFS in the range of 25–92 %.

19.5 Complications and Adverse Events

Salvage therapy for prostate cancer has a higher complication rate. The incidence of rectal injuries is higher for salvage radical prostatectomies as compared to radical prostatectomies. Salvage prostatectomy is still considered to have better oncologic results than some of the other salvage focal therapies. A comparison of the adverse events after salvage focal therapy with that seen after salvage RP (Table 19.3, last row) gives an idea of the relative risks of adverse events between the modalities.

Complications after salvage cryoablation are more common and more serious when compared to primary cryoablation, but in appropriately identified patients, the relatively favorable long-term results may outweigh the risks [30].

Refinement in techniques of salvage focal therapies, improved imaging, and better targeting options are some of the reasons that explain why complication rates are dropping. The incidence of complications with salvage cryoablations is lower now than what was seen with the previous generations of machines. Table 19.3 summarizes the results from two systematic reviews [19, 35].

Rectourethral Fistula RUF: This is by far the most troublesome complication after any salvage treatment performed on the prostate. Although conservative treatment of fistulas is an option in select cases, the presence of fibrosis, radiation proctitis, and endarteritis obliterans seen after RT virtually precludes the use of conservative techniques to treat RUF. The use of diverting colostomies and urinary diversions often becomes necessary and can cause significant patient inconvenience thereby leading to dissatisfaction with outcomes. The overall fistula rates are in the range of 2–4 %.

Incontinence: This is exceedingly common after salvage prostatectomy and can be seen in up to half the patients (Table 19.3). Salvage brachytherapy series have reported on incontinence rates of around 6 %, but it is much more common after salvage cryoablation or HIFU.

Brachytherapy also increases the risk of significant (grade 3 or 4) rectal and genitourinary toxicities, from the collateral damage to adjacent organs from the radiation. Strictures after salvage focal therapies are seen in 4–17 %. With the use of urethral warming and multiprobe temperature monitoring, the incidence of urethral sloughing, urethral mucosal injuries, and subsequent strictures after cryoablation will continue to improve.

Patients undergoing salvage cryoablation can also develop pelvic pain syndromes and can have urinary retention. Rarer complications like prostatic abscesses or perirectal abscesses are anecdotal.

Table 19.3 Complications and adverse events

Author (year) reference	# Patients range	Fistula % (range)	Incontinence % (range)	Stricture and urethral complications % (range)	Rectal toxicity % (range)	Genitourinary toxicity % (range)	Others % (range)	Comments
Salvage brachytherapy								
Parekh (2013) [19]	7–49	3.1 (0–12)	6.2 (0–30.8)	7.5 (0–71.4)	4.7 (0–20)	12.9 (0–30.8)		
Nguyen (2007) [35]	13–49	3.4 (0–8)	6 (0–24)	NA	5.6 (0–24)	17 (0–47)		
Salvage cryoablation								
Parekh (2013) [19]	18–279	1.6 (0–11.1)	16.4 (0–91.3)	4.2 (0–44.4)	–	8.2 (0–52.2) tissue slough	15.6 (0–39.5) 9.9 (0–21.4)	Retention
Nguyen (2007) [35]	18–131	2.6 (0–11)	36 (4.3–83)	17 (0–28) bladder neck stricture/retention	–	11 (0–55) tissue slough	36 (5.6–44)	Perineal pain
Salvage HIFU								
Parekh (2013) [19]	31–167	3.6 (0–6.5)	36.9 (0–49.7)	17.2 (0–35.5) bladder neck stricture	2.1 (0–2.8) rectal injury	NA	–	–
Salvage radical prostatectomy								
Parekh (2013) [19]	6–404	2.4 (0–7.1)	49.7 (15.4–78.1)	26.1 (0–33.3) bladder neck stricture	5.3 (2–11.1) rectal injury	–	Mortality 0.2 %	From 24 studies reviewed
Nguyen (2007) [35]	6–199	NA	41 (17–67)	24 (0–30) bladder neck stricture	4.7 (0–8) rectal injury	–	Mortality 0.2 %	From 14 studies

Conclusions

Salvage cryoablation and other salvage focal therapy options may be inferior to salvage prostatectomy, and some authors recommend that younger, healthy patients should be offered salvage RP as it offers superior biochemical disease-free survival and may potentially offer the best chance of cure [56]. However, the convenience and the minimally invasive nature of salvage focal therapy make it an attractive option. It, currently, has a definite role in the management of patients with BF after RT, and with continued evolution in technology and imaging, salvage focal therapy may become the treatment of choice in a select group of patients.

References

1. Finley DS, Belldegrun AS. Salvage cryotherapy for radiation-recurrent prostate cancer: outcomes and complications. Curr Urol Rep. 2011;12(3):209–15.
2. Kupelian PA, et al. Radical prostatectomy, external beam radiotherapy <72 Gy, external beam radiotherapy > or =72 Gy, permanent seed implantation, or combined seeds/external beam radiotherapy for stage T1-T2 prostate cancer. Int J Radiat Oncol Biol Phys. 2004;58(1):25–33.
3. Kupelian PA, et al. Effect of increasing radiation doses on local and distant failures in patients with localized prostate cancer. Int J Radiat Oncol Biol Phys. 2008;71(1):16–22.
4. Babaian RJ, et al. Best practice statement on cryosurgery for the treatment of localized prostate cancer. J Urol. 2008;180(5):1993–2004.
5. Rukstalis DB, et al. Prostate cryoablation: a scientific rationale for future modifications. Urology. 2002;60(2 Suppl 1):19–25.
6. Leibovich BC, et al. Proximity of prostate cancer to the urethra: implications for minimally invasive ablative therapies. Urology. 2000;56(5):726–9.
7. Huang WC, et al. The anatomical and pathological characteristics of irradiated prostate cancers may influence the oncological efficacy of salvage ablative therapies. J Urol. 2007;177(4):1324–9; quiz 1591.
8. Touma NJ, Izawa JI, Chin JL. Current status of local salvage therapies following radiation failure for prostate cancer. J Urol. 2005;173(2):373–9.
9. Shuman BA, et al. Histological presence of viable prostatic glands on routine biopsy following cryosurgical ablation of the prostate. J Urol. 1997;157(2):552–5.
10. Izawa JI, et al. Incomplete glandular ablation after salvage cryotherapy for recurrent prostate cancer after radiotherapy. Int J Radiat Oncol Biol Phys. 2003;56(2):468–72.
11. Consensus statement: guidelines for PSA following radiation therapy. American Society for Therapeutic Radiology and Oncology Consensus Panel. Int J Radiat Oncol Biol Phys. 1997;37(5):1035–41.
12. Horwitz EM, et al. Definitions of biochemical failure that best predict clinical failure in patients with prostate cancer treated with external beam radiation alone: a multi-institutional pooled analysis. J Urol. 2005;173(3):797–802.
13. Roach 3rd M, et al. Defining biochemical failure following radiotherapy with or without hormonal therapy in men with clinically localized prostate cancer: recommendations of the RTOG-ASTRO Phoenix Consensus Conference. Int J Radiat Oncol Biol Phys. 2006;65(4):965–74.
14. Stephenson AJ. Is the Phoenix definition superior to ASTRO for predicting clinical outcomes in prostate cancer? Nat Clin Pract Urol. 2008;5(7):356–7.
15. Chin JL, et al. Results of salvage cryoablation of the prostate after radiation: identifying predictors of treatment failure and complications. J Urol. 2001;165(6 Pt 1):1937–41; discussion 1941–2.

16. Bahn DK, et al. Salvage cryosurgery for recurrent prostate cancer after radiation therapy: a seven-year follow-up. Clin Prostate Cancer. 2003;2(2):111–4.
17. Levy DA, Pisters LL, Jones JS. Prognostic value of initial prostate-specific antigen levels after salvage cryoablation for prostate cancer. BJU Int. 2010;106(7):986–90.
18. Shinohara K, et al. Cryosurgical ablation of prostate cancer: patterns of cancer recurrence. J Urol. 1997;158(6):2206–9; discussion 2209–10.
19. Parekh A, Graham PL, Nguyen PL. Cancer control and complications of salvage local therapy after failure of radiotherapy for prostate cancer: a systematic review. Semin Radiat Oncol. 2013;23(3):222–34.
20. Blana A, et al. High-intensity focused ultrasound for prostate cancer: comparative definitions of biochemical failure. BJU Int. 2009;104(8):1058–62.
21. Tatsutani K, et al. Effect of thermal variables on frozen human primary prostatic adenocarcinoma cells. Urology. 1996;48(3):441–7.
22. Shinohara K, et al. Cryosurgical treatment of localized prostate cancer (stages T1 to T4): preliminary results. J Urol. 1996;156(1):115–20; discussion 120–1.
23. Pisters LL, et al. The efficacy and complications of salvage cryotherapy of the prostate. J Urol. 1997;157(3):921–5.
24. Wong WS, et al. Cryosurgery as a treatment for prostate carcinoma: results and complications. Cancer. 1997;79(5):963–74.
25. Chaussy C, et al. Technology insight: high-intensity focused ultrasound for urologic cancers. Nat Clin Pract Urol. 2005;2(4):191–8.
26. Uchida T, et al. Transrectal high-intensity focused ultrasound for treatment of patients with stage T1b-2n0m0 localized prostate cancer: a preliminary report. Urology. 2002;59(3):394–8; discussion 398–9.
27. Lerner SE, Blute ML, Zincke H. Critical evaluation of salvage surgery for radio-recurrent/resistant prostate cancer. J Urol. 1995;154(3):1103–9.
28. Crook J, et al. Postradiotherapy prostate biopsies: what do they really mean? Results for 498 patients. Int J Radiat Oncol Biol Phys. 2000;48(2):355–67.
29. Bostwick DG, Egbert BM, Fajardo LF. Radiation injury of the normal and neoplastic prostate. Am J Surg Pathol. 1982;6(6):541–51.
30. Chin JL, Lim D, Abdelhady M. Review of primary and salvage cryoablation for prostate cancer. Cancer Control. 2007;14(3):231–7.
31. Levy DA, Li J, Jones JS. Disease burden predicts for favorable post salvage cryoablation PSA. Urology. 2010;76(5):1157–61.
32. Spiess PE, et al. Presalvage prostate-specific antigen (PSA) and PSA doubling time as predictors of biochemical failure of salvage cryotherapy in patients with locally recurrent prostate cancer after radiotherapy. Cancer. 2006;107(2):275–80.
33. D'Amico AV, et al. Preoperative PSA velocity and the risk of death from prostate cancer after radical prostatectomy. N Engl J Med. 2004;351(2):125–35.
34. D'Amico AV, et al. Pretreatment PSA velocity and risk of death from prostate cancer following external beam radiation therapy. JAMA. 2005;294(4):440–7.
35. Nguyen PL, et al. Patient selection, cancer control, and complications after salvage local therapy for postradiation prostate-specific antigen failure: a systematic review of the literature. Cancer. 2007;110(7):1417–28.
36. Pucar D, et al. Prostate cancer: correlation of MR imaging and MR spectroscopy with pathologic findings after radiation therapy-initial experience. Radiology. 2005;236(2):545–53.
37. Roy C, et al. Comparative sensitivities of functional MRI sequences in detection of local recurrence of prostate carcinoma after radical prostatectomy or external-beam radiotherapy. AJR Am J Roentgenol. 2013;200(4):W361–8.
38. Donati OF, et al. Multiparametric prostate MR imaging with T2-weighted, diffusion-weighted, and dynamic contrast-enhanced sequences: are all pulse sequences necessary to detect locally recurrent prostate cancer after radiation therapy? Radiology. 2013;268:440–50.

39. Hofer C, et al. Fluorine-18-fluorodeoxyglucose positron emission tomography is useless for the detection of local recurrence after radical prostatectomy. Eur Urol. 1999;36(1):31–5.

40. Chang CH, et al. Detecting metastatic pelvic lymph nodes by 18F-2-deoxyglucose positron emission tomography in patients with prostate-specific antigen relapse after treatment for localized prostate cancer. Urol Int. 2003;70(4):311–5.

41. Seltzer MA, et al. Comparison of helical computerized tomography, positron emission tomography and monoclonal antibody scans for evaluation of lymph node metastases in patients with prostate specific antigen relapse after treatment for localized prostate cancer. J Urol. 1999;162(4):1322–8.

42. Oyama N. Editorial comment on: detection of lymph-node metastases with integrated [11C] choline PET/CT in patients with PSA failure after radical prostatectomy: results confirmed by open pelvic-retroperitoneal lymphadenectomy. Eur Urol. 2007;52(2):429.

43. Greco C, Cascini GL, Tamburrini O. Is there a role for positron emission tomography imaging in the early evaluation of prostate cancer relapse? Prostate Cancer Prostatic Dis. 2008;11(2):121–8.

44. de Jong IJ, et al. 11C-choline positron emission tomography for the evaluation after treatment of localized prostate cancer. Eur Urol. 2003;44(1):32–8; discussion 38–9.

45. Oyama N, et al. 11C-acetate PET imaging of prostate cancer: detection of recurrent disease at PSA relapse. J Nucl Med. 2003;44(4):549–55.

46. Sandblom G, et al. Positron emission tomography with C11-acetate for tumor detection and localization in patients with prostate-specific antigen relapse after radical prostatectomy. Urology. 2006;67(5):996–1000.

47. de Jong IJ, et al. Preoperative staging of pelvic lymph nodes in prostate cancer by 11C-choline PET. J Nucl Med. 2003;44(3):331–5.

48. Scattoni V, et al. Detection of lymph-node metastases with integrated [11C] choline PET/CT in patients with PSA failure after radical retropubic prostatectomy: results confirmed by open pelvic-retroperitoneal lymphadenectomy. Eur Urol. 2007;52(2):423–9.

49. Boukaram C, Hannoun-Levi JM. Management of prostate cancer recurrence after definitive radiation therapy. Cancer Treat Rev. 2010;36(2):91–100.

50. Gleave ME, et al. Ability of serum prostate-specific antigen levels to predict normal bone scans in patients with newly diagnosed prostate cancer. Urology. 1996;47(5):708–12.

51. Luboldt W, et al. Prostate carcinoma: diffusion-weighted imaging as potential alternative to conventional MR and 11C-choline PET/CT for detection of bone metastases. Radiology. 2008;249(3):1017–25.

52. Mosavi F, et al. Whole-body diffusion-weighted MRI compared with (18)F-NaF PET/CT for detection of bone metastases in patients with high-risk prostate carcinoma. AJR Am J Roentgenol. 2012;199(5):1114–20.

53. Gomez-Veiga F, et al. Brachytherapy for the treatment of recurrent prostate cancer after radiotherapy or radical prostatectomy. BJU Int. 2012;109 Suppl 1:17–21.

54. Grado GL, et al. Salvage brachytherapy for localized prostate cancer after radiotherapy failure. Urology. 1999;53(1):2–10.

55. Pisters LL, et al. Salvage prostate cryoablation: initial results from the cryo on-line data registry. J Urol. 2008;180(2):559–63; discussion 563–4.

56. Pisters LL, et al. Locally recurrent prostate cancer after initial radiation therapy: a comparison of salvage radical prostatectomy versus cryotherapy. J Urol. 2009;182(2):517–25; discussion 525–7.

57. Chen CP, et al. Salvage HDR brachytherapy for recurrent prostate cancer after previous definitive radiation therapy: 5-year outcomes. Int J Radiat Oncol Biol Phys. 2013;86(2):324–9.

58. Kimura M, et al. Current salvage methods for recurrent prostate cancer after failure of primary radiotherapy. BJU Int. 2010;105(2):191–201.

59. Peters M, et al. Patterns of outcome and toxicity after salvage prostatectomy, salvage cryosurgery and salvage brachytherapy for prostate cancer recurrences after radiation therapy: a multicenter experience and literature review. World J Urol. 2013;31(2):403–9.
60. Autran-Gomez AM, Scarpa RM, Chin J. High-intensity focused ultrasound and cryotherapy as salvage treatment in local radio-recurrent prostate cancer. Urol Int. 2012;89(4):373–9.
61. Mouraviev V, Spiess PE, Jones JS. Salvage cryoablation for locally recurrent prostate cancer following primary radiotherapy. Eur Urol. 2012;61(6):1204–11.
62. Ahmed HU, et al. Focal salvage therapy for localized prostate cancer recurrence after external beam radiotherapy: a pilot study. Cancer. 2012;118(17):4148–55.
63. Sountoulides P, Theodosiou A, Finazzi-Agro E. The current role of high-intensity focused ultrasound for the management of radiation-recurrent prostate cancer. Expert Rev Med Devices. 2012;9(4):401–8.

Focal Therapy: Current Status and Future Directions

Behfar Ehdaie, Jonathan A. Coleman, and Peter T. Scardino

20.1 Introduction

The widespread practice of screening for prostate cancer among asymptomatic men using the prostate-specific antigen (PSA) test is largely responsible for the dramatic rise in prostate cancer detection and survival [1, 2]. In the United States, the age-adjusted incidence of prostate cancer has increased considerably over the past two decades, rising from 92 cases per 100,000 men in 1975 to a peak of 240 cases per 100,000 men in 1992. Although the incidence of prostate cancer has remained stable at 180 cases per 100,000 men since 2001, annual age-adjusted mortality rates in the United States have drastically decreased, by more than 40 % [1]. Similarly, in the United Kingdom the incidence of prostate cancer has more than doubled, from 47.4 to 102.9 per 100,000 men, while the disease-specific mortality rate has decreased by 11 %, from 26.8 to 23.8 per 100,000 men [3].

B. Ehdaie
Urology Service, Department of Surgery,
Memorial Sloan-Kettering Cancer Center, New York, USA

Health Outcomes Group, Department of Epidemiology and Biostatistics,
Memorial Sloan-Kettering Cancer Center, New York, USA

J.A. Coleman
Urology Service, Department of Surgery,
Memorial Sloan-Kettering Cancer Center, New York, USA

P.T. Scardino (✉)
Urology Service, Department of Surgery,
Memorial Sloan-Kettering Cancer Center, New York, USA

Department of Surgery, Memorial Sloan-Kettering Cancer Center,
1275 York Avenue, Box 65, New York, NY 10065, USA
e-mail: scardinp@mskcc.org

© Springer-Verlag France 2015
E. Barret, M. Durand (eds.), *Technical Aspects of Focal Therapy
in Localized Prostate Cancer*, DOI 10.1007/978-2-8178-0484-2_20

Despite worldwide improvement in mortality trends across continents, prostate cancer remains a lethal malignancy. In the United States, prostate cancer has been the second or third leading cause of cancer mortality in men in each of the last 75 years. In the European Union, prostate cancer was the third most commonly occurring cancer, causing an estimated 92,200 deaths in 2012 [4]. And although prostate cancer mortality in Asia remains lower than in Western countries, the rate of cancer mortality in Asian countries has been markedly increasing over the last 40 years [5]. Given these data, a diagnosis of prostate cancer continues to indicate a serious medical condition, regardless of the patient's age, health status, or disease risk, and management decisions for localized disease are complex, owing to the paucity of evidence comparing various treatment options.

20.2 Overdetection of Prostate Cancer

The adoption of recommended prostate cancer screening strategies has successfully shifted the detection of prostate cancer to an earlier stage of localized disease, at which point tumors are small and often identified as low-grade. This staging improvement has paradoxically highlighted the limitations in our ability to differentiate biologically aggressive tumors from low-risk, indolent tumors that may be discovered incidentally, using diagnostic techniques designed primarily to detect the presence of any prostate cancer. The lack of a more discriminating test that would distinguish indolent from aggressive cancers, coupled with the risk of treatment-related morbidities and societal costs associated with indiscriminate radical treatment of patients regardless of the threat posed by the disease, has increased awareness of the risks of overtreatment of prostate cancer. This heightened scrutiny has occasionally been taken to an extreme, with some questioning the utility of serum PSA-based prostate cancer screening, despite existing data that document the benefits associated with screening [6]. New, "smarter" screening approaches based on the best clinical and biological data are needed to accurately characterize prostate tumors and to guide appropriate therapies with less risk of overtreatment.

Overtreatment is a key concern in prostate cancer care [7]. Among men treated conservatively, those with moderately differentiated tumors and clinical stage <T2b cancer have less than a 10 % risk of dying from prostate cancer at 20 years and 57 % risk of dying from other causes, on average [8]. However, there has been a significant increase in the use of radical therapy with advanced treatment technologies, such as robotic-assisted surgical procedures and intensity-modulated radiation therapy, between 2004 and 2009, among men who have both low-risk cancer and a high risk of death from other causes [9]. A workshop convened by the FDA and composed of experts representing multiple stakeholders, including urologists, medical oncologists, radiation oncologists, industry representatives, and patient advocates, evaluated potential trial designs for the development of therapies for localized prostate cancer. The consensus recommendation on focal treatment strategies was that future clinical trials should investigate men with low-volume intermediate- and high-risk localized prostate cancer with life expectancy exceeding 10 years.

20.3 Treatment of Localized Prostate Cancer

Prostate cancer management is evolving in response to our improved understanding of the natural history and clinical features of this disease. Standard curative treatments have included radical prostatectomy and whole-gland radiation therapy. Although these treatments are clinically effective in eradicating tumors, patients risk a significant reduction in quality of life and increased posttreatment morbidity, including incontinence, erectile dysfunction, and bowel urgency [10–12]. The results of two recent clinical trials have demonstrated the safety – in the intermediate time frame – of active surveillance in men with localized prostate cancer, with delayed treatment occurring at the time of disease progression [13, 14]. The PIVOT trial reported no difference in cancer-specific and overall mortality at 12 years in men with prostate cancer randomized to radical prostatectomy or observation [14]. Although men on observation incurred an increased risk of bone metastases, especially in patients with high-risk disease, radical prostatectomy was associated with a significant increase in the rates of incontinence (17.1 % vs 6.3 %) and erectile dysfunction (55.9 % vs 18.9 %). Today active surveillance is widely recommended for primary management in men with low-risk prostate cancer (Gleason pattern 6 or less, PSA less than 10 ng/mL, and clinical stage T1c or T2a).

The challenge to clinicians is to accurately risk-stratify patients to distinguish between those who would benefit from immediate treatment and those who could safely be treated expectantly. The current approach to prostate cancer diagnosis is susceptible to systematic sampling errors, in which many tumors detected are low-risk, yet some high-risk tumors are missed, especially when they are located in the anterior and apical areas of the prostate. Prostate needle biopsy using transrectal ultrasound guidance has a false-negative rate (missing a high-grade cancer) of up to 30 %. In the absence of reliable techniques to accurately characterize tumors, it is difficult for physicians to reassure patients that their cancer poses minimal risk, and most urologists recommend immediate radical treatment. In a national registry study across 36 urology practices in the United States conducted in 2010, less than 7 % of patients chose active surveillance among 11,892 men diagnosed with prostate cancer [15]. The explanations for the apparent underuse of active surveillance are speculative, but presumably reflect an assessment of risk by physicians and patients who accept treatment-related morbidity as preferable to uncertainty about the risk of metastatic progression.

The desire to achieve cancer control with minimal side effects has driven current research into minimally invasive, innovative focal treatment modalities that ablate the local tumor without affecting surrounding structures crucial to normal bowel, urinary, and sexual function. Despite the recommendations of previous consensus panels on focal therapy to treat patients with very low-risk disease, today the most promising role for focal therapy is for intermediate-risk tumors, because active surveillance has been shown to be an effective management strategy for most patients with low-risk prostate cancer. The major advantage of focal therapy for intermediate-risk cancers is the reduction in treatment-related adverse effects, compared with radical prostatectomy and radiation therapy. It is unlikely that a trial of focal therapy in low-risk prostate cancer could demonstrate a clinical benefit compared with active surveillance, in terms of reduced morbidity or better cancer control. The barriers to adopting focal therapy for treatment of intermediate- and high-risk prostate tumors include: accurate identification of the location of the high-grade lesions, appropriate management of incidental multifocal lesions (treat associated high-grade lesions but monitor low-grade lesions), and developing an effective way to monitor patients after treatment to be able to initiate timely whole-gland therapy when necessary to prevent metastases. Future research efforts should seek to identify molecular, genetic, and imaging characteristics that distinguish aggressive prostate tumors from indolent lesions. Recently, a study of men treated conservatively for prostate cancer identified cell cycle progression signatures on needle biopsy specimens as useful predictors of the risk of death from prostate cancer in men managed conservatively [16, 17]. Molecular profiles, along with optimal imaging and biopsy techniques, are valuable tools for prospective clinical trials using improved risk stratification and tumor localization to demonstrate the clinical utility of focal ablation of aggressive tumors and observation of indolent lesions.

20.4 Pretreatment Cancer Classification

To individualize treatment successfully for men with prostate cancer, it is essential to develop reliable methods for accurately identifying tumor location and characterizing biology. Diagnostic magnetic resonance imaging (MRI) is a promising tool for evaluating the location and extent of cancer within the prostate. MR imaging has also been used to direct focal therapy, assess treatment effect, and monitor for disease recurrence or progression. Currently multiparametric MRI (mpMRI) is the best studied modality; it is considered the most accurate imaging technique for detecting aggressive, clinically important cancer [18], and it has been used in risk stratification of low-risk prostate cancer when the image is normal or nearly normal [19, 20]. Using MRI to target lesions for biopsy may prove to be a particularly useful way to identify appropriate candidates for focal therapy [21]. If the negative predictive value of MRI in men with low-risk tumors who have a confirmatory biopsy is >90 %, then the best candidates for focal therapy would be those with a focal area of cancer on systematic biopsy with an MRI that shows no other suspicious areas [19]. The Prostate MRI Imaging Study (PROMIS) is a clinical trial currently accruing patients in the United Kingdom to evaluate the value of MRI in identifying cancer prior to prostate needle biopsy using a systematic template saturation biopsy to compare biopsy histology to imaging characteristics [22].

20.5 Rationale for Focal Therapy

Many urologic cancers (e.g., kidney or bladder) can be treated effectively with focal resection or ablation, in selected cases, as effectively as with whole-gland extirpation with radical surgery [23–25]. Prostate cancer may also be amenable to organ-sparing focal therapies. The prostate is easily accessible through the perineum and the rectum, and many urologists are experienced in performing image-guided procedures in the gland to obtain diagnostic needle biopsies. The focal therapy's ability to preserve critical structures, including the neurovascular bundle posterolaterally and the rhabdosphincter at the apex of the prostate, could also preserve the patients' quality of life, compared with radical surgery. This therapeutic improvement may be most marked in patients undergoing salvage procedures for recurrent tumors after radiation therapy. Although the potential quality of life benefits of focal therapy makes it an attractive treatment option, future clinical trials are needed to demonstrate effective cancer control.

The most appropriate patients for focal therapy today are not those with low-risk disease that can be effectively managed with active surveillance but those with intermediate-risk lesions. Any biopsy-proven lesion that contains Gleason pattern 4 or 5 cancer, if limited in size and extent, can be treated by ablating the sector of the prostate that harbors the disease, offering patients an opportunity to defer or avoid radical therapy. The challenge for focal therapy is to demonstrate accurate targeting of the index lesion while avoiding serious understaging and subsequent undertreatment.

20.6 Understaging

Eighty-five percent of all prostate cancers are multifocal. Variations in reported rates of multifocality are probably related to patient selection and pathology sectioning technique [26]. However, index lesions account, on average, for 80 % of the total tumor volume and almost always represent the highest-grade lesion within the prostate, as well as 90 % of all lesions with extraprostatic extension [27]. The non-index foci tend to be smaller than 0.5 cm^3, low grade, and confined to the prostate – cancers that, in themselves, would be suitable for monitoring on an active surveillance protocol [28, 29]. In addition, the overall risk of disease progression is mainly associated with the characteristics of the index lesion rather than of the secondary tumor. In contemporary patients, the rate of unifocality appears to be increasing; 38 % of radical prostatectomy specimens contain a single disease site [30], albeit sometimes far too large for focal ablation.

The current diagnostic approach to prostate cancer is susceptible to sampling errors associated with systematic, regionally directed, nontargeted biopsies of the periphery of the prostate gland. Characterization of prostate cancer by stage, grade, and PSA level alone is insufficient to individualize patient management or to select patients appropriate for active surveillance, focal therapy, or radical treatment.

The role of systematic mapping biopsies has been investigated in a prospective study of men who underwent a three-dimensional prostate mapping biopsy after initial transrectal biopsy detected unifocal disease [21]. Among 180 men, 61 % had cancer detected bilaterally and 22 % had an increase in Gleason grade, including pattern 4 or 5. This study demonstrated that the complication rate was 7.7 %, reporting prolonged catheterization in 14 patients and hematuria requiring bladder irrigation in two patients. Although sampling errors in a standard transrectal ultrasound-guided biopsy are reduced with mapping biopsy, this approach is burdensome for many patients and requires general anesthesia. Therefore, incorporating advanced imaging into the diagnostic approach for prostate cancer would be a useful noninvasive technique, if studies prove the accuracy of MRI to target significant tumors.

Multiparametric MRI demonstrates promising performance characteristics to identify clinically important prostate tumors – those larger than 0.5 cm or high-grade (Gleason $\geq 4+3$). Targeting needle biopsy to lesions identifiable by MR imaging, either alone or in combination with a 12-core systematic biopsy, promises greater accuracy and is currently being widely explored [31]. Integrating multiparametric MRI-guided targeted biopsies (with or without systematic biopsies) with standard clinical and pathologic characteristics may add additional prognostic information and improve risk classification by distinguishing indolent from aggressive tumors [31].

The accurate assessment of disease risk remains imperfect with current biopsy and imaging modalities. Despite improvements in characterizing prostate cancer with confirmatory biopsies [32] or multiparametric MRI [33], more studies are needed to determine the accuracy of MR imaging and of MR plus targeted biopsies. These studies will require prospective reporting of MRI data, consistent criteria for identifying which patients to biopsy, and the use of systematic three-dimensional mapping biopsy as the diagnostic standard. Data from these studies will add to the evidence from landmark studies evaluating the accuracy of MRI compared with whole-mount radical prostatectomy specimens. Previous reports were limited by studying only patients who had been selected to undergo radical prostatectomy; therefore, the role of MRI in men with low-risk disease or no previous diagnosis of prostate cancer is unknown [33–35].

If targeted biopsy proves accurate, focal therapy may become an effective intermediate form of treatment for men with more aggressive disease who are ineligible for active surveillance to prevent the progression of disease requiring radical treatment. Refinements in targeted biopsy techniques will be vital for characterizing higher-risk tumors. The selection of patients for focal therapy should be able to extend beyond those with low-risk cancers who are reluctant to accept active surveillance. In the future, clinical trials should include patients with limited size intermediate- or high-risk disease, evaluating clinically significant endpoints, such as local progression or metastases, including time to intervention with radical or systemic therapy for documented progression. For phase III trials, a comparative cohort could include men treated with whole-gland radiation therapy, with the intermediate end points being sustained fall in serum PSA, periodic posttreatment MRI, and confirmatory systematic and targeted biopsies. In the focal therapy arm, re-treatment should be permitted if studies continue to show its low morbidity.

The patient best suited for a focal therapy clinical trial today would have a targetable region of disease or a clearly localized, Gleason $3+4$ or higher lesion of relatively small volume amenable to focal ablation, who accepts the necessity of long-term follow-up with periodic imaging and repeat prostate biopsies. At baseline, patients would be characterized by a multivariable risk model that includes PSA, Gleason grade, and clinical stage and extent of disease on biopsy and imaging. The ideal ablative technology would allow real-time visualization of the area of ablation during treatment, eradicate the tumor with minimal damage to surrounding structures, and not complicate future radical therapy, if needed. One caution is the effect of focal ablation on the accuracy of imaging during follow-up. Without evidence to support the superiority of any particular ablative technology, there is room to study a variety of approaches. Currently treatment strategies are largely based on the risk of side effects and the avoidance of potential damage to surrounding structures.

20.7 Thermal Tissue Ablation

Thermal tissue ablation devices create extreme temperature changes within tissue, freezing or heating it to cause necrosis. The effectiveness of hypothermic and hyperthermic forms of treatment is governed by the laws of thermodynamics and affected by tissue-dependant factors, including conductivity, vascularity, and the heat-sink effect.

Cryotherapy has evolved, with the advent of thermal monitoring probes and third-generation cryoprobes that use argon-based gas systems. The use of compressed argon gas rather than liquid nitrogen led to greater precision and mitigation of complications by achieving equivalent low temperatures critical for tissue ablation while enabling the freezing process to start and stop instantaneously, thereby decreasing damage to adjacent organs. Treatments can be delivered even more precisely with real-time ultrasound guidance, improving effectiveness and decreasing treatment-related morbidity. The extreme low temperature required to achieve tumor cryolysis and the surrounding temperature gradient remain disadvantages for focal cryotherapy because the area of ablation must be extended beyond the tumor. The necessity of extending the visualized leading edge of the ice ball at the periphery to achieve tumor ablation exposes surrounding structures to damage [36]. Therefore, achieving effective tumor ablation while limiting side effects such as erectile dysfunction, urethral strictures, and rectal injures has proved challenging [37, 38]. Unfortunately, the lack of rigorous clinical trials of focal cryosurgery prevents an adequate evaluation of oncologic efficacy and side effects. In selected cohorts of men, small retrospective studies report negative posttreatment biopsy rates of 75 % and potency rates ranging from 74 to 90 % [39, 40]. The advantages of focal cryotherapy include real-time assessment of treatment location using transrectal ultrasound and the ability to perform re-treatment safely. However, disadvantages include the inability to assess histologic changes during treatment, lack of precision at the leading edge of the ice ball to prevent collateral damage to surrounding structures, and destruction of local tissue anatomy, which complicates the planning and performance of subsequent radical surgery, should it become necessary. Although most patients recover erectile function with unilateral ablation, the effects of bilateral ablation are greater, should cancer appear in the contralateral lobe in the future.

High-intensity focused ultrasound (HIFU) produces thermal ablation with temperatures above 75 °C to achieve coagulative necrosis within the targeted tissue [41]. The effectiveness of treatment may be limited by interference from tissue factors, including prostate volume (specifically related to the distance from the probe to the anterior tumor) and calcifications. MRI integration with HIFU permits imaging of the tumor for accurate localization and targeting of malignant lesions for ablation. MRI technology permits real-time thermography as treatment proceeds and gadolinium contrast assessment of histologic effect by delineating areas of ischemia or necrosis so the treatment area can be extended or modified to ensure complete ablation of the target [42]. HIFU has been used as focal treatment in primary prostate cancer therapy and in salvage treatment following radiation, with patient outcomes significantly associated with pretreatment tumor characteristics, the patient's functional status, and whether the treatment is primary or salvage therapy [43].

The oncologic efficacy of focal HIFU treatment is difficult to evaluate, given the short follow-up periods in published reports. Recent studies have confirmed that focal HIFU is associated with fewer side effects, compared with whole-gland treatment [44–46]. Preservation of erectile function sufficient for intercourse was reported in 90 % of patients 1 year after treatment; however, larger studies are needed to evaluate the poorer outcomes described on subscales for orgasmic function and erectile satisfaction [45]. In addition, the Clavien classification of complications may underestimate the impact of side effects, including urinary retention or hematuria, especially in patients who are asymptomatic at baseline. Finally, reports of rectal-urethral fistulas in the early experience with focal HIFU suggest a significant learning curve that may limit the broad dissemination of this technology among urologists [46].

20.8 Nonthermal Tissue Ablation

Damage to surrounding structures by thermal tissue ablation spurred the development of chemical ablative treatments. Tumors are selectively targeted by the injection of chemical compounds that produce tissue necrosis without appreciable temperature change. The effectiveness of these treatments relies on the specificity of the compound for the targeted tissue and on sparing surrounding structures from the effects of therapy.

Vascular-targeted photodynamic (VTP) therapy for prostate cancer involves the intravenous injection of a light-sensitive compound that localizes in the targeted tissue and is activated by near-infrared illumination delivered by optical fibers. The treatment effect is mediated through the production of reactive oxygen species and the secondary activation of nitrogen species that initiate rapid necrosis and apoptosis of cells [47]. The advantage of VTP is the minimal toxicity profile reported in initial phase I and phase II studies [48]. The disadvantages of VTP include the inability to monitor treatment during therapy and uncertainty in identifying and retreating recurrences during follow-up. Phase III studies completed in Europe should provide more data to evaluate the efficacy of VTP in men with prostate cancer.

Electroporation transmits pulses of direct electrical current through localized tissue, at levels sufficient to damage cell membranes while sparing surrounding structures [49]. Studies of the use of electroporation in prostate cancer are preliminary at present; however, this treatment has been evaluated in diseases of other organ systems [50]. The main disadvantage of electroporation, as with VTP, is the inability to monitor treatment effect with imaging; the concern is damage to surrounding structures and difficulty monitoring the extent of injury during treatment.

Conclusions

Advances in understanding the natural history of prostate cancer have refined the recommendations for risk-stratified treatment, especially for men with low-risk localized disease. However, the sharp rise in the detection of prostate cancer attributable to routine screening of asymptomatic men ushered in an era of increased use of radical whole-gland treatments. Subsequently, less invasive therapies have emerged that selectively target prostate cancer lesions using organ-sparing techniques that could bring prostate cancer management into line with treatments used for many other solid-organ malignancies. Currently, the clinical experience in focal therapy is limited, and focal prospective trials are few. And although risks seem low, it is difficult to assess benefits. As focal ablative technologies continue to advance, the development of standardized treatment protocols and outcomes reporting will be essential to the accurate assessment of treatment efficacy. Clinical trials are needed to evaluate the benefits and risks of focal therapy for men with intermediate- or high-risk prostate cancer because active surveillance has been found to be a sufficient way to manage low-risk cancers. In this era of overtreatment, coordinated research is needed to personalize patient management by improving risk stratification and providing safe, reasonable, and effective treatment alternatives appropriate to the nature of each man's cancer and the risk it poses to life and health.

Acknowledgments The Thompson Foundation, the Skirball Foundation, and the Sidney Kimmel Center for Prostate and Urologic Cancers

References

1. Siegel R, Naishadham D, Jemal A. Cancer statistics, 2012. CA Cancer J Clin. 2012;62(1): 10–29.
2. Potosky AL, Miller BA, Albertsen PC, Kramer BS. The role of increasing detection in the rising incidence of prostate cancer. JAMA. 1995;273(7):548–52.
3. Bray F, Lortet-Tieulent J, Ferlay J, Forman D, Auvinen A. Prostate cancer incidence and mortality trends in 37 European countries: an overview. Eur J Cancer. 2010;46(17):3040–52.
4. Ferlay J, Steliarova-Foucher E, Lortet Tieulent J, Rosso S, Coebergh JWW, Comber H et al. Cancer incidence and mortality patterns in Europe: estimates for 40 countries in 2012. Eur J Cancer. 2013;49:1374–1403.
5. Marugame T, Mizuno S. Comparison of prostate cancer mortality in five countries: France, Italy, Japan, UK and USA from the WHO mortality database (1960–2000). Jpn J Clin Oncol. 2005;35(11):690–1.

6. Moyer VA. Screening for prostate cancer: U.S. Preventive Services Task Force recommendation statement. Ann Intern Med. 2012;157(2):120–34.

7. Ellison LM, Heaney JA, Birkmeyer JD. Trends in the use of radical prostatectomy for treatment of prostate cancer. Eff Clin Pract. 1999;2(5):228–33.

8. Albertsen PC, Hanley JA, Fine J. 20-year outcomes following conservative management of clinically localized prostate cancer. JAMA. 2005;293(17):2095–101.

9. Jacobs BL, Zhang Y, Schroeck FR, Skolarus TA, Wei JT, Montie JE, et al. Use of advanced treatment technologies among men at low risk of dying from prostate cancer. JAMA. 2013;309(24):2587–95.

10. Sanda MG, Dunn RL, Michalski J, Sandler HM, Northouse L, Hembroff L, et al. Quality of life and satisfaction with outcome among prostate-cancer survivors. N Engl J Med. 2008;358(12):1250–61.

11. Hu JC, Gu X, Lipsitz SR, Barry MJ, D'Amico AV, Weinberg AC, et al. Comparative effectiveness of minimally invasive vs open radical prostatectomy. JAMA. 2009;302(14):1557–64.

12. Resnick MJ, Koyama T, Fan KH, Albertsen PC, Goodman M, Hamilton AS, et al. Long-term functional outcomes after treatment for localized prostate cancer. N Engl J Med. 2013;368(5):436–45.

13. Klotz L, Zhang L, Lam A, Nam R, Mamedov A, Loblaw A. Clinical results of long-term follow-up of a large, active surveillance cohort with localized prostate cancer. J Clin Oncol. 2010;28(1):126–31.

14. Wilt TJ, Brawer MK, Jones KM, Barry MJ, Aronson WJ, Fox S, et al. Radical prostatectomy versus observation for localized prostate cancer. N Engl J Med. 2012;367(3):203–13.

15. Cooperberg MR, Broering JM, Carroll PR. Time trends and local variation in primary treatment of localized prostate cancer. J Clin Oncol. 2010;28(7):1117–23.

16. Cuzick J, Berney DM, Fisher G, Mesher D, Moller H, Reid JE, et al. Prognostic value of a cell cycle progression signature for prostate cancer death in a conservatively managed needle biopsy cohort. Br J Cancer. 2012;106(6):1095–9.

17. Cuzick J, Swanson GP, Fisher G, Brothman AR, Berney DM, Reid JE, et al. Prognostic value of an RNA expression signature derived from cell cycle proliferation genes in patients with prostate cancer: a retrospective study. Lancet Oncol. 2011;12(3):245–55.

18. Nagarajan R, Margolis D, Raman S, Sheng K, King C, Reiter R, et al. Correlation of Gleason scores with diffusion-weighted imaging findings of prostate cancer. Adv Urol. 2012;2012:374805.

19. Vargas HA, Akin O, Afaq A, Goldman D, Zheng J, Moskowitz CS, et al. Magnetic resonance imaging for predicting prostate biopsy findings in patients considered for active surveillance of clinically low risk prostate cancer. J Urol. 2012;188(5):1732–8.

20. Vargas HA, Akin O, Shukla-Dave A, Zhang J, Zakian KL, Zheng J, et al. Performance characteristics of MR imaging in the evaluation of clinically low-risk prostate cancer: a prospective study. Radiology. 2012;265(2):478–87.

21. Onik G, Miessau M, Bostwick DG. Three-dimensional prostate mapping biopsy has a potentially significant impact on prostate cancer management. J Clin Oncol. 2009;27(26):4321–6.

22. UK Clinical Research Network Study Portfolio, PROMIS Prostate MRI Imaging Study (MRC PRII) http://public.ukcrn.org/uk/search/StudyDetail.aspx?StudyID=9941 Accessed 12 Nov 2014.

23. Huang WC, Levey AS, Serio AM, Snyder M, Vickers AJ, Raj GV, et al. Chronic kidney disease after nephrectomy in patients with renal cortical tumours: a retrospective cohort study. Lancet Oncol. 2006;7(9):735–40.

24. Holzbeierlein JM, Lopez-Corona E, Bochner BH, Herr HW, Donat SM, Russo P, et al. Partial cystectomy: a contemporary review of the memorial Sloan-Kettering Cancer Center experience and recommendations for patient selection. J Urol. 2004;172(3):878–81.

25. De Stefani S, Isgro G, Varca V, Pecchi A, Bianchi G, Carmignani G, et al. Microsurgical testis-sparing surgery in small testicular masses: seven years retrospective management and results. Urology. 2012;79(4):858–62.

26. Arora R, Koch MO, Eble JN, Ulbright TM, Li L, Cheng L. Heterogeneity of Gleason grade in multifocal adenocarcinoma of the prostate. Cancer. 2004;100(11):2362–6.

27. Ohori M, Eastham J, Koh H, Kuroiwa K, Slawin K, Wheeler T. Is focal therapy reasonable in patients with early stage prostate cancer- an analysis of radical prostatectomy specimens. J Urol Suppl. 2006;175(507). Abstract 1574.
28. Karavitakis M, Winkler M, Abel P, Livni N, Beckley I, Ahmed HU. Histological characteristics of the index lesion in whole-mount radical prostatectomy specimens: implications for focal therapy. Prostate Cancer Prostatic Dis. 2011;14(1):46–52.
29. Wise AM, Stamey TA, McNeal JE, Clayton JL. Morphologic and clinical significance of multifocal prostate cancers in radical prostatectomy specimens. Urology. 2002;60(2):264–9.
30. Simma-Chiang V, Horn JJ, Simko JP, Chan JM, Carroll PR. Increased prevalence of unifocal prostate cancer in a contemporary series of radical prostatectomy specimens: implications for focal ablation. J Urol. 2006;175:374.
31. Wysock JS, Rosenkrantz AB, Huang WC, Stifelman MD, Lepor H, Deng FM, et al. A prospective, blinded comparison of magnetic resonance (MR) imaging-ultrasound fusion and visual estimation of performance of MR-targeted prostate biopsy: the PROFUS trial. Eur Urol. 2014;66:343–51.
32. Berglund RK, Masterson TA, Vora KC, Eggener SE, Eastham JA, Guillonneau BD. Pathological upgrading and up staging with immediate repeat biopsy in patients eligible for active surveillance. J Urol. 2008;180(5):1964–7. discussion 7–8.
33. Shukla-Dave A, Hricak H, Akin O, Yu C, Zakian KL, Udo K, et al. Preoperative nomograms incorporating magnetic resonance imaging and spectroscopy for prediction of insignificant prostate cancer. BJU Int. 2012;109(9):1315–22.
34. Wang L, Mazaheri Y, Zhang J, Ishill NM, Kuroiwa K, Hricak H. Assessment of biologic aggressiveness of prostate cancer: correlation of MR signal intensity with Gleason grade after radical prostatectomy. Radiology. 2008;246(1):168–76.
35. Zakina KL, Sircar K, Hircak H, Chen HN, Shukla-Dave A, Eberhardt S. Correlation of proton MR spectroscopic imaging with Gleason score based on step-section pathologic analysis after radical prostatectomy. Radiology. 2005;234(3):804–14.
36. Baust J, Gage AA, Ma H, Zhang CM. Minimally invasive cryosurgery–technological advances. Cryobiology. 1997;34(4):373–84.
37. Janzen NK, Han KR, Perry KT, Said JW, Schulam PG, Belldegrun AS. Feasibility of nerve-sparing prostate cryosurgery: applications and limitations in a canine model. J Endourol. 2005;19(4):520–5.
38. Hubosky SG, Fabrizio MD, Schellhammer PF, Barone BB, Tepera CM, Given RW. Single center experience with third-generation cryosurgery for management of organ-confined prostate cancer: critical evaluation of short-term outcomes, complications, and patient quality of life. J Endourol. 2007;21(12):1521–31.
39. Onik G, Vaughan D, Lotenfoe R, Dineen M, Brady J. The "male lumpectomy": focal therapy for prostate cancer using cryoablation results in 48 patients with at least 2-year follow-up. Urol Oncol. 2008;26(5):500–5.
40. Bahn D, de Castro Abreu AL, Gill IS, Hung AJ, Silverman P, Gross ME, et al. Focal cryotherapy for clinically unilateral, low-intermediate risk prostate cancer in 73 men with a median follow-up of 3.7 years. Eur Urol. 2012;62(1):55–63.
41. Vaezy S, Andrew M, Kaczkowski P, Crum L. Image-guided acoustic therapy. Annu Rev Biomed Eng. 2001;3:375–90.
42. Kim YS, Trillaud H, Rhim H, Lim HK, Mali W, Voogt M, et al. MR thermometry analysis of sonication accuracy and safety margin of volumetric MR imaging-guided high-intensity focused ultrasound ablation of symptomatic uterine fibroids. Radiology. 2012;265(2):627–37.
43. Cordeiro ER, Cathelineau X, Thuroff S, Marberger M, Crouzet S, de la Rosette JJ. High-intensity focused ultrasound (HIFU) for definitive treatment of prostate cancer. BJU Int. 2012;110(9):1228–42.
44. Ahmed HU, Cathcart P, McCartan N, Kirkham A, Allen C, Freeman A, et al. Focal salvage therapy for localized prostate cancer recurrence after external beam radiotherapy: a pilot study. Cancer. 2012;118(17):4148–55.

45. Ahmed HU, Hindley RG, Dickinson L, Freeman A, Kirkham AP, Sahu M, et al. Focal therapy for localised unifocal and multifocal prostate cancer: a prospective development study. Lancet Oncol. 2012;13(6):622–32.
46. Barret E, Ahallal Y, Sanchez-Salas R, Galiano M, Cosset JM, Validire P, et al. Morbidity of focal therapy in the treatment of localized prostate cancer. Eur Urol. 2013;63(4):618–22.
47. Ashur I, Goldschmidt R, Pinkas I, Salomon Y, Szewczyk G, Sarna T, et al. Photocatalytic generation of oxygen radicals by the water-soluble bacteriochlorophyll derivative WST11, noncovalently bound to serum albumin. J Phys Chem A. 2009;113(28):8027–37.
48. Azzouzi A. Results of 3-year phase 2 program with Tookad Soluble. 4th International Symposium on Focal Therapy and Imaging in Prostate and Kidney Cancer. Noordwijk, 2012.
49. Onik G, Mikus P, Rubinsky B. Irreversible electroporation: implications for prostate ablation. Technol Cancer Res Treat. 2007;6(4):295–300.
50. Kingham TP, Karkar AM, D'Angelica MI, Allen PJ, Dematteo RP, Getrajdman GI, et al. Ablation of perivascular hepatic malignant tumors with irreversible electroporation. J Am Coll Surg. 2012;215(3):379–87.